LIPPINCOTT'S REVIEW SERIES

Maternal-Newborn Nursing

FOURTH EDITION

Barbara R. Stright, RN, PhD
Associate Professor, Division of
Nursing Education
Baccalaureate Nursing Program
University of the Virgin Islands
St. Thomas
U.S. Virgin Islands

LIPPINCOTT WILLIAMS & WILKINS
A **Wolters Kluwer** Company
Philadelphia • Baltimore • New York • London
Buenos Aires • Hong Kong • Sydney • Tokyo

STAFF

Executive Publisher
Judith A. Schilling McCann, RN, MSN

Editorial Director
William J. Kelly

Clinical Director
Joan M. Robinson, RN, MSN

Senior Art Director
Arlene Putterman

Art Director
Mary Ludwicki

Editorial Project Manager
Ann Houska

Copy Editor
Karen C. Comerford

Designers
Lesley Weissman-Cook (book design), Lynn Foulk (project manager)

Digital Composition Services
Diane Paluba (manager), Joyce Rossi Biletz, Donna S. Morris

Manufacturing
Patricia K. Dorshaw (director), Beth J. Welsh

Editorial Assistants
Megan L. Aldinger, Tara L. Carter-Bell, Linda K. Ruhf

Librarian
Wani Z. Larsen

Indexer
Deborah K. Tourtlotte

The clinical treatments described and recommended in this publication are based on research and consultation with nursing, medical, and legal authorities. To the best of our knowledge, these procedures reflect currently accepted practice. Nevertheless, they can't be considered absolute and universal recommendations. For individual applications, all recommendations must be considered in light of the patient's clinical condition and, before administration of new or infrequently used drugs, in light of the latest package insert information. The authors and publisher disclaim any responsibility for any adverse effects resulting from the suggested procedures, from any undetected errors, or from the reader's misunderstanding of the text.

LRSMNN – D N O
07 06 05 04 10 9 8 7 6 5 4 3 2 1

Library of Congress Cataloging-in-Publication Data

Stright, Barbara R.
Maternal newborn nursing / Barbara R. Stright. — 4th ed.
p. ; cm. — (Lippincott's review series)
Includes bibliographical references and index.
1. Maternity nursing — Examinations, questions, etc.
2. Maternity nursing — Outlines, syllabi, etc. I. Title. II. Series.
[DNLM: 1. Maternal-Child Nursing — Examination Questions. 2. Maternal-Child Nursing--Outlines. WY 18.2 S916m 2005]
RG951.L57 2005

618.2'0231'076--dc22
ISBN 1-58255-359-9 (alk. paper) 2004013780

DEDICATION

For Norman, my husband, my life-long love, and my best friend.

He has always encouraged me and supported my every effort.

He is a strong yet kind and gentle man, and with his love I can't go wrong.

CONTRIBUTORS

Joan Pasadino Bruno, RNC, MSN, NNP
Neonatal Nurse Practitioner
Department of Pediatrics
Staten Island University Hospital
Staten Island, New York

Laurie Gasperi Kaudewitz, RN, BSN, MSN, RNC
Assistant Professor
East Tennessee State University
College of Nursing
Johnson City, Tennessee

Celesta Kirk, RN, CS, MA, MSN, FNP
Associate Professor
East Tennessee State University
Department of Family-Community Nursing
Johnson City, Tennessee

Linda J. Kobokovich, MScN, RNC
Director of Nursing Practice
Dartmouth-Hitchcock Medical Center
Lebanon, New Hampshire

Francine M. Pasadino, CNM, MA
Staff Nurse and Midwife
Department of Obstetrics & Gynecology
Maimonides Medical Center
Brooklyn, New York

INTRODUCTION

Lippincott's Review Series is designed to help you in your study of the key subject areas in nursing. The series consists of six books, one in each core nursing subject area:

Medical-Surgical Nursing
Mental Health and Psychiatric Nursing
Pediatric Nursing
Pathophysiology
Maternal-Newborn Nursing
Fluids and Electrolytes

Lippincott's Review Series was planned and developed in response to your requests for comprehensive outline review books that address each major subject area and also contain a self-test mechanism. These books meet the need for strong and weak areas of knowledge. Each book is a complete source for review and self-assessment of a single core subject — all six together provide an excellent comprehensive review of entry-level nursing.

Each book is all-inclusive of the content addressed in major textbooks. The content outline review uses a consistent nursing process format throughout and addresses nursing care for well and ill clients. Also included are necessary teaching and other concepts, such as growth and development, nutrition, pharmacology, body structures and functions, and pathophysiology. Special features include:

- **Nursing process overview sections** review each step of the nursing process for the system or group of disorders in discussion. These reviews improve your ability to apply principles to practice by highlighting common assessment findings, diagnoses, goals, interventions, and outcomes.
- **Nursing process overview icons** remind you to refer back to the nursing process overview section for in-depth discussion of relevant nursing interventions.
- **Nursing alerts** are fundamental guidelines you can follow to ensure safe and effective care.
- **Drug charts** provide quick reference for medications that are commonly used in treating the disorders discussed within a given chapter. The drug classification, indications, and selected nursing interventions are provided.
- **Client and family teaching boxes** detail health teaching information that may be applied in the clinical setting.
- **Chapter study questions** help you chart your progress through each chapter. Answer keys are provided, with rationales for correct and incorrect responses.
- **Comprehensive examination** mimics the NCLEX and allows you to assess your strengths and weaknesses. An answer key is provided with rationales for correct and incorrect responses.
- **Accompanying CD-ROM** provides 200 additional NCLEX-style questions so you can practice computer-adaptive test-taking skills. Answers are provided, with rationales for correct and incorrect responses.

You can use the books in this series in several different ways. Overall, you can use them as subject reviews to augment general study throughout your basic nursing program and as a review to prepare for the National Council Licensure Examination (NCLEX-RN). How you use each book depends on your individual needs and preferences and on whether you review each chapter systematically or concentrate only on those chapters whose subject areas are particularly problematic or challenging. You may instead choose to use the comprehensive examination as a self-assessment opportunity to evaluate your knowledge base before you review the content outline. Likewise, you can use the study questions for pretesting or posttesting after study, followed by the comprehensive examination as a means of evaluating your knowledge and competencies of an entire subject area. Regardless of how you use the books, one of the strengths of the series is the self-assessment opportunity it offers, in addition to guidance in studying and reviewing content. The chapter study questions and comprehensive examination questions have been carefully developed to cover all topics in the outline review.

Unlike the NCLEX, which tests the cumulative knowledge needed for safe practice by an entry-level nurse, these practice tests systematically evaluate the knowledge base that serves as the building block for the entire nursing educational process. In this way, you can prepare for the NCLEX throughout your course of study. Good study habits throughout your educational program not only are the best way to ensure ongoing success but also will prove the most beneficial way to prepare for the licensing examination.

Keep in mind that these books are not intended to replace formal learning. They cannot substitute for textbook reading, discussion with instructors, or class attendance. Every effort has been made to provide accurate and current information, but class attendance and interaction with an instructor will provide invaluable information not found in books. Used correctly, these books will help you increase understanding, improve comprehension, evaluate strengths and weakness in areas of knowledge, increase productive study time, and, as a result, help you improve your grades.

MONEY-BACK GUARANTEE — Lippincott's Review Series will help you study more effectively during coursework throughout your educational program, and help you prepare for quizzes and tests, including the NCLEX. If you buy and use any of the six volumes in Lippincott's Review Series and fail the NCLEX, simply send verification of your exam results and your copy of the review book to the address below. We will promptly send you a check for our suggested list price.

Lippincott's Review Series
Marketing Department
Lippincott Williams & Wilkins
530 Walnut Street
Philadelphia, PA 19106

ACKNOWLEDGMENTS

I would like to thank everyone at Lippincott Williams & Wilkins who helped make this fourth edition of the *Lippincott Review Series: Maternal-Newborn Nursing* possible. I would especially like to express my appreciation to Elizabeth Nieginski and Joan Robinson for their encouragement and support. I believe nursing students, returning nurses, and others who desire a thorough review of maternal and infant nursing will find this review text a useful and complete tool for boosting their knowledge.

BRS

CONTENTS

1 Introduction to Maternal-Newborn Nursing

I. FAMILY-CENTERED MATERNAL-NEWBORN NURSING

A. Description

1. Family-centered maternal-newborn nursing is the term used to describe the provision of safe, quality nursing care that recognizes, focuses on, and adapts to the physical and psychosocial needs of the pregnant woman, her family, and the newborn.
2. Family-centered nursing care fosters family unity and promotes and protects the physiologic well-being of the mother, fetus, and newborn.
3. Family-centered nursing care is culturally competent; incorporates into policy and practice recognition and respect for cultural diversity, strengths, and individuality across all families, and includes ethnic, racial, spiritual, social, economic, eographic, and educational diversity.
4. Family-centered nursing care ensures that all hospital, home, and community services and support systems are flexible, accessible, and comprehensive in their responses to individual needs.
5. Family-centered nursing care is research-oriented, and nursing theory and evidence-based practice provide the foundation for nursing care.

B. Development.

Several significant activities set the stage for a change in how care was provided for both mother and baby.

1. It was discovered that puerperal infection was preventable by implementing hygienic practices such as frequent hand washing.
2. Research indicated that the benefits of early, extended parent-newborn contact significantly outweighed the risk of infection.
3. In the late 1950s, a coalition of consumers, health care professionals, and childbirth educators began challenging the routine use of analgesics and anesthetics for childbirth.
4. Childbirth preparation and participation of the father in labor and birth were introduced.
5. Several researchers studied the effects of maternal attachment, separation, and deprivation on the mother and the newborn.
6. St. Mary's Hospital in Evansville, Indiana established the first family-centered maternity care program, and this approach quickly spread across the nation.
7. By 2000, 98% of births occurred in hospitals; however, this trend is changing as families choose alternative environments for the birth experience.
8. A growing trend toward health care consumerism has made childbearing families active participants in their own health care. This same trend has enabled the movement of health care from hospitals to community sites and from long hospital stays to shortened stays with increased dependence on home care.

C. Philosophy

1. The following statements summarize the principles of family-centered maternal-newborn nursing:
   a. Pregnancy and childbirth are usually normal healthy events within the family.
   b. Childbirth affects the entire family and marks the beginning of a new set of important relationships.
   c. Families are able to make decisions about care if given the proper information.
   d. A maternal-newborn nurse serves as an advocate for the rights of all family members, including the fetus.
   e. Personal, cultural, and religious attitudes influence the meaning of pregnancy and birth within the family.

f. Promoting health through role modeling, teaching, and counseling is important to the future health of the community in which the family lives.

2. Important features of family-centered maternal-newborn nursing include:

a. Prenatal and parent education classes
b. Family participation in all aspects of the pregnancy and birth
c. Presence of support person for complicated births or cesarean section
d. Use of homelike birth setting
e. Flexible policies regarding routine procedures
f. Early extended parent-newborn contact
g. Flexible rooming-in policy
h. Family involvement in care of the mother and newborn
i. Early postbirth discharge with close follow-up at home
j. Nontraditional labor and birth settings (birth centers or home birth)
k. Single-room maternity systems, which may be called labor, delivery, and recovery (LDR) rooms or labor, delivery, recovery, and postpartum (LDRP) rooms.

TABLE 1-1
Sample nursing practice standards and guidelines related to maternal-newborn care

Standard	Interpretation
Standard I Quality of care	The nurse systematically evaluates the quality and effectiveness of nursing practice.
Standard II Performance appraisal	The nurse evaluates his or her own nursing practice in relation to professional practice standards and relevant statutes and regulations.
Standard III Education	The nurse acquires and maintains current knowledge in nursing practice.
Standard IV Collegiality	The nurse contributes to the professional development of peers, colleagues, and others.
Standard V Ethics	The nurse's decisions and actions on behalf of patients are determined in an ethical manner.
Standard VI Collaboration	The nurse collaborates with the patient, significant others, and health care providers in providing patient care.
Standard VII Research	The nurse uses research findings in practice.
Standard VIII Resource utilization	The nurse considers factors related to safety, effectiveness, and cost in planning and delivering patient care.
Standard IX Practice environment	The nurse contributes to the environment of care delivery within the practice setting.
Standard X Accountability	The nurse is professionally and legally accountable for his or her practice. The professional registered nurse may delegate to and supervise qualified personnel who provide patient care.

Adapted from Association of Women's Health, Obstetric, and Neonatal Nurses. (2003). *Standards for the nursing care of women and newborns.* 6th ed. Washington, DC: Association of Women's Health, Obstetric, and Neonatal Nurses.

TABLE 1-2
Definition of statistical terms used to report maternal-infant health

Statistical term	Definition
Birth rate	The number of births per 1,000 population
Fertility rate	The number of pregnancies per 1,000 women of childbearing age
Fetal death rate	The number of fetal deaths occurring in infants weighing over 500 g per 1,000 live births
Perinatal death rate	The number of deaths per 1,000 live births occurring between birth and the first 28 days of life
Neonatal death rate	The number of deaths per 1,000 live births of fetuses weighing more than 500 g and in the first 28 days of life
Maternal mortality	The number of maternal deaths per 100,000 live births that occur as a direct result of the childbearing process
Infant mortality	The number of deaths per 1,000 live births occurring at birth or in the first 12 months of life
Child mortality	The number of deaths per 1,000 population in children from 1 to 14 years of age

D. Standards of care

1. Nursing organizations develop standards of care to promote consistency and ensure the quality of care in their specific area of nursing practice. Standards of practice provide important guidelines for planning care and identifying outcome criteria for evaluation of nursing care.
2. In maternal-newborn nursing, standards of practice have been developed by the American Nurses Association (ANA) and the Association of Women's Health, Obstetric and Neonatal Nurses (AWHONN) to serve as guides (*Table* 1-1, page 3).
3. Understanding the range of services that can be provided by the nurse, and the standards of care for the practice of nursing, can help the nurse stay within legal parameters.

II. MATERNAL-NEWBORN HEALTH

A. Measuring maternal-newborn health

1. The maternal and newborn population is continuously changing as a result of variations in social structure, family lifestyles, increased health care costs, inadequate distribution of resources, and advances in technology.
2. In order to provide a descriptive picture of the health of mothers and babies, compare outcomes, and plan for future health care, the systematic, accurate collection and interpretation of data are required.
   a. The statistical data collected can indicate the general health of a group, the value of health care within the group, the availability and access to health care experienced by the group, and gaps in health care for a group.
   b. A number of statistical terms are used to describe the outcome of pregnancy and birth (*Table* 1-2). The values attached to these statistical terms can vary widely with-

in the United States (from state to state and among ethnic groups) and from country to country. However, the infant mortality rate of a country is regarded as an indicator of the general health of that country. This rate is the standard used to compare a nation's health care with previous years and to that of other countries.
- When compared with other developed countries, the United States has an infant mortality rate that is higher than 27 other countries. One reason for this is the lack of equity in the distribution of health care among diverse populations. Other reasons include shrinking family size, increasing number of single-parent families, lack of financial resources, the need for cost containment in health care, and maternal age.
- The main causes of infant death are problems occurring at birth or shortly thereafter. These problems may include congenital anomalies, very low to low birth weight, short gestation, sudden infant death, maternal complications of pregnancy, and complications of placenta, cord, and membranes.

B. Programs and trends in maternal-newborn health care

1. Both federal and state governments support several programs aimed at improving the health of mothers, infants, and children (*Table* 1-3).

TABLE 1-3
Government interventions related to maternal-child care

Intervention	Purpose
Title V of Social Security Act (1935)	Provides government funds for maternal-child programs
National Institute of Child Health and Human Development (1962)	Supports research and education for health care personnel required for maternal-child health programs
Title V Amendment of the Public Health Service Act (1964)	Established the Maternal Infant Care (MIC) projects to provide comprehensive prenatal and infant care in public clinics
Title XIX of Medicaid (1965)	Provides funds to enable women and children to have access to health care
Head Start (1968)	Provides educational opportunities for preschool-age children of low-income families
National Center for Family Planning (1969)	Provides contraceptive information and education
Women, Infants, and Children (1975)	Provides nutrition information and supplemental food to mothers, infants, and children
Human Genome Project (1990)	Explores and maps human genetic material
Federal Fertility Clinic Success Rate and Certification Act (1992)	Requires clinics performing assisted reproductive technology to report their success rates annually to the Centers for Disease Control and Prevention
Newborn's and Mother's Health Protection Act (1996)	Provides for a postpartum stay of up to 48 hours after vaginal birth and 96 hours after cesarean birth at the discretion of the mother and her health care provider; effective January 1998
Presidents Council on Bioethics (2001)	Oversees all federally funded embryonic stem cell research; studies the range of ethical issues in the biomedical and behavioral sciences

TABLE 1-4
Examples of diagnosis-related groups (DRGs) in maternal-newborn care

Code	Diagnosis
370	Cesarean section with complications
371	Cesarean section without complications
372	Vaginal delivery with complications
373	Vaginal delivery without complications
375	Vaginal delivery with operative procedures
379	Therapeutic abortion
382	False labor
386	Prematurity with respiratory distress syndrome
387	Prematurity without other complications
388	Premature with other complications
389	Full-term neonate with complications

2. In response to the need for resource management and cost containment, several alternative methods of providing health care while containing costs are in use today.

a. **Diagnosis-related groups (DRGs)** provide a method of classifying related medical diagnoses based on the amount of resources required by the client. The length of stay in the hospital is also determined (*Table* 1-4).

b. **Managed care** is an alternative to the DRG as a health care system. Examples of this type of delivery system are **health maintenance organizations (HMOs)** and **preferred provider organizations (PPOs).**
- The HMO, in return for a set fee, is responsible for providing fairly comprehensive health care for the persons enrolled.
- PPOs are groups of health care providers who agree to provide health services to a specific group of clients on a discounted basis. They may require arranged payments or preadmission authorization for a procedure or treatment.

c. **Outcomes management** is a systematic method of collaborative clinical practice that will identify client outcomes and focus on the interventions needed to accomplish the outcome. Guidelines for care are developed by each health care facility.

d. **Clinical pathways** also are called critical paths, care paths, or multidisciplinary action plans (MAPs). In general, they define expected client outcomes, length of stay, and specific interventions needed to accomplish the stated outcomes. These guidelines are intended to provide collaborative care and are developed by each health care facility.

e. Since 1990, **home care** of mothers and infants has experienced a dramatic increase. The expansion of these services is due to actual cost benefit and increased reimbursement by both state and federal governments.

f. Since 2000, an increasing number of families are choosing birth at home or in settings other than the hospital. In response to this trend, hospitals have created labor, delivery, and recovery (LDR) rooms and labor, delivery, recovery, and postpartum (LDRP) rooms. Mother and infant stay in one room for the length of their hospitalization. Family members are encouraged to visit and to participate in the care of the mother and newborn.

III. ADVANCED PRACTICE ROLES IN MATERNAL-NEWBORN NURSING

A. A **women's health nurse practitioner** is a nurse with advanced study in health promotion and health maintenance of women.

B. A **family nurse practitioner (FNP)** is a nurse in an advanced practice role who provides care not only to women but to clients across the life span.

C. A **pediatric nurse practitioner (PNP)** and a **neonatal nurse practitioner (NNP)** are nurses in advanced practice roles who provide skilled care to children and infants.

D. A **certified nurse-midwife** is a nurse who has completed an intensive program of study combined with extensive clinical experience. She holds licensure as a registered nurse and is tested and certified by the American College of Nurse Midwives. She provides complete care during an uncomplicated pregnancy, labor, and birth.

E. A **clinical nurse specialist** is prepared at the master's degree level and functions as a consultant in her area of expertise. She is a role model, researcher, and teacher of quality nursing care.

F. A **certified registered nurse (RNC)** is a nurse who has shown expertise in a particular field of nursing, such as labor and delivery, by taking and passing a national certification examination.

IV. ETHICAL AND LEGAL ISSUES IN MATERNAL-NEWBORN NURSING

A. Ethical issues

1. Ethics involves determining the best course of action, what is morally right and reasonable, in a given situation. **Bioethics** is the application of ethics to health care situations. Ethical nursing behavior has been described in codes set forth by various nursing organizations.
2. Ethical issues have become more complex with advanced technology, which allows the family more options. They are also controversial because there may be support for more than one action, or none of the actions may be desirable.
3. Complex ethical questions are related to maternal versus fetal rights, widely varying standards of viability, abortion, mandated contraception, use of fetal tissue for research, length of time resuscitation should be continued, cord blood banking, and the use and protection of genetic information. Conception issues, particularly those related to in vitro fertilization, embryo transfer, ownership of frozen oocytes or sperm, and surrogate mothers, are current critical issues.

B. Professional liability

1. Nurses are legally responsible and accountable for the quality of nursing care they give. They may also be held accountable for care given by other members of the health care team.
   a. Accurate assessment data and careful documentation are essential in protecting the nurse and justifying a course of action. Documentation is the best evidence of the quality of care received by the client. It must be accurate and reflect the care given.

b. Crucial areas of concern are establishing who may give consent for health care, providing care for the fetus, and caring for clients not of legal age.

c. Nurses are legally responsible for reporting the following:
- Suspected cases of child abuse
- Inappropriate or incomplete care provided by other health care workers
- Professionals impaired by substance abuse

2. Malpractice claims against both physicians and nurses have escalated during the past few years.

a. Perinatal nursing is the area in which most lawsuits occur. The most common problems occurring at birth or shortly after are prematurity, low birth weight, congenital anomalies, respiratory distress syndrome, and early infant death. These unexpected complications of a normal process are a tragic outcome for the parents, and they may look for someone to blame.

b. To avoid malpractice claims, nurses are expected to provide care within the context of nurse practice acts, standards of care, and policies developed by the agency in which they practice.

c. Documentation is essential to protecting the nurse and justifying her actions. A nursing note written during labor and birth or during the newborn's hospital stay may need to be defended as many as 21 years in the future. A child who feels he was wronged during this time by health care personnel can bring a lawsuit when he reaches legal age. If an action is not documented, it is not done.

NURSING PROCESS OVERVIEW

V. MATERNAL-NEWBORN NURSING

A. Overview

1. The nursing process is a proven process of problem-solving based on the scientific method that applies equally to all of nursing care. It consists of five steps.

a. Assessment

b. Nursing diagnoses

c. Planning and outcome identification

d. Implementation

e. Outcome evaluation

2. When caring for mothers and infants, the nurse must adapt the nursing process for a population that is basically healthy and engaged in a normal life event that has a potential for growth as well as risks. This is somewhat confusing when using the mostly problem-oriented lists of nursing diagnoses developed by the North American Nursing Diagnosis Association (NANDA).

3. **Critical thinking,** in nursing, is crucial in order to make the best clinical judgment in a given situation. It is based on reason and analysis, rather than preference and prejudice. Nurses must examine thinking in this manner in order to prevent poor clinical judgment and inappropriate actions.

4. Accurate and careful **documentation** of each step of the nursing process may help prevent professional liability by confirming sound clinical judgment and appropriate interventions.

B. Assessment

1. Nursing assessment is a systematic, organized manner of data collection that includes not only physiologic data but also psychological, social, and cultural data. Three levels

of nursing assessment are used to collect data—comprehensive assessment, focused assessment, and emergency assesment.

a. **Comprehensive assessment** is usually performed on initial contact with the woman. Its purpose is to collect information about all aspects of her health. It is also referred to as baseline data. It describes the woman's health status before intervention begins.

b. **Focused assessment** is used to collect information that is related to an actual health problem or a potential health risk.

c. **Emergency assessment** is used to gather data in specific critical situations, such as drowning, choking, or cardiopulmonary failure.

2. Nursing assessment of the client and family is accomplished through:
   a. Interview and observation
   b. Nursing health history
   c. Measurement of vital signs
   d. Other physiologic indicators
   e. Review of medical records
   f. Use of various standardized tools to measure growth and development
   g. Physical examination
3. Data gathered during the assessment are either **subjective data,** which the client must tell the nurse, or **objective data,** which the nurse can observe or measure. Data are then grouped and analyzed so that problems, potential problems, and risks can be identified.

C. Nursing diagnoses

1. Health problems that the nurse is responsible for treating independently are called nursing diagnoses. More than 100 nursing diagnoses have been identified by NANDA. Each diagnosis consists of three parts—the problem, defining characteristics, and the etiology.
2. An actual nursing diagnosis indicates that the problem exists, whereas a potential for risk indicates that the client or family may develop the problem later. Nursing diagnoses that may apply to maternal-newborn nursing include:
   a. Anxiety
   b. Breast-feeding: Effective, Ineffective, or Interrupted
   c. Body Image Disturbance
   d. Constipation
   e. Decisional Conflict
   f. Altered Family Process
   g. Fatigue
   h. Risk for Infection
   i. Pain
   j. Altered Parent/Infant Attachment
   k. Altered Role Performance
   l. Situational Low Self-esteem
   m. Sleep Pattern Disturbance
   n. Ineffective Thermoregulation
   o. Altered Urinary Elimination

D. Planning and outcome identification

1. The third step of the nursing process involves planning care for the problems that were identified in the assessment and are reflected in the applicable nursing diagnosis.

2. In this phase, the nurse determines priorities and develops goals. Outcomes state what is to be accomplished by when.

E. Implementation

1. Interventions are developed and implemented to accomplish the goals or outcomes that have been identified.
2. Nursing intervention in maternal-newborn care involves activities designed to promote positive adaptation and high-level wellness.
   a. Interventions encompass everything from comfort measures to counseling and health education.
   b. Client teaching for self-care is an example of a primary nursing intervention with healthy childbearing families. It is based on client or family learning needs, principles of teaching and learning, sociocultural factors, and the physical and psychological condition of the client and family.
3. Written interventions must be specific in their description of the following:
   a. What is to be done or given
   b. How much or how long it is to be done or given
   c. How it is to be done or given
   d. At what time it is to be done or given
   e. Why it is to be done or given
4. Dissemination of the written plan for care to others responsible for providing care is essential to promote safety and continuity.

F. Outcome evaluation

1. This step determines how well the goals or outcomes were met and the effectiveness of the plan.
2. Appropriate evaluation involves establishing criteria for measurement and observation (goals and outcomes), assessing current client responses for evidence of progress, and comparing current responses to the established criteria.
3. The nurse, based on the evaluation, makes a decision to continue, change, or discontinue the existing plan of care.
4. Because the nursing process is dynamic, the evaluation usually results in the collection of additional assessment data, new nursing diagnoses, or both, which may result in modification of the plan.

Study questions

1. Which of the following was accomplished by Title V of the Social Security Act?
1. Organization of nurse-midwifery in the United States
2. Provision of contraceptive information and education
3. Comprehensive prenatal and newborn care in public clinics
4. Federal funding for maternal-child health programs

2. Which of the following identifies a method used to classify clients according to the amount of resources and length of hospital stay?
1. Health maintenance organizations
2. Preferred provider organizations
3. Diagnosis-related groups
4. Managed care

3. Which of the following acronyms identifies an important program that provides supplemental food to low-income families?
1. CHAP
2. EPSDT

3. CNM
4. WIC

4. In maternal-infant care, the **most** commonly filed lawsuits involve claims related to which of the following?
1. Perinatal complications
2. Maternal injury
3. Maternal death
4. Newborn death

5. Which of the following terms is regarded as an indicator of a country's general health?
1. Birth rate
2. Infant mortality rate
3. Maternal mortality rate
4. Fertility rate

6. Family-centered nursing care for women and newborns focuses on which of the following?
1. Assisting individuals and families to achieve their optimal health
2. Diagnosing and treating problems promptly
3. Preventing further complications from developing
4. Conducting nursing research to evaluate clinical practice

7. In which of the following advanced practice roles would the nurse provide complete care during an uncomplicated birth?
1. Women's health nurse practitioner
2. Certified nurse midwife
3. Clinical nurse specialist
4. Case manager

8. When reviewing the ethical dilemmas facing maternal-newborn nurses today, which of the following has contributed to their complexity?
1. Limitation of available options
2. Support for one viable action
3. Advancements in technology
4. Consistent desirable standards

9. The nurse is caring for a 38-year-old unmarried woman. She is 38 weeks pregnant and has two school-age children at home. She has gained 4 pounds in the last week and she states her "rings are tight and won't come off." Her significant other, who is not the father of this baby or the other children, attends prenatal clinic with her to provide support and share information. Based on the philosophy of family-centered maternal-newborn nursing, which of the following principles apply to the care of this family? Select all that apply.
1. Pregnancy and childbirth are usually normal, healthy events in the family.
2. Pregnancy and childbirth affect the entire family.
3. Families are able to make decisions about care if given the proper information.
4. Personal and cultural attitudes influence the meaning of pregnancy and birth in the family.
5. The family may choose a nontraditional birth setting.

Answer key

1. The answer is 4.
Title V of the Social Security Act of 1935 provided federal funding for maternal-child health programs. Organized nurse-midwifery grew out of the activities of the Maternity Center Association in New York City. The National Center for family planning provides contraceptive information and education. The MIC projects emphasized comprehensive prenatal and newborn care in public clinics.

2. The answer is 3.
Diagnosis-related groups (DRG) provide a method of classifying related medical diagnoses based on the amount of resources required by the client. The length of stay (LOS) is also determined. Health maintenance or-

ganizations (HMOs) are an example of managed health care systems. In return for a set fee, they are responsible for providing fairly comprehensive health care for persons enrolled. Preferred provider organizations (PPOs) are also examples of managed health care systems. They are groups of health care providers who agree to provide health services to a specific group of clients at a discounted rate. They may require arranged payments or preadmission authorization for a procedure or treatment. Managed care, which includes HMOs and PPOs, is an alternative to the DRG as a health care system.

3. The answer is **4.**
WIC, which stands for Women, Infants, and Children, is the program that provides supplemental food to low-income families. In 1977, CHAP (Child Health Assessment Act) and the EPSDT (Early Periodic Screening, Diagnostic, and Testing) program provided eligible children with regular health screening and treatment through federal funding. CNM are the letters signifying that a registered nurse with advanced education has met the requirements and successfully completed the examination as a certified nurse-midwife.

4. The answer is **1.**
The perinatal period comprises the period of time beginning when the fetus weighs 500 g through the first 28 days of extrauterine life. Complications occurring during this time are a tragic surprise for the parents, and they may look for someone to blame. Maternal injury, maternal death, and newborn death may result in lawsuits, but they are not as frequent.

5. The answer is **2.**
The infant mortality rate of a country is regarded as an indicator of the general health of that country. This rate is the standard used to compare a nation's health care with that of previous years and with that of other countries. The birth, maternal mortality, and fertility rates are all statistical terms used to report various aspects of maternal and child health, but they are not considered the standard indicator.

6. The answer is **1.**
Family-centered nursing care for women and newborns focuses on helping individuals and families achieve their optimal health. This reflects the standards developed by American Nurses Association (ANA) and the Association of Women's Health, Obstetric, and Neonatal Nurses (AWHONN). Prompt diagnosis and treatment, prevention of further complications, and performance of nursing research, also commonly found in the standards of practice formulated by the ANA and AWHONN, are accomplished through the use of the nursing process, critical thinking, and selection of appropriate interventions. Together, these activities form the basis for the ultimate goal of optimal health achievement.

7. The answer is **2.**
Certified nurse-midwives, nurses who have completed an intensive program of study combined with extensive clinical experience holding licensure as a registered nurse and being tested and certified by the American College of Nurse Midwives, provide complete care during uncomplicated pregnancy, labor, and birth. A women's health nurse practitioner is a nurse with advanced study in health promotion and health maintenance of women. Clinical nurse specialists are prepared at the master's degree level and are able to function as consultants in their area of expertise. They are role models, researchers, and teachers of quality nursing care. A case manager is a graduate-level nurse who supervises a group of clients from the time they enter the health care setting until they are discharged. They monitor the effectiveness, cost, and level of satisfaction of the care received.

8. The answer is **3.**
Ethical issues have become more complex with advanced technology, which allows the family more options from which to choose.

Adding to this complexity is the fact that ethical issues are also controversial because there may be support for more than one action, or none of the actions may be desirable. Complex ethical questions are related to maternal versus fetal rights, widely varying standards of viability, abortion, mandated contraception, use of fetal tissue for research, and length of time resuscitation should be continued. Conception issues, particularly those related to in vitro fertilization, embryo transfer, ownership of frozen oocytes or sperm, and surrogate mothers, are current critical issues.

9. The answer is **2, 3, 4.**
In this nontraditional family, the applicable philosophy of family-centered maternal-newborn nursing includes the statements "childbirth affects the entire family," "families are able to make decisions about care if given the proper information," and "personal and cultural attitudes influence the meaning of pregnancy and birth in the family." The statement "pregnancy and childbirth are usually normal healthy events within the family" does not apply because the mother has a weight gain of 4 pounds, which is excessive for this time in pregnancy, and she states that her "rings are tight and won't come off." These may be signs and symptoms of pregnancy-induced hypertension, a complication of pregnancy. The statement "The family may choose a nontraditional birth setting" does not apply because the potential complication means this family is not a candidate for a home birth or birthing center.

2 Reproduction and Sexuality

I. STRUCTURE AND FUNCTION OF THE FEMALE AND MALE REPRODUCTIVE SYSTEMS

A. Female reproductive system

1. External organs
   a. The **mons pubis** is a mound of fatty tissue over the symphysis pubis that cushions and protects the bone.
   b. The **labia majora** are longitudinal folds of pigmented skin extending from the mons pubis to the perineum.
   c. The **labia minora** are soft longitudinal skin folds between the labia majora.
   d. The **clitoris** is erectile tissue located at the upper end of the labia minora. It is the primary site of sexual arousal.
   e. The **urethral meatus** (urethral orifice) is a small opening of the urethra. It is located between the clitoris and the vaginal orifice for the purpose of urination.
   f. **Skene** or **paraurethral glands** are small mucus-secreting glands that open into the posterior wall of the urinary meatus and lubricate the vagina.
   g. The **vestibule** is an almond-shaped area between the labia minora containing the vaginal introitus, hymen, and Bartholin glands.
   h. The **vaginal introitus** is the external opening of the vagina.
   i. The **hymen** is a membranous tissue ringing the vaginal introitus.
   j. **Bartholin** or **vulvovaginal glands** are mucus-secreting glands located on either side of the vaginal orifice.
   k. The **perineal body** is composed of muscles and fascia that support pelvic structures.
   l. The **perineum** is the area of tissue between the anus and vagina; an episiotomy is performed here.
2. Internal organs
   a. The **vagina** is the female organ of copulation and also serves as the birth canal. It is a tubular musculomembranous organ that lies between the rectum and the urethra and bladder (*Figure* 2-1, page 16).
   b. The **uterus** is a hollow, muscular organ with three muscle layers (perimetrium, myometrium, and endometrium). It is located between the bladder and rectum, and consists of the fundus, body (corpus), and cervix. Uterine functions include:
   - Menstruation, the sloughing away of spongy layers of endometrium with bleeding from torn vessels.
   - Environment for pregnancy; the embryo and fetus develop in the uterus after fertilization.
   - Labor, consisting of powerful contractions of the muscular uterine wall that result in expulsion of the fetus.

   c. Uterine ligaments include:
   - Broad and round ligaments that provide upper support for the uterus.
   - Cardinal, pubocervical, and uterosacral ligaments that are suspensory and provide middle support.
   - Pelvic muscular floor ligaments that provide lower support.

   d. The **fallopian tubes** extend from the upper outer angles of the uterus and end near the ovary. These tubes serve as the passageway for the ovum to travel from the ovary to the uterus and for the sperm to travel from the uterus to the ovary.
   e. The **ovaries** are female sex glands located on each side of the uterus. The two functions of the ovaries are

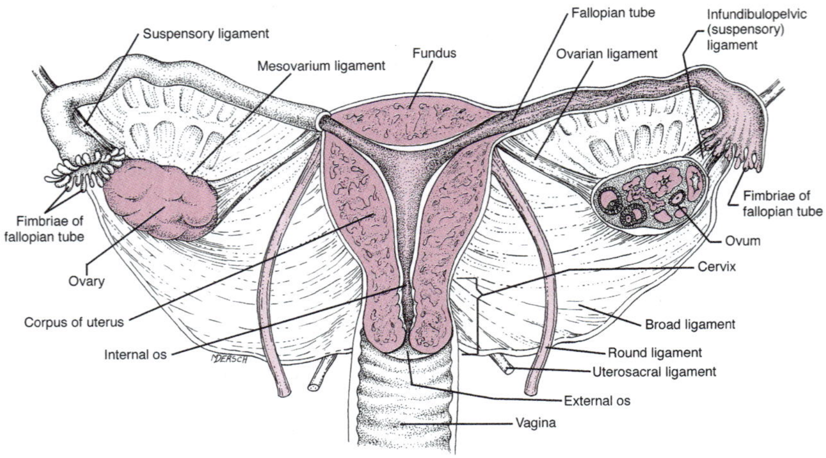

FIGURE 2-1

Anterior view of the uterus and related structures.

- Ovulation (release of ovum)
- Secretion of hormones (estrogen and progesterone)

3. Pelvis

a. The pelvis is a bony ring in the lower portion of the trunk. It consists of three parts (ilium, ischium, and pubis) and four bones (two innominate bones or hipbones, sacrum, and coccyx).

b. The pelvic bones are held together by four joints (articulations)—symphysis pubis, two sacroiliac, and sacrococcygeal. Fibrocartilage between these joints provides movability.

c. Types of pelves include:

- **Gynecoid,** a typical female pelvis with a rounded inlet.
- **Android,** a normal male pelvis with a heart-shaped inlet.
- **Anthropoid,** an "apelike" pelvis with an oval inlet.
- **Platypelloid,** a flat, female-type pelvis with a transverse oval inlet.

d. **Pelvimetry** (the process of measuring the internal or external pelvis) is performed with radiography or by internal examination.

- Internal pelvic inlet measurement measures the diagonal conjugate, which is the lower margin of the symphysis pubis to the promontory of the sacrum; it is normally 11.5 cm or more.
- Internal midpelvic measurement measures the distance between ischial spines and prominence or bluntness of spines; it is normally 10.5 cm.
- Internal pelvic outlet measurement is an estimation of the angle of the pubic arch (90 degrees), mobility of coccyx, intertuberous diameter (11 cm), and posterior sagittal diameter (7.5 cm).

e. Pelvic size and structural irregularities can alter labor and birth.

4. Breasts

a. The female breasts (mammary glands) are specialized sebaceous glands that produce milk after childbirth (lactation).

b. Internal breast structures include:
- **Glandular tissue** (parenchyma is composed of acini milk-producing) cells that cluster in groups of 15 to 20 to form the lobes of the breast.
- **Lactiferous ducts or sinuses,** which form passageways from the lobes to the nipple.
- **Fibrous tissue,** also called Cooper ligaments, which provide support to the mammary glands.
- **Adipose and fibrous tissues** (stroma), which provide the relative size and consistency of the breast.

c. External structures include:
- The **nipple,** a raised, pigmented area of the breast.
- The **areola,** pigmented skin around the nipple.
- **Montgomery tubercles,** sebaceous glands of the areola.

d. The breasts change in size and nodularity in response to cyclic ovarian hormonal changes, including:
- Estrogen stimulation, which produces tenderness
- Progesterone (postovulation), which causes increased tenderness and breast enlargement

e. Physical changes in breast size and activity are at a minimum 5 to 7 days after menstruation stops; this is the best time to detect pathologic changes through breast self-examination.

5. Menstrual cycle and hormones

a. **Menarche** (onset of menstruation) typically occurs between 9 and 17 years of age, with average age of onset at 12 or 13 years.

b. The **menstrual cycle** is a monthly pattern of ovulation and menstruation.
- **Ovulation** is the discharge of a mature ovum from the ovary.
- **Menstruation** is the periodic shedding of blood, mucus, and epithelial cells from the uterus; average blood loss is 30 to 80 ml.

c. The ovaries produce mature gametes and secrete the following hormones:
- **Estrogen,** which contributes to female characteristics (such as female body build and breast growth)
- **Progesterone** (hormone of pregnancy), which quiets or decreases the contractility of the uterus
- **Prostaglandins,** which regulate the reproductive process by stimulating the contractility of uterine and other smooth muscles

d. The menstrual cycle occurs on four levels — central nervous system (CNS) or hypothalmic-pituitary, ovarian, endometrial (menstrual), and cervical.
- **CNS response.** The hypothalamus stimulates the anterior pituitary gland by secreting gonadotropin-releasing hormone (GnRH). The anterior pituitary secretes two gonadotropins — follicle-stimulating hormone (FSH) and luteinizing hormone (LH).
  - FSH prompts the ovary to develop ovarian follicles; the developing follicles secrete estrogen, which feeds back to the anterior pituitary to suppress FSH and trigger a surge of LH (*Figure* 2-2, page 18).
  - LH acts with FSH to cause ovulation and enhance corpus luteum formation.
- **Ovarian response** (two phases). An oocyte grows within the primordial follicle in two phases — follicular and luteal.
  - In the follicular phase (days 1 to 14), the follicle matures as a result of FSH.

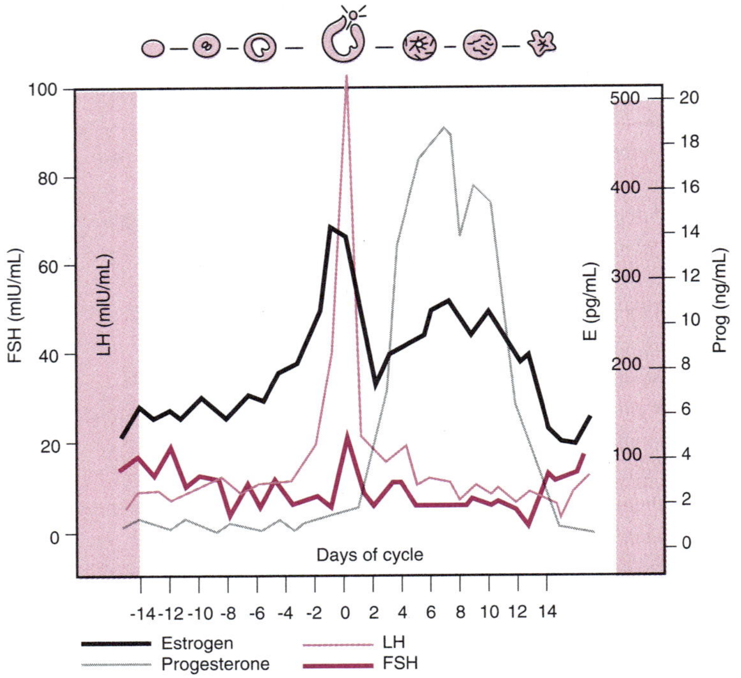

FIGURE 2–2
Plasma hormones in the normal female reproductive cycle.

- In the luteal phase (days 15 to 22), the corpus luteum develops from a ruptured follicle (*Figure* 2-3).

– **Endometrial response** (four phases)
  - In the menstrual phase (days 1 to 5), the estrogen level is low and cervical mucus is scanty.
  - In the proliferative (follicular) phase (days 6 to 14), the estrogen level is high, the endometrium and myometrium thicken, and changes in cervical mucosa occur (see later). (Note: Variations in the menstrual cycle are due to variations in the number of days in this phase.) On average, ovulation occurs on day 14 of a 28-day cycle.
  - In the secretory phase (days 14 to 26), after release of the ovum, the estrogen level drops, the progesterone level is high, increased uterine vascularity occurs, and tissue glycogen levels increase.
  - In the ischemic phase (days 27 to 28), estrogen and progesterone levels recede, arterial vessels constrict, the endometrium prepares to shed, the blood vessels rupture, and menstruation begins.

– **Cervix and cervical mucus response**
  - Before ovulation, estrogen levels rise, causing cervical os dilation, abundant liquid mucus, high spinnbarkeit, and excellent sperm penetration.
  - After ovulation, progesterone levels rise, resulting in cervical os constriction, scant viscous mucus, low spinnbarkeit, no ferning, and poor sperm penetration.
  - During pregnancy, cervical circulation (blood supply) increases and a protective mucus plug forms.

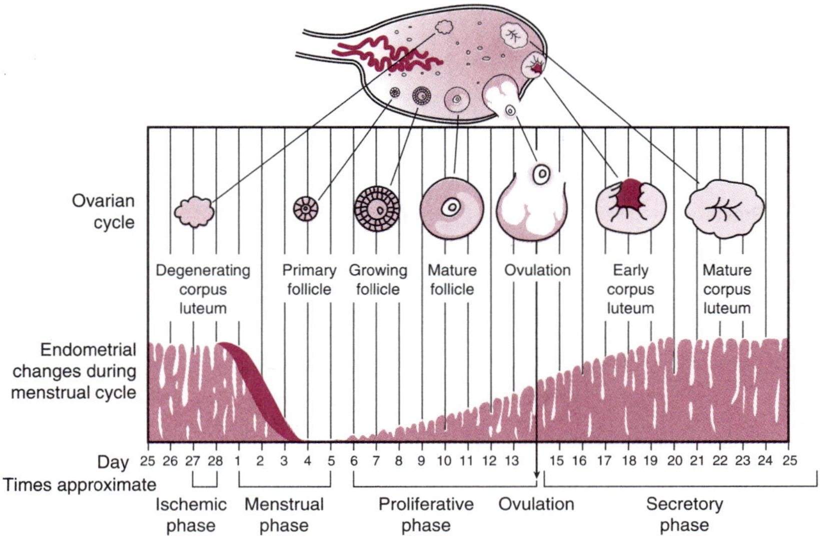

FIGURE 2-3

Schematic representation of one ovarian cycle and the corresponding changes in the thickness of the endometrium

e. **Climacteric period and menopause**

- The climacteric is a transitional period during which ovarian function and hormonal production decline.
- Menopause refers to a woman's last menstrual period; the average age of menopause is 51.4 with an age range of 40 to 55 years. However, it is important to note that women may ovulate after menopause and thus can become pregnant.
- The earlier the age of menarche the earlier menopause tends to occur.

B. Male reproductive system

1. External structures

a. The **penis** is the male organ of copulation (*Figure* 2-4, page 20). This cylindrical shaft consists of the following:
- Two lateral columns of erectile tissue (corpora cavernosa)
- A column of erectile tissue on the underside of the penis (corpus spongiosum) that encases the urethra
- The glans penis, a cone-shaped expansion of the corpus spongiosum that is highly sensitive to sexual stimulus
- The prepuce, or foreskin, a skin flap that covers the glans penis in uncircumcised men

b. The **scrotum** is a pouch hanging below the penis that contains the testes. Internally, the medial septum divides the scrotum into two sacs, each of which contains a testicle.

2. Internal structures

a. The **testes** are two solid, ovoid organs 4 to 5 cm long, divided into lobes containing seminiferous tubules. The two functions of the testes are production of testosterone and spermatogenesis (sperm production).

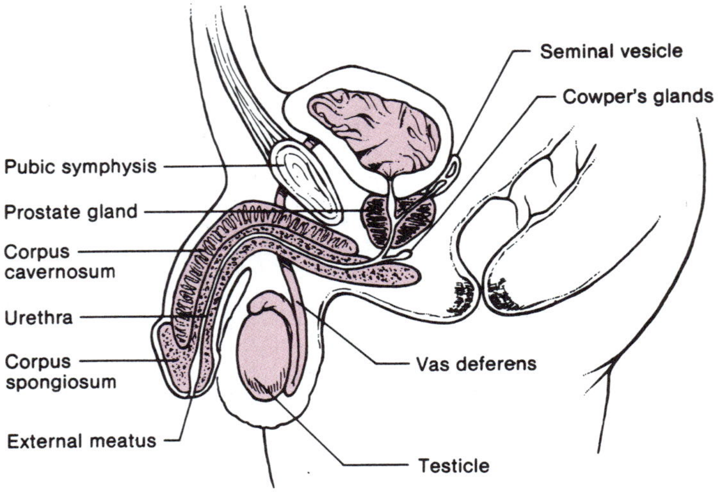

FIGURE 2–4

Lateral cross section of male reproductive structures.

b. The **epididymis** is a tubular sac located next to each testis that is a reservoir for sperm storage and maturation.

c. The **vas deferens** is a duct extending from the epididymis to the ejaculatory duct, which provides a passageway for sperm.

d. The **ejaculatory duct** is the canal formed by the union of the vas deferens and the excretory duct of the seminal vesicle. It enters the urethra at the prostate gland.

e. The **urethra** is the passageway for urine and semen that extends from the bladder to the urethral meatus.

3. **Accessory glands.** Other structures in the male reproductive system produce secretions that facilitate transportation of spermatozoa along the urethra during ejaculation and provide a temporary safe milieu for the fragile sperm. The function of the accessory glands is maintained by testosterone. The accessory glands include:

   a. **Seminal vesicles,** which are located behind the bladder and in front of the rectum, deliver secretions to the urethra through the ejaculatory ducts.

   b. The **prostate gland,** which surrounds the base of the urethra and the ejaculatory duct, secretes a clear fluid with a slightly acid pH rich in acid phosphatase, citric acid, zinc, and proteolytic enzymes.

   c. **Bulbourethral** and **urethral glands** (Cowper glands) lie at the base of the prostate and on either side of the membranous urethra. They produce a clear, alkaline mucinous substance that lubricates the urethra and coats its surface. The alkalinity assists in neutralizing acidic female vaginal secretions, which otherwise would be detrimental to sperm survival.

4. Semen

   a. Semen is a thick, whitish fluid ejaculated by the man during orgasm. It contains spermatozoa and fructose-rich nutrients. During ejaculation, semen receives contributions of fluid from the seminal vesicles and the prostate gland.

   b. Semen is alkaline (average pH, 7.5) and the average amount of semen released during ejaculation is 2.5 to 3.5 ml.

5. Male breasts
   a. Male mammary tissue remains dormant throughout life, but the breasts are a site of sexual excitation and arousal.
   b. Although rare (accounting for less than 1% of all breast cancers in the United States), male breast cancer occurs frequently enough to warrant routine inspection of the breasts for dimpling, discharge, or nipple inversion.
6. Neurohormonal control of the male reproductive system
   a. At puberty, the hypothalamus stimulates the pituitary gland to produce FSH and LH.
      - FSH stimulates germ cells within the testes to manufacture sperm.
      - LH stimulates the production of testosterone in the testes. Although LH stimulates the Leydig cells to produce testosterone from cholesterol, testosterone inhibits the secretion of LH by the anterior pituitary.
   b. **Testosterone,** one of several androgens (and the most potent) produced in the testes, is responsible for the development of secondary sex characteristics at puberty.
      - Testosterone production occurs in the interstitial Leydig cells in the seminiferous tubules. Leydig cells are abundant in the newborn and pubescent boy, and testosterone is abundant during these periods.
      - Testosterone production slows after 40 years of age; by 80 years of age, production is only about one-fifth peak level.
   c. **Spermatogenesis** occurs continually after puberty, providing large numbers of sperm for unlimited ejaculations during the mature life span.
      - Spermatozoa are released from the epithelial wall of the seminiferous tubules. Meiosis occurs during the process, and the number of chromosomes in each cell is reduced by one-half (haploid number).
      - Spermatogenesis is a heat-sensitive process; the 2° to 3° F difference between scrotal and abdominal temperatures allows spermatogenesis to proceed in the cooler environment.
      - The entire period of spermatogenesis, from germinal cell to mature sperm, takes about 75 days.

C. Female and male reproductive potentials

1. Female reproductive potential
   a. A woman's reproductive life span is finite; it begins shortly after menarche (between 9 and 17 years of age), declines somewhat during the late reproductive years, and terminates with menopause. The average age of naturally occurring menopause is 51.4 years, with an age range of 40 to 55 years
   b. The large initial store of germ cells (primordial ova) present at birth represents the total ova formed during the life span. By way of atresia, these germ cells decrease in number; by puberty, only 300,000 of the 6 to 7 million fetal germ cells remain. A woman releases no more than 500 ova during ovulation throughout her lifetime.
   c. A woman's capacity to reproduce may be disassociated from sexual excitement or receptivity.
2. Male reproductive potential
   a. Reproductive activity in men begins with sperm production at the onset of puberty and continues throughout his lifetime.
   b. New sperm cells are generated about every 75 days, and billions of mature sperm are produced during a man's normal lifetime.
   c. A man's capacity to reproduce is associated with sexual excitement, penile erection, and ejaculation.

II. HUMAN SEXUAL FUNCTION

A. Sexual response cycles. The human sexual response cycle, or how the human body responds to sexual arousal, is composed of four distinct phases.

1. Excitement phase
   a. In **women,** the following occur:
   - Vaginal lubrication increases.
   - The inner two-thirds of the vagina begins to lengthen and distend, the outer one-third undergoes slight thickening, and the body of the uterus is pulled upward. The vaginal walls become congested with blood and darken in color, and the clitoris increases in diameter, possibly with slightly increased tumescence of the glans clitoris.
   - The labia minora become engorged with blood and increase in size.
   - The labia majora flatten somewhat and retract away from the middle of the vulva.
   - The nipples become erect, and breast size increases.
   - Flushing occurs in approximately 75% of women.
   - Overall muscle tension increases.

   b. In **men,** the following occur:
   - Penile erection begins.
   - Scrotal skin becomes congested and thick.
   - Testes elevate into the scrotal sac.
   - Some nipple erection may occur.
   - Flushing may occur.
   - Heart rate and blood pressure begin to increase.
   - Generalized muscle tension increases, with a tendency toward involuntary muscle contractions.

2. Plateau phase
   a. In **women,** the following occur:
   - The walls of the outer one-third of the vagina become further engorged with blood, decreasing the internal vaginal diameter.
   - The labia minora become further engorged with blood and darken and swell.
   - The clitoris retracts and is covered by the clitoral hood; the clitoral body decreases in size by about 50%.
   - The nipples become further engorged.
   - Flushing may spread to the abdomen, thighs, and back.
   - Muscle tension increases. Breathing becomes deeper; heart rate and blood pressure increase markedly as tension rises toward orgasm.

   b. In **men,** the following occur:
   - The penis further enlarges, sometimes undergoing color changes corresponding to reddening of the female labia.
   - Preorgasmic emission may occur from Cowper glands.
   - The testes continue to be elevated, enlarge, and rotate (approximately 30 degrees).
   - Heart rate, blood pressure, and respiratory rate continue to increase.
   - Muscle tension increases.

3. Orgasmic phase
   a. In **women,** the following occur:
   - Strong muscular contractions occur in the outer one-third of the vagina, and the inner two-thirds expands.
   - The uterine muscles contract.
   - No observable changes occur in the labia majora, labia minora, clitoris, or breasts.
   - Flushing reaches a peak of color intensity and distribution.
   - Possibly strong muscular contractions, both voluntary and involuntary, may occur in many parts of the body, including the rectal sphincter muscle.
   - Respiratory rate may reach a peak of two to three times normal, heart rate may double, and blood pressure may increase as much as one-third above normal.

   b. In **men,** the following occur:
   - Rhythmic contractions expel semen from the epididymis through the vas deferens, seminal vesicles, prostate gland, urethra, and urethral meatus.
   - Testes are at maximum elevation, size, and rotation.
   - Flushing reaches its peak.
   - Heart and respiratory rates also peak.
   - A general loss of voluntary control occurs.
   - A refractory period begins as the final contractions of the urethral walls occur.

4. Resolution phase
   a. In **women,** the following occur:
   - Blood engorging the walls of the outer one-third of the vagina disperses rapidly.
   - The inner two-thirds of the vagina gradually shrinks, and color returns to pre-excitement shade.
   - The uterus descends, and the cervix dips into the seminal pool.
   - The labia minora and majora return to unstimulated thickness and close toward the midline.
   - The clitoris protrudes from under the clitoral hood, and eventually returns to prestimulated size.
   - Flushing disappears.
   - Muscles relax quickly.
   - Heart rate and blood pressure return to normal.

   b. In **men,** the following occur:
   - More than 50% of the erection is lost rapidly in the first stage of resolution, with the penis gradually returning to its unstimulated size during the second stage.
   - The scrotum gradually loses its congested and thick status.
   - The testes descend and return to normal size.
   - Nipple erection subsides.
   - Flushing disappears.
   - Heart rate, blood pressure, and respiratory rate return to normal.
   - General muscle relaxation occurs.

B. Differences in male and female sexual response

1. Women have three identifiable sexual response patterns.
   a. Rapid progression to plateau stage with some peaks and valleys, and one intense orgasm, followed by rapid resolution; resembles the male pattern
   b. Steady progression to plateau stage, followed by an intense orgasm and possibly subsequent orgasms, with slower resolution
   c. Slower progression to plateau stage, followed by minor surges toward orgasm, causing prolonged pleasurable feelings without definitive orgasm

2. Men have one basic sexual response pattern — excitement progresses steadily to plateau stage, with one intense orgasm, followed by resolution.
3. In general, women experience orgasms in a wider range of duration and intensity than do men.
4. Female orgasmic contractions last twice as long as the man's contractions; however, the strength of the contractions is not as markedly concentrated in the first few pulsations.

C. Sexual concerns related to pregnancy

1. During pregnancy, the woman's desire for sex may be altered owing to fatigue, nausea, and other discomforts of pregnancy.
2. Breasts may be painful to touch, especially during the first trimester.
3. Some men may find the normal increase in the amount and odor of vaginal discharge during pregnancy a "turn off"; others do not.
4. Other sexual concerns during pregnancy include dyspareunia and male erectile dysfunction.
5. Some women and couples need "permission" to be sexually active during pregnancy, along with reassurance that female orgasm will not harm the fetus.
6. For a couple who cannot have or who choose not to have intercourse during pregnancy, kissing, hugging, and oral or manual genital stimulation can be satisfying expressions of closeness and intimacy.

III. SEXUALITY, GENDER IDENTITY, AND SEXUAL ORIENTATION

A. Sexuality

1. A person's sexuality encompasses complex emotions, attitudes, preferences, and behaviors related to expression of the sexual self and eroticism.
2. Sexual relationships are a dynamic aspect of life and are intertwined with biological and psychosocial components.
3. Nurses commonly are resource people for clients seeking information related to human sexuality and functioning during the reproductive years.
4. Responsible sexuality involves commitment to a relationship, responsible reproductive health care, and rational decisions about childbearing.

B. Gender identity and gender roles

1. **Gender identity** is a person's sense of his or her own masculinity or femininity. Gender identity is thought to be established in part by how the individual was treated by his or her parents as a child, by hormonal influences in utero, and by psychosocial factors.
2. **Gender roles** are composed of behaviors, attributes, and attitudes an individual conveys about being male or female.
3. Born a sexual being, a child's gender identity and gender role behavior usually develop from, and conform to, cultural norms and expectations.
4. **Biologic gender** is the term used to denote chromosomal sexual development.
5. In any individual, biologic gender, gender identity, and gender role may not be the same.

C. Sexual orientation and expression

1. Sexual orientation refers to a person's preference for heterosexual, homosexual, or bisexual relationships. Preference may vary during a person's lifetime and is probably shaped by a complex interaction of several factors, including prenatal hormone envi-

ronment, early parental interactions, social mores and values, family dynamics, and imitation of the most valued parent.

2. Sexual expression refers to the activities that the individual chooses to give and receive physical love and gratification.
   a. There are many ways to experience sexual gratification, such as coitus, masturbation, celibacy, and fetishism.
   b. One's culture determines acceptable forms of sexual expression.
   c. What is considered normal may vary greatly among cultures.
   d. Acceptable sexual activity includes the elements of privacy, consent, and lack of force.
   e. Adolescence is an especially confusing and difficult time because adolescents need to feel comfortable with their own sexuality before they can reach out to others.

NURSING PROCESS OVERVIEW

IV. REPRODUCTION AND SEXUALITY

A. Assessment

1. Before interacting with any client regarding sexuality and reproduction, the nurse must perform a self-assessment; personal attitudes and values will greatly influence the nursing care provided.
2. A sexual history involves gathering information about the client or couple, such as:
   a. Past and current experiences with sexual activity
   b. Sexual knowledge and how it was obtained
   c. Attitudes toward sexuality
   d. Current problems, if any
   e. Number of sexual partners in the last 6 months
   f. History of sexually transmitted diseases
   g. Knowledge and use of "safer" sex practices
   h. Menstrual and obstetric history
   i. Method of birth control used
   j. Specific concerns related to sex and sexuality

B. Nursing diagnoses

1. Knowledge Deficit
2. Sexual Dysfunction
3. Altered Sexual Function
4. Anxiety

C. Planning and outcome identification

1. The client and her partner will be knowledgeable about reproduction and sexuality.
2. The client and her partner will resume a mutually satisfying sexual relationship.
3. The client and her partner will experience reduced anxiety related to their sexual relationship.

D. Implementation

1. Provide education regarding reproduction and sexuality.
   a. Provide the client or couple with specific information about the reproductive system's structure and function.
   b. Suggest ways to alleviate reproductive system discomforts and to prevent reproductive disease.
   c. Discuss risk and potential effects of sexual activity.

2. Promote optimal sexual functioning.
   a. Plan interventions to strengthen gender identity or role behavior.
   b. Design care that demonstrates equal acceptance of all lifestyle choices.
   c. Provide information about alternative means of sexual expression.
   d. Discuss perceptions and expectations of sexual functioning.
   e. Refer clients with complex problems to professionals specializing in sexuality issues.
3. Provide support to relieve anxiety. Allow the client or couple to discuss sexual feelings and concerns openly.

E. Outcome evaluation

1. The client or couple reports decreased anxiety related to their sexual relationship.
2. The client or couple verbalizes positive sexual contact.
3. The client or couple reports engaging in sexual intercourse and pleasurable noncoital activities.

Study questions

1. Which of the following terms refers to the tissue lying between the vaginal orifice and the anus?
1. Mons pubis
2. Perineum
3. Hymen
4. Vestibule

2. Which of the following reproductive organs contains the perimetrium, myometrium, and endometrium?
1. Decidua
2. Ovaries
3. Uterus
4. Vagina

3. Which of the following breast structures is responsible for milk production?
1. Acini cells
2. Areola
3. Lactiferous ducts
4. Nipple

4. A client asks, "How much blood do I lose during menstruation?" Which of the following would be the nurse's **best** response?
1. "Normal blood loss can be a little or a lot."
2. "Normal blood loss is about 1 cup."
3. "Normal blood loss is about $^1/_4$ cup."
4. "Normal blood loss is about $^1/_8$ cup."

5. Which of the following hormones stimulates the ovary to produce estrogen during the menstrual cycle?
1. Follicle-stimulating hormone (FSH)
2. Gonadotropin-releasing hormone (GnRH)
3. Luteinizing hormone (LH)
4. Human chorionic gonadotropin (HCG)

6. Days 6 through 14 of the menstrual cycle constitute which of the following phases?
1. Estrogen
2. Proliferative
3. Luteal
4. Secretory

7. Variations in the length of the menstrual cycle are due to variations in the number of days in which of the following phases?
1. Proliferative phase
2. Luteal phase
3. Ischemic phase
4. Secretory phase

8. During the menstrual cycle, ovulation generally occurs at which of the following times?
1. 7 days after the last day of menstruation
2. 14 days after the last day of the menstrual cycle

3. 7 days before the end of menstruation
4. 14 days before the end of the menstrual cycle

9. When providing sexual care to clients, the nurse knows that the most common nursing diagnosis is which of the following?
1. Sexual dysfunction related to psychological factors
2. Self-esteem disturbance related to guilt
3. Body image disturbance related to negative feelings
4. Knowledge deficit related to altered sexual function

10. When taking a sexual history, which of the following denotes the **correct** manner from which the nurse would proceed?
1. Specific to general problems
2. Common to unusual problems
3. Physical to psychological problems
4. Simple to complex problems

11. Which of the following should the nurse do **first** when dealing with a couple having sexual problems after 20 years of marriage?
1. Provide the couple with information about common sexual problems.
2. Arrange a physical examination for both partners.
3. Refer the couple to a support group for sexual dysfunction.
4. Allow the couple to talk about their sexual problems.

12. A young woman expresses concern about her partner's desire for sexual intercourse during her menstrual period. The nurse explains that during menses:
1. sexual intercourse is not contraindicated.
2. the male partner should wear a condom to avoid contact with blood.
3. orgasm may increase menstrual flow.
4. intercourse should be avoided to prevent infection.
5. the woman's emotional response to intercourse should guide the couple.

Answer key

1. The answer is 2.
The perineum is the tissue lying between the vaginal orifice and the anus. The mons pubis is fatty tissue over the symphysis pubis. The hymen is the membranous tissue circling the vaginal introitus. The vestibule is the area between the labia minora.

2. The answer is 3.
The uterus contains the perimetrium, myometrium, and the endometrium. The decidua is the mucous lining of the uterus during pregnancy. The ovaries are female sex glands located on each side of the uterus. The vagina, or birth canal, is a tubular organ lying between the rectum and the urethra.

3. The answer is 4.
Acini cells in the breast are responsible for milk production. The areola is the pigmented area around the nipple. Lactiferous ducts in the breast transport milk to the nipple. The nipple is the raised pigmented area in the areola through which milk passes.

4. The answer is 3.
Normal blood loss during menstruation is about 50 ml, or approximately $^1/_4$ cup. Telling the client that the blood loss can be a little or a lot is too vague and provides no useful information. Blood loss of one cup, or 240 ml, is excessive, whereas blood loss of approximately $^1/_8$ cup, or 30 ml, is a scant amount.

5. The answer is 1.
FSH is a pituitary hormone that stimulates the ovary to develop ovarian follicles that secrete estrogen. GnRH is released by the hypothalamus, which stimulates the anterior pituitary to secrete FSH and LH. LH is released by the anterior pituitary, which acts with FSH to cause ovulation and enhance de-

velopment of the corpus luteum. HCG is secreted by the placenta, which stimulates the ovaries to produce estrogen and progesterone to maintain a healthy pregnancy.

6. The answer is **2.**
Days 6 through 14 are the proliferative phase of the menstrual (endometrial) cycle. During this phase, the estrogen level is high and the uterine lining is thick. Estrogen is a hormone produced by the ovaries, not a phase of the menstrual cycle. During the luteal phase, days 15 through 22 of the ovarian cycle, the corpus luteum develops. The secretory phase, days 14 through 26 of the endometrial cycle, follows release of the ovum. During this phase, the progesterone level is high.

7. The answer is **1.**
Variation in the proliferative phase affects the length of the menstrual cycle. During this time, the estrogen level is high, the endometrium and myometrium thicken, and changes in cervical mucosa occur. The luteal phase is part of the ovarian response. In the ischemic phase (days 27 to 28), estrogen and progesterone levels recede, arterial vessels constrict, the endometrium prepares to shed, the blood vessels rupture, and menstruation begins. In the secretory phase (days 14 to 26), after release of the ovum, the estrogen level drops, the progesterone level is high, increased uterine vascularity occurs, and tissue glycogen levels increase. In the secretory phase (days 14 to 26), after release of the ovum, the estrogen level drops, the progesterone level is high, increased uterine vascularity occurs, and tissue glycogen levels increase.

8. The answer is **4.**
During the menstrual cycle, ovulation usually occurs on day 14 of a 28-day cycle. This is 14 days before the menstrual cycle ends.

9. The answer is **4.**
Lack of knowledge and misinformation are the most common problems. Sexual dysfunction may apply, but this diagnosis usually signifies a problem that is beyond the nurse's ability to intervene. The client should be referred to a specialist. Self-esteem and body image disturbance may result from lack of knowledge or misinformation.

10. The answer is **4.**
When taking a sexual history, it is important for the nurse to start out with simple questions, gathering general information, and then proceed to more complex, specific areas. In doing so, the nurse is able to obtain information in a nonthreatening atmosphere. Because the area of sexual function often is a difficult topic to address with clients, the client may feel embarrassed, inadequate, and self-consciousness. Thus the nurse must be sure to present a nonjudgmental, listening attitude. Focusing on specific common or physical problems first could overwhelm the client and add to his or her current feelings.

11. The answer is **4.**
When dealing with a couple having sexual problems, determine the problem by letting the couple discuss their problems to reveal any misconceptions about sexual functioning or communication problems from which to develop an appropriate plan for them. Once this baseline is obtained, providing the couple with information about common sexual problems, arranging for physical examinations, or referring them to a support group may be appropriate.

12. The answer is **1235.**
When teaching a client about menstrual health, the nurse should discuss exercise, sexual relations, activities of daily living, relief of discomfort, rest, and nutrition. In view of the client's specific concern, the nurse should explain that sexual intercourse is not contraindicated during menses, the client's male partner should wear a condom to avoid contact with blood and body fluids, that the client may experience increased or decreased sexual arousal, and that orgasm may increase menstrual flow. However, if the client is uncomfortable or "turned off" by the activity, her partner should respect her feelings.

3 Family Planning and Contraception

I. OVERVIEW

A. Family planning

1. Family planning is the conscious process by which a couple decides on the number and spacing of children and the timing of births.
2. Specific objectives of family planning include:
   a. Avoiding unwanted pregnancies through contraception
   b. Regulating intervals between pregnancies
   c. Deciding on the number of children that will be in the family
   d. Controlling the time at which births occur
   e. Preventing pregnancy for women with serious illness in whom pregnancy would pose a health risk
   f. Providing the option of avoiding pregnancy to women who are carriers of genetic disease
3. The overall goal of nursing intervention in family planning is to improve general maternal, neonatal, and family health.
4. Preconception planning — an ideal that is not always realized — offers couples an opportunity to enhance the probability of having a healthy newborn. It involves examining the health history and physical health of both partners and providing appropriate instruction relative to physical, psychological, and financial preparation for pregnancy and childbirth.
5. The nurse assists the couple in choosing a method of family planning by describing the methods available for reproductive planning, explaining the advantages and disadvantages of the various methods, and discussing the risk factors associated with each method.

B. Contraception

1. Contraception is the voluntary prevention of pregnancy. The decision to practice contraception has individual and social implications.

BOX 3-1
Culturally competent contraceptive care

Nurses recognize that decisions and attitudes about birth control may be influenced by cultural factors. Although it is impossible to attribute one attitude to an entire group of people, the following general information may provide a helpful point of reference when working with women from a particular ethnic group :

- The IUD is the most popular form of birth control among women from China. Sterilization is also a common practice.
- Oral contraceptives are the most common form of birth control among African-American women.
- Some African-American women who wish to avoid pregnancy or space children may see contraception as a blessing; others may view contraception as a form of genocide.
- Many African-Americans are opposed to abortion because of religious or cultural beliefs; the high rate of teen pregnancies has slightly decreased this opposition.
- Among Hispanic women, abstinence and rhythm may be the only acceptable methods. Abortion is considered morally wrong. Prolonged breast-feeding may be used as protection against pregnancy.
- Among many Native Alaskans and American Indians, large families are valued and, traditionally, birth control is not used.

From Cefalo and Dominguez. (2002). *Culture, Women, and Health Care: A Multicultural Approach to Patients. A Continuing Education Monograph.* New York: New York Medical Education Collaborative and Creative 4 Media, Inc.

2. When choosing an appropriate contraceptive method, the client must consider many factors, including:
   a. Religious orientation
   b. Social and cultural values (*Box* 3-1)
   c. Medical contraindications
   d. Psychological contraindications
   e. Individual sexual expression
   f. Cost
   g. Availability of bathroom facilities and privacy
   h. Partner's support and willingness to cooperate
   i. Personal lifestyle
3. The ideal contraceptive method is the one that is the most comfortable and natural for the partners, and the one that they will use correctly and consistently. (*Box* 3-2)
4. Contraceptive effectiveness is defined in terms of maximal effectiveness and typical effectiveness.
   a. Maximal effectiveness is a method's effectiveness under ideal conditions (that is, when it is completely understood and used as recommended).
   b. Typical effectiveness is a method's effectiveness under actual use, in which some people use the method correctly and others use it carelessly or incorrectly.

C. Nursing responsibilities

1. Assisting the couple in selecting and using an effective contraceptive method is an important part of the nurse's role.
2. Understanding one's own philosophy, beliefs, and standards is important to avoid presenting biased information.
3. Educating the individual or couple about the complete range of contraceptive possibilities is a key factor in helping the client make an informed and satisfactory contraceptive choice.
4. Understanding and teaching about available contraceptive methods and their use, effectiveness, advantages, disadvantages, and side effects are vital nursing roles in reproductive health care.
5. Providing a comfortable, factual, nonjudgmental attitude when discussing contraception and sexuality is a significant element of effective nursing care.
6. Compiling a thorough health history and assessment data is essential to planning appropriate contraception teaching.

BOX 3-2

Characteristics of the ideal contraceptive method

For any couple, an *ideal* contraceptive should be:
- Safe
- 100% effective (with consistent use)
- Free of undesirable side effects
- Easily obtainable
- Affordable
- Acceptable to the user and sexual partner
- Free of effects on future pregnancies

II. CONTRACEPTIVE METHODS

A. Natural or fertility awareness methods. These methods consist of identifying particular days during each menstrual cycle when sexual intercourse is most likely to result in pregnancy, and avoiding sexual intercourse during these days. Methods 2 through 6 below offer no protection from sexually transmitted diseases (STDs).

1. Abstinence
   - *a.* Abstinence is the most effective method for preventing conception (0% failure rate).
   - *b.* It is also the most effective way to prevent STDs.
   - *c.* Individuals or couples may find compliance with this method difficult or may completely overlook it as an option.
2. Calendar method
   - *a.* The calendar (rhythm) method relies on abstinence from intercourse during fertile periods.
   - *b.* Fertile periods are calculated by recording 12 consecutive menstrual cycles, then subtracting 18 days from the end of the shortest cycle and subtracting 11 days from the end of the longest cycle to determine the fertile period.
   - *c.* The typical user pregnancy rate is about 13%.
   - *d.* Advantages are that it is inexpensive and convenient, has no side effects, encourages communication, is ethically and morally noncontroversial, and is appropriate for sexual education programs.
   - *e.* Disadvantages are that, in general, it requires long periods of abstinence and self-control, correct calculations, and regular menstrual periods to be effective. In addition, confusing irregular uterine bleeding with a menstrual period may lead to incorrect calculations. Effectiveness is unreliable and depends on many variables.
3. Basal body temperature (BBT) method
   - *a.* Contraception by the BBT method uses the single sign of a rise in BBT to predict ovulation (signaling the fertile period) and to begin abstinence. In general, abstinence begins with the first days of menses and continues until the third day of temperature elevation.
   - *b.* BBT is measured by taking and recording the temperature orally or rectally each morning before arising after at least 3 hours of sleep. BBT drops before ovulation and rises 0.4° to 0.8° F with ovulation (in response to progesterone production from the corpus luteum).
   - *c.* During typical use, the pregnancy rate is about 20%.
   - *d.* Advantages are that it is inexpensive, has no side effects, encourages communication, is ethically and morally noncontroversial, and is appropriate for sexual education programs.
   - *e.* Disadvantages are that it is not as effective as other methods, temperature elevation may result from conditions other than ovulation, it requires regular and accurate record keeping, and it calls for partners to have intercourse only in the postovulatory period (usually about 10 days of the month).
4. Cervical mucus method
   - *a.* This method uses the appearance, characteristics, and amount of cervical mucus to identify ovulation. Because of the activity of estrogen and progesterone in the ovulatory period, cervical mucus is clear and slippery (like an egg white) and more abundant. In the preovulatory and postovulatory periods, cervical mucus is yellowish, less abundant, and thick and sticky, thereby inhibiting sperm motility.

  b. The probability of pregnancy during typical use is about 20%.
  c. Advantages are that it is inexpensive, has no side effects, and is noncontroversial.
  d. The disadvantage is that it is not as effective as other methods.

5. Symptothermal method
  a. The couple uses a combination of the above-mentioned techniques to determine the fertile period.
  b. The probability of pregnancy can range from 13% to 20% among typical users.
  c. Advantages are that it is inexpensive, provides the couple with more information, encourages communication, and has no side effects.
  d. Disadvantages are that it is more complex and difficult to learn, and requires regular and daily effort.

6. Mittelschmerz
  a. Between menstrual cycles, some women experience pain when the ovary releases an egg. Rarely, the pain may be accompanied by scant vaginal spotting. Some couples use this symptom as the signal of the beginning of the fertile period and avoid sexual intercourse until the fertile period passes.
  b. Advantages are that it is convenient and inexpensive.
  c. Disadvantages are that it requires reliable and identifiable pain and differentiation among like symptoms, and it is not as reliable as other methods.

B. Coitus interruptus

1. This method requires withdrawal of the penis from the vagina before ejaculation.
2. It is highly ineffective because sperm exist in preejaculatory fluid. Effectiveness depends on the man's ability to withdraw before ejaculation. Among typical users during the first year, the pregnancy rate is about 19%.
3. Advantages are that it is inexpensive and medically safe.
4. Disadvantages are that it is unreliable, interrupts sexual excitation or plateau, and diminishes satisfaction. It also does not eliminate the risk of STDs.

C. Spermicides

1. Vaginal jelly, cream, suppository, or foam preparations interfere with sperm viability and prevent sperm from entering the cervix. Nonoxynol-9, the active chemical ingredient, destroys the sperm cell membrane (*Drug Chart* 3-1, pages 34 and 35).
2. Pregnancy rate among typical users ranges from 5% to 50%.
3. Advantages are that spermicides are available without prescription, are useful when other methods are inappropriate or contraindicated, and have few or no side effects. They also may provide moderate protection (up to 25%) against some STDs, including gonorrhea and chlamydial infection.
4. Disadvantages are that they have a lower effectiveness than other methods, may irritate tissues (most products contain alum), and are esthetically unpleasant. One dose of most spermicides is effective for 1 hour. If a longer time has passed, a new application of spermicide is required.

D. Barrier methods

1. Female condom (vaginal pouch)
  a. This is a long polyurethane sheath that inserts manually into the vagina with a flexible internal ring forming the cervical barrier and a wide outer ring extending to cover the perineum; it is lubricated with spermicide (nonoxynol-9). It can be inserted up to 8 hours before intercourse and is available over the counter (OTC).
  b. It is about 80% effective.

(Text continues on page 36.)

DRUG CHART 3-1

Medications used for contraception

Classifications	Uses	Selected interventions
Hormones		
Monophasic oral Nelova 150/M, Norinyl 1 +50, Ortho-Novum, Lo/Ovral, Loestrin 21 1.5/30 **Biphasic oral** Ortho-Novum 10/11 Nelova 10/11 **Triphasic oral** Tri-Norinyl, Triphasil Ortho-Novum 7/7/7 Ortho Tri-Cyclen **Progestin-only oral** Micronor, Nor-QD, Overtte	▪ To prevent pregnancy ▪ To regulate menstrual cycle ▪ Most suppress FSH and LH ▪ May alter cervical mucus and the endometrial environment ▪ To prevent penetration by the sperm ▪ To prevent implantation of the egg ▪ May also suppress ovulation	▪ Explain to the client that oral contraceptives are effective only in the month they are taken; Depo-Provera (IM) is effective for 3 months after injection, and the Norplant System (implants) is effective for 5 years. ▪ Assess blood pressure before and regularly during therapy. ▪ Monitor hepatic function throughout therapy (glucose, triglycerides, prothrombin, and sodium). ▪ Encourage the client to take oral contraceptives with food to reduce nausea. Instruct the client to take oral medications at the same time daily. Explain what to do if a pill is missed. ▪ Stress the importance of an annual physical and pelvic examination, Pap smear, and mammography. ▪ Explain to the client that cigarette smoking significantly increases the risk of thromboembolic phenomena (estrogen only). ▪ Advise the client that chronic alcohol use may decrease the efficacy of oral contraceptives.
Contraceptive implant Norplant System (levonorgestrel)	▪ To prevent pregnancy	▪ Norplant is inserted subdermally in the midportion of the upper arm about 8 to 10 cm above the elbow crease. Six implantable capsules are inserted at one time.
Injectable contraceptives Depo-Provera (medroxyprogesterone)	▪ To prevent pregnancy	▪ Vigorously shake the vial containing the I.M. injection (Depo-Provera) before use to ensure uniform suspension. Administer deep I.M. into gluteal or deltoid muscle. If the time between injections is >14 weeks, determine that the client is NOT pregnant before administering the dose. ▪ Advise the client to report any of the following side effects: Migraine headache, depression, contact lens intolerance, pulmonary embolism, coronary thrombosis, cerebral hemorrhage, hypertension, edema, nausea, vomiting, spotting, breakthrough bleeding, rash, hyperglycemia, weight change, dysmenorrhea.
Lunelle injection Combination of medroxyprogesterone acetate and estradiol	▪ To prevent pregnancy	▪ Explain to the clilent that an I.M. injection is administered every 28 to 30 days (may not exceed 33 days). ▪ Advise the client that fertility returns promptly when medication is discontinued. ▪ Tell the client that the injection has the same side effects and contraindications as do oral contraceptives.

DRUG CHART 3-1
Medications used for contraception *(continued)*

Classifications	Uses	Selected interventions
Hormones (continued)		
Transdermal patch Ortho-Evra Combined hormonal contraceptive patch	■ To prevent pregnancy	■ Tell the client to apply one patch weekly for three weeks. ■ Advise the client to use one of four sites—abdomen, buttocks, upper outer arm, or trunk. ■ Caution the client not to apply over breast. ■ Explain to the client that during fourth week no patch is applied and menses occurs. ■ Advise the client that the patch is highly effective in women weighing <198 pounds and that it is safe and has a high rate of user compliance. ■ Tell the client that she may apply the patch on Sunday (she may require a back-up contraceptive method the first month of use) or day 1 of cycle (prevents ovulation with the first cycle). ■ Help the client develop a calendar with reminders for application and removal of the patch.
NuvaRing Vaginal contraceptive ring Sustained-release combined hormonal contraceptive	■ To prevent pregnancy	■ This is a soft, flexible vaginal ring; one size fits most women ■ Explain to the client that one ring is inserted monthly and left in place for 21 days and then removed for 7 days. A new ring is inserted for the next month. ■ Caution the client with vaginal prolapse to check for expulsion of the ring during early use ■ Help the client develop a calendar for insertion and reminders for removal of the ring.
Spermicide		
nonoxynol-9	■ To prevent pregnancy ■ Cause death of the sperm before they enter the cervix ■ Change vaginal pH to a strong acid level	■ Explain the following to the client and her partner: ■ Spermicides must be inserted into the vagina before intercourse. ■ These products should be inserted no more than 1 hour before intercourse. ■ Suppositories are usually inserted at least 15 minutes before intercourse. ■ The woman should not douche for 6 hours after intercourse. ■ Application must be renewed before each act of intercourse. ■ These products do not require a prescription and may be used with other methods. ■ They are contraindicated if pregnancy must not occur or if the woman has acute cervicitis. ■ They are not adequate for women experiencing menopause because of decreased vaginal moisture during this time (they depend on vaginal moisture to be activated). ■ Explain to the client that vaginal or penile irritation may occur.

c. Advantages are that it protects against STDs and conception, allows the woman to control protection, is inexpensive for single use, and is disposable.
d. Disadvantages are that it is esthetically unappealing, requires dexterity, is expensive for frequent use, may cause sensitivity to sheath material, and decreases spontaneity.

2. Male condom
a. This is a rubber sheath that fits over the erect penis and prevents sperm from entering the vagina.
b. The condom is about 86% effective.
c. Advantages are that it helps prevent conception and transmission of STDs (thereby preserving fertility), is available OTC, and has no side effects. In addition, the condom helps men maintain erections longer, prevents premature ejaculation, prevents sperm allergies, and is easily and discretely carried by men and women.
d. Disadvantages are that it may decrease spontaneity and sensation, and should be used with vaginal jelly if the condom or vagina is dry. The male condom cannot be used in cases of latex allergy in the man or woman.
e. "Natural" (animal skin) condoms are available, but they are expensive and do not protect against most STDs.

3. Cervical cap
a. This is a small rubber or plastic dome that fits snugly over the cervix.
b. Effectiveness depends on parity. In parous women, effectiveness is about 60%; in nulliparous women, effectiveness is about 80%.
c. The advantage is that it provides continuous protection for 48 hours, no matter how many times intercourse occurs. Additional spermicide is not necessary for repeated acts of intercourse.
d. Disadvantages are that it may dislodge, must be filled with spermicide, must be fitted individually by a health care provider, and may not be used if the woman has anatomic abnormalities or an allergy to plastic, rubber, or spermicide. Wearing for longer than 48 hours is not recommended because of the risk of toxic shock syndrome.
e. Side effects include trauma to the cervix or vagina, pelvic infection, cervicitis, and abnormal Pap test results. Odor problems may occur with prolonged use.

4. Diaphragm
a. This is a flexible ring covered with a dome-shaped rubber cap that inserts into the vagina and covers the cervix. The posterior rim rests on the posterior fornix and the anterior rim fits snugly behind the pubic bone. It is used with spermicide in the dome and around the rim, is applied no more than 2 hours before intercourse, and is left in place for 6 hours after coitus, but no longer than 12 (and never more than 24) hours (*Client and Family Teaching* 3-1). Additional spermicide must be applied for repeated intercourse.
b. Effectiveness is about 80% with typical use.
c. Advantages are that it is reusable and inexpensive with use over several years.
d. Disadvantages are that it requires dexterity to insert, it must be fitted individually, and it must be refitted after childbirth or after a weight loss of 15 lb or more. Wearing for longer than 24 hours is not recommended because of the risk of toxic shock syndrome (see *Client and Family Teaching* 3-1).
e. Side effects include toxic shock syndrome, cystitis, cramps or rectal pressure, and allergic reactions to spermicide or rubber.

CLIENT AND FAMILY TEACHING 3-1

Preventing toxic shock syndrome (TSS) associated with diaphragm and cervical cap use

Explain to the client and her partner that there is a risk of TSS while using a diaphragm or cervical cap. Teach the client the following ways to lower her risk:

- Wash your hands thoroughly before inserting or removing a diaphragm or cervical cap.
- Never leave a diaphragm or cervical cap in place for longer than 24 hours (preferably, remove after 12 hours).
- Never use a diaphragm or cervical cap during menstruation.
- Never use a diaphragm or cervical cap if you have a history of TSS.
- Notify your physician if any of the following symptoms of TSS occur:
  - Fever (temperature above 102° F [38.9° C])
  - Vomiting
  - Diarrhea
  - Severe muscle aches
  - Rash that develops 1 to 2 weeks after other symptoms
  - Severe headache, confusion, disorientation

E. Intrauterine device (IUD)

1. This is a flexible device inserted into the uterine cavity. It alters tubal and uterine transport of sperm so that fertilization does not occur.
2. Estimates of effectiveness vary between 93% (typical effectiveness) and 97% (maximal effectiveness).
3. Advantages are that it is inexpensive for long-term use, is reversible, has no systemic side effects, may be used in breast-feeding women, and requires no attention other than checking that it is in place (by feeling for the attached string in the vaginal canal). An ideal candidate for an IUD is a parous woman in a mutually monogamous relationship.
4. Disadvantages are that there are possibly serious side effects. The device is available only through a health care provider and cannot be used if the woman has an active or chronic pelvic infection, postpartum infection, endometrial hyperplasia or carcinoma, or uterine abnormalities. It should not be used by women who have an increased risk of STDs and women with multiple sexual partners.
5. Side effects include dysmenorrhea, increased menstrual flow, spotting between periods, uterine infection or perforation, and ectopic pregnancy. Danger signs to report to the health care provider include late or missed menstrual period, severe abdominal pain, fever and chills, foul vaginal discharge, and spotting, bleeding, or heavy menstrual periods. Spontaneous expulsions occur in 2% to 10% of users in the first year.

F. Pharmacologic methods

1. Oral contraceptives
   a. Combined estrogen and progesterone preparation in tablet form inhibits the release of FSH, LH, and an ovum. The tablets are taken daily and are available in numerous hormone combinations (and as a progesterone-only preparation; see section II, F, 4). Biphasic and triphasic contraceptives closely mirror normal hormonal fluctuations of the menstrual cycle (see *Drug Chart* 3-1, pages 34 and 35).

   b. They are about 97% effective.

   c. Advantages are that they are among the most reliable contraceptive methods and are convenient to use. In addition, they are protective against ovarian and endometrial cancer, benign breast disease, ovarian cysts, ectopic pregnancy, pelvic inflammatory disease (PID), and anemia. Oral contraceptives also tend to decrease menstrual cramps and pain.

   d. Disadvantages are that they should not be used by women who smoke or by women with a history of thrombophlebitis, circulatory disease, varicosities, diabetes, estro-

BOX 3-3
Absolute and possible contraindications to oral contraceptive use

Absolute
- Breast-feeding
- Family history of cerebrovascular accident or coronary artery disease
- History of thromboembolic disease
- History of liver disease
- Undiagnosed vaginal bleeding

Possible
- Age 40+
- Breast or reproductive tract malignancy
- Diabetes mellitus
- Elevated cholesterol or triglycerides
- High blood pressure
- Mental depression
- Migraine or other vascular-type headache
- Obesity
- Pregnancy
- Seizure disorders
- Sickle cell or other hemoglobinopathies
- Smoking
- Use of medication or drug with interaction effect

From Pillitteri, A. (2003). *Maternal and Child Health Nursing—Care of the Childbearing and Childrearing Family,* 4th ed. Philadelphia: Lippincott Williams & Wilkins, p. 106.

gen-dependent carcinomas, or liver disease. Reassessment and reevaluation are essential every 6 months. Oral contraceptives offer no protection against STDs.

e. Side effects include breakthrough bleeding, nausea, vomiting, susceptibility to vaginal infections, thrombus formation, edema, weight gain, irritability, and missed periods. Danger signs indicating complications include abdominal pain, chest pain or shortness of breath, headaches, blurred or loss of vision, and pain in the calf or thigh.

f. Contraindications and possible contraindications include breast-feeding and diabetes mellitus (*Box* 3-3).

2. Minipills

a. These contraceptive pills contain progestin but no estrogen. A pill must be taken each day and preferably at the same time each day to achieve maximal effectiveness (see *Drug Chart* 3-1, pages 34 and 35).

b. The use of minipills results in a thin atrophic endometrium and a thick cervical mucus, which inhibits permeability of sperm. Minipills do not suppress ovulation consistently; 40% of women will ovulate normally.

c. Typical user failure rate is 3%.

d. Advantages are that they may be used immediately postpartum if the client is not breast-feeding and 6 weeks postpartum if she is exclusively breast-feeding; they are highly effective when combined with breast-feeding; they have no estrogen side effects; fertility immediately returns when they are discontinued; and there is a decreased risk of PID and iron-deficiency anemia.

e. Disadvantages include irregular bleeding, increased risk of functional ovarian cysts, increased risk of ectopic pregnancy (if pregnancy does occur), and they must be taken at the same time each day.

f. There are no data to suggest that minipills increase the risk of cardiovascular disease or malignancy.

3. Subdermal implants

a. Six, soft, Silastic rods filled with synthetic progesterone are implanted into the woman's arm. The progesterone leaks into the bloodstream, inhibiting ovulation, making cervical mucus hostile to sperm and inhibiting implantation in the endometrium. The implants are known as Norplant (see *Drug Chart* 3-1, pages 34 and 35).

b. Estimates of effectiveness vary from 0.04% failure to 99% effective within 24 hours (dropping to 96% effective after 5 years).

c. Advantages are that they are long-acting (effective for up to 5 years), are not coitus-dependent, are reversible, are inexpensive over the life of the drug, and require little attention other than health care visits for problems or scheduled health maintenance. Production of thick cervical mucus confers a protective effect against PID.

d. Disadvantages are that they require surgical insertion through a half-inch incision on the inside surface of the nondominant arm, may be difficult to remove, and should not be used by a woman who has active thrombophlebitis, unexplained bleeding, active liver disease or tumor, or known or suspected breast cancer.

e. Side effects include tenderness and bruising at the insertion site, irregular bleeding, headaches, acne, weight change, and breast tenderness. Signs of reportable complications include infection, bleeding, and pain at the insertion site; subdermal rod breaking through the skin; heavy vaginal bleeding; severe abdominal pain; and sudden menstrual irregularity after a regular cycle has been established. Any pregnancy that does occur is likely to be ectopic.

4. Subcutaneous injection

a. Medroxyprogesterone (DMPA or Depo-Provera) is an intramuscular injection given every 3 months that works like subdermal implants (see *Drug Chart* 3-1, pages 34 and 35).

b. Effectiveness is similar to subdermal implants.

c. Advantages are that it is highly effective and requires little attention except for returning to the health care provider for injection every 3 months. Also, it may be used by breast-feeding women.

d. Disadvantages are similar to those for subdermal implants. In addition, the risk of breast cancer and osteoporosis may be increased, there may be a delayed return to fertility (up to 18 months), and bone density may decrease (reversible).

e. Side effects are similar to those for subdermal implants, primarily spotting, headache, and weight gain. DMPA is likely to cause amenorrhea, particularly after the first year.

5. The two newest forms of contraception are the transdermal patch (Ortho-Evra) and the contraceptive vaginal ring (NuvaRing) (see *Drug Chart* 3-1, pages 34 and 35).

G. Sterilization

1. Vasectomy

a. Surgical ligation of the vas deferens terminates sperm passage through the vas completely after residual sperm clear the male reproductive tract.

b. It is almost 100% effective (the nurse should point out the finality of the procedure).

c. Advantages are that it is highly effective and usually permanent.

d. Disadvantages are that it requires surgery and may be irreversible. Reversal success rates vary; anatomic success is 40% to 90%; clinical success is 18% to 60%. Vasectomy offers no protection against STDs.

2. Tubal ligation

a. The fallopian tubes are surgically ligated or cauterized through either minilaparotomy or laparoscopy.

b. It is almost 100% effective (the nurse should stress the finality of the procedure).

c. Advantages are that it is highly effective and usually permanent. May be performed immediately postpartum.

d. Disadvantages are that it is an invasive procedure and may be irreversible. Tubal reconstruction has a 50% to 70% successful reversal rate; however, there is a high risk of ectopic pregnancy after reversal. In addition, no protection is conferred against STDs.

H. Emergency postcoital contraception

1. Emergency contraception is an hormonal method to prevent fertilization, implantation, or both. It temporarily disrupts ovarian hormone production, causing an inadequate luteal phase, an endometrium unable to support implantation, inadequate tubal transport, and capitation.
2. Research indicates that emergency contraception used within 72 hours after a single act of unprotected intercourse is about 75% to 89% effective.
3. It may be used at the request of the client. It is indicated if the woman is worried about pregnancy resulting from rape or possible contraceptive failure. The client must have no contraindications to hormonal contraception.
4. Combined oral contraceptives are given as two Ovral pills (or four Lo-Ovral pills) within 72 hours of unprotected coitus. The dose is then repeated 12 hours later.
5. The Food and Drug Administration has approved two kits for emergency contraception. **Preven** is a combined hormonal approach (levonorgestrel and ethinyl estradiol) and **Plan B** is a progestin (levonorgestrel) only. Although emergency contraception is frequently referred to as the "morning after pill," the woman actually takes two pills as soon as possible after unprotected intercourse and two more pills 12 hours later.
6. Plan B is more effective than other emergency contraceptives and has a much lower incidence of nausea and vomiting.
7. The regimen must be started within 72 hours of unprotected intercourse. Emergency contraceptives are safe for almost all women.
8. The only contraindication is a diagnosed pregnancy because the method will not be effective.
9. Currently, there is much debate concerning how best to improve access to information about emergency contraception and how to improve access to the method.
10. Information about postcoital emergency contraception is available through the Emergency Contraception Hotline (1-888-NOT-2-LATE), or on the World Wide Web at http://opr.princeton.edu/ec/.

I. Postpartum contraception considerations

1. Breast-feeding
   a. When a woman chooses to breast-feed her newborn exclusively, the return to normal ovulatory and menstrual cycles will be delayed for weeks and even months.
   b. Sometimes, women rely on breast-feeding as a contraceptive method. It is most effective if the woman is exclusively breast-feeding with no supplementation and no pacifier use by the infant.
   c. The client must be amenorrheic. This is not a reliable form of birth control because ovulation may occur without menstruation.
   d. The pregnancy rate at 6 months postpartum is 2.9%.
2. **Fertility awareness** is not a reliable method until menstrual cycles are reestablished. Most non-breast-feeding women will resume menstruation by 4 to 6 weeks postpartum. Breast-feeding women may not resume menstruation for months, although they may ovulate sooner.
3. **Barrier methods** (cervical cap and diaphragm). The woman must wait until involution is completed to ensure a proper fitting (about 6 weeks).

4. **IUD.** The woman must wait a minimum of 6 to 8 weeks to ensure that involution is complete.
5. Pharmacologic methods
   a. Combined oral contraceptives. Breast-feeding is not necessarily a contraindication; the pills may be used after 6 weeks postpartum so that the mother has an opportunity to establish a good milk supply.
   b. Minipills may be used while the client is breast-feeding. Negligible amounts are secreted in the breast milk.
   c. Norplant and DMPA. Breast feeding is not a contraindication; negligible amounts are secreted in the breast milk. Some clinicians advise waiting until 6 weeks postpartum, when the milk supply should be well established.

NURSING PROCESS OVERVIEW

III. FAMILY PLANNING AND CONTRACEPTION

A. Assessment

1. Health history
   a. Determine the type of contraception the woman or couple desires.
   b. Obtain a thorough medical, surgical, menstrual, and obstetric history to identify any contraindications to the desired method.
2. **Physical examination.** Perform a precontraception physical examination to include breast and pelvic examination, vital signs, and other aspects as appropriate.
3. Laboratory and diagnostic studies
   a. A **Pap smear** is used to detect cervical cancer or to validate that lesions from infections are healing.
   b. **Serologic test** is used to detect syphilis or gonorrhea.
   c. **Cultures** are used to detect gonorrhea or other sexually transmitted infections.
   d. **Urinalysis** is used to detect urinary tract infections.
   e. **Complete blood count** is used to determine anemia or infection and to estimate clotting ability.

B. Nursing diagnoses

1. Knowledge Deficit
2. Decisional Conflict
3. Spiritual Distress
4. Health-Seeking Behavior
5. Powerlessness
6. Ineffective Sexuality Pattern

C. Planning and outcome identification

1. The woman or couple will identify possible methods of contraception that will fit their lifestyle.
2. The woman or couple will choose an appropriate contraceptive method (see *Box* 3-2, page 31).

D. Implementation

1. Provide client and family education.
   a. Evaluate the woman's or couple's knowledge of available contraceptive methods; provide information to correct misconceptions.

b. Teach the woman or couple about the chosen method, including, as appropriate:
- Insertion and removal (for example, diaphragm)
- Application and removal (for example, condom)
- Dosage schedule for oral contraceptives
- Techniques for natural methods

c. Discuss possible side effects and steps to take if they occur.

2. Assist the woman or couple in choosing an appropriate method of contraception.
   a. Counsel the couple about safer sex practices such as using a condom during intercourse.
   b. Provide an atmosphere of nonjudgmental discussion and information sharing.
   c. Because this is a highly personal decision, obtain the couple's view of contraception, and their beliefs and attitudes.
   d. Discover the couple's fears and concerns related to birth control.
   e. Educate the couple about the correct use of the various methods available.

E. Outcome evaluation

1. The woman or couple explains how to use the selected method, and any danger signs associated with the method selected.
2. The woman or couple demonstrates the correct use of the contraceptive method chosen.
3. The woman or couple verbalizes satisfaction with the selected contraceptive method.

Study questions

1. When reviewing contraceptive methods before teaching a class, the nurse would keep in mind which of the following methods **most** likely to be the least effective for most couples?
1. Cervical cap
2. Coitus interruptus
3. Subdermal implant
4. Condom and foam

2. Which of the following would the nurse use as the basis for explaining how an IUD prevents conception?
1. Alteration in the fallopian tube environment
2. Change in the endometrial environment
3. Alteration in the tubal transport of sperm
4. Direct destruction of the sperm cell membrane

3. A client who is using a diaphragm for contraception and who is currently participating in a weight loss program asks the nurse about the need to refit the diaphragm. The nurse should instruct the client to have the diaphragm refitted after a weight loss of at least which of the following amounts?
1. 5 lb
2. 10 lb
3. 15 lb
4. 20 lb

4. When using the basal body temperature (BBT) for contraception, the nurse would instruct the couple to abstain from intercourse during which of the following times?
1. From the first day of temperature elevation until the temperature returns to normal
2. From the first days of menses to the third day of temperature elevation
3. Once cervical mucus becomes thick and yellowish until it becomes slippery
4. From the first day of menses until the woman experiences mittelschmerz

5. Which of the following methods would be avoided for a woman who is 38 years old, has three children, and smokes one pack of cigarettes per day?

1. Oral contraceptive
2. Cervical cap
3. Diaphragm
4. Intrauterine device

6. A woman using a diaphragm for contraception should be instructed to leave it in place for at least how long after intercourse?

1. 1 hour
2. 6 hours
3. 12 hours
4. 28 hours

7. A client pregnant with her third child is deciding about having tubal ligation after she delivers. When evaluating a client's teaching plan about tubal ligation, which of the following client statements would indicate the need for additional teaching?

1. "I can have the procedure reversed if we change our mind and want more children."
2. "The procedure requires a small surgical incision in my abdomen."
3. "I can have the procedure done immediately after I deliver my baby."
4. "I still have to be careful about sexually transmitted diseases even after the procedure."

8. After the nurse teaches a couple about contraceptive methods, the couple is asked to identify fertility awareness methods. Which of the following identified by the couple would indicate the need for additional instruction?

1. Calendar method
2. Symptothermal method
3. Cervical mucus method
4. Female condom method

9. Which of the following would the nurse identify as an advantage to using a cervical cap for contraception?

1. Provides continuous protection for 48 hours
2. Is disposable and available over the counter
3. Allows spermicide application 2 hours before intercourse
4. Minimizes risk of allergic reaction to plastic

10. The transdermal patch is replaced once every ______ days for _____ weeks.

Answer key

1. The answer is 2.

Coitus interruptus is the withdrawal of the penis from the vagina before ejaculation occurs. It is highly ineffective because sperm is contained in the preejaculatory fluid. Effectiveness depends on the man's ability to withdraw before ejaculation. Among typical users during the first year, the pregnancy rate is about 19%. The cervical cap's effectiveness depends on parity. In parous women, effectiveness is about 60%; in nulliparous women, effectiveness is about 80%. Subdermal implants are estimated to be highly effective, ranging from 0.04% failure to 99% effective within 24 hours (dropping to 96% effective after 5 years). Condoms are considered 86% effective.

2. The answer is 3.

An IUD prevents conception by altering the tubal transport of sperm so that fertilization does not occur. The environments of the fallopian tube and endometrium are not affected. Spermicides directly destroy the sperm cell membrane.

3. The answer is 3.

A diaphragm needs to be refitted after a weight loss of 15 lb or more. Refitting is not necessary with weight loss of less than 15 lb.

4. The answer is 2.

When using the BBT for contraception, because a rise in temperature signals ovulation, a couple should engage in abstinence from the first days of menses until the third day of temperature elevation. The first day of temperature rise indicates ovulation and places the woman at risk for conception should intercourse occur. Cervical mucus changes indicating ovulation involve a change from thick yellowish discharge to clear slippery discharge. Therefore, abstinence should occur when the mucus changes to this clear slippery discharge. Mittelschmerz indicates ovulation. Thus abstinence should occur just before and after the woman experiences the sensation.

5. The answer is **1.**
For the female client who smokes cigarettes, oral contraceptives are avoided because of the increased risk of embolism formation. Cervical cap, diaphragm, and IUD are appropriate contraceptive choices for an older woman who smokes. In fact, an ideal candidate for an IUD is a parous woman in a mutually monogamous relationship.

6. The answer is **2.**
The diaphragm should remain in place for at least 6 hours after intercourse but not longer than 12 hours to avoid the possibility of toxic shock syndrome.

7. The answer is **1.**
A tubal ligation is a sterilization procedure that is highly effective and usually permanent. However, tubal reconstruction has a 50% to 70% successful reversal rate and there is a high risk of ectopic pregnancy after reversal. Therefore, the client needs additional teaching about the "irreversible" nature of the procedure. Tubal ligation, an invasive procedure, is performed by surgically ligating or cauterizing the tubes, through either a minilaparotomy or laparoscopy. It is advantageous because it can be performed immediately postpartum.

8. The answer is **4.**
The female condom is a barrier method of contraception. Therefore, if the couple identifies this method, they need additional teaching. Fertility awareness methods (identifying particular days during each menstrual cycle when sexual intercourse is most likely to result in pregnancy, and avoiding sexual intercourse during these days) include the calendar method, basal body temperature, symptothermal, cervical mucus method, and mittelschmerz.

9. The answer is **1.**
The cervical cap is a small rubber or plastic dome that fits snugly over the cervix. It provides continuous protection for 48 hours, no matter how many times intercourse occurs. Additional spermicide is not necessary for repeated acts of intercourse. The cervical cap is not disposable or available over the counter, as is the female condom. A cervical cap must be fitted to the individual by a health care provider. There is a risk of allergic reaction if the woman develops allergies to plastic, rubber, or spermicide.

10. The answer is **7,3.**
The transermal patch is removed and replaced with a new patch once every 7 days for a total of 3 weeks each month. No patch is applied the fourth week, when menses occurs.

4 Infertility

I. OVERVIEW

A. Fertility

1. The reproductive potential of men and women depends on multiple factors, including age, sex, and overall health status.
2. Under optimal conditions, about 50% of couples who try to conceive will do so within 6 months. An additional 35% of couples who try to conceive will do so within 12 months. This brings the total to 85% over a 12-month period.
3. See Chapters 2 and 6 for discussions of fertility and conception.

B. Infertility

1. Description
   a. Infertility is the inability to conceive after at least 1 year of sexual intercourse at least four times per week without contraception.
   - **Primary infertility** refers to no previous history of either partner conceiving or impregnating.
   - **Secondary infertility** is the inability to conceive after a previous successful pregnancy.

   b. Although infertility implies that some potential for conception exists, sterility denotes a total and irreversible inability to become pregnant or to impregnate.

   c. In the United States, the incidence of infertility is 10% to 15% of couples in their reproductive years. Although the general public may perceive that the incidence of infertility has increased, the fact is there has been no significant change in the proportion of infertile couples in the United States. However, the diagnosis of infertility has increased in the 25- to 44-year-old age-group.

   d. Infertility results from a problem for the woman 45% of the time; a problem for the man 35% of the time; and a problem for both partners or an unidentified cause about 20% of the time. Professional intervention can help approximately 65% of infertile couples achieve pregnancy.
2. Etiology
   a. Factors contributing to **female infertility** include:
   - **Vaginal problems** include vaginal infections, anatomic abnormalities, sexual dysfunction that prevents penetration by the penis, a highly acidic vaginal environment, which markedly decreases sperm survival, and use of coital lubricants.
   - **Cervical problems** include:
     - A disruption in any of the **physiologic changes** that normally occur during the preovulatory and ovulatory period that make the cervical environment conducive to sperm survival (such as opening of the cervical os, increased alkalinity, increased secretions, ferning, and antisperm antibodies).
     - **Mechanical problems,** such as cervical incompetence associated with women whose mothers were treated with diethylstilbestrol (DES) during pregnancy
   - **Uterine problems** may be:
     - **Functional** (such as an unfavorable environment for the movement of sperm up the uterus into the fallopian tubes or for implantation after fertilization)
     - **Structural** (such as uterine myomas or leiomyomas)
   - **Tubal problems**
     - Infertility due to tubal problems is becoming more prominent with the increased incidence of pelvic inflammatory disease (PID). PID leads to scarring that blocks the fallopian tubes. The increased use of intrauterine devices (IUDs) contributes

to the rise in PID because 40% of infections associated with IUD use are asymptomatic and remain untreated.
- Endometriosis also can contribute to tubal obstruction.

- **Ovarian problems** include anovulation, oligo-ovulation, and polycystic ovary syndrome. Secretory malfunctions also contribute; for example, inadequate progesterone secretion or an inadequate luteal phase will interfere with the ability of a fertilized ovum to be maintained.

b. Factors contributing to **male infertility** include:
- **Congenital factors** include maternal history of DES ingestion during pregnancy and absence of the vas deferens or the testes.
- **Ejaculation problems** include retrograde ejaculation associated with diabetes, nerve damage, medications, or surgical trauma.
- **Sperm abnormalities** include inadequate sperm production or maturation, inadequate motility, blockage of sperm along the male reproductive tract, and an inability to deposit sperm in the vagina.
- **Testicular abnormalities** include those due to illness (for example, orchitis associated with mumps after puberty), cryptorchidism, trauma, or irradiation.
- **Coital difficulties** may occur owing to obesity or spinal nerve damage.
- **Drugs** (such as methotrexate, amebicides, sex hormones, and nitrofurantoin) may interfere with spermatogenesis.
- **Other factors** that interfere with sperm or semen production include infections (such as sexually transmitted diseases), stress, inadequate nutrition, excessive alcohol intake, and nicotine.

c. **Interactive problems**, resulting from causes specific to each couple, include:
- Insufficient frequency of sexual intercourse
- Poor timing of intercourse
- Development of antibodies against a partner's sperm
- Use of potentially spermicidal lubricants, such as petroleum jelly and some water-soluble lubricants
- Inability of the sperm to penetrate the egg

II. DIAGNOSTIC EVALUATION

A. Initial assessment

1. Evaluation of infertility must begin with a complete health history and physical examination of both partners, and basic laboratory tests, including complete blood count (CBC), thyroid function tests, and urinalysis (see section IV).
2. If these results are negative, an infertility work-up consisting of more invasive and intensive diagnostic studies begins.

B. Diagnostic studies

1. Semen analysis
   a. The test is performed after 48 to 72 hours of abstinence from orgasm to avoid false low readings.
   b. Repeated serial analysis is done 74 days apart.
   c. Sperm count, volume of ejaculate, infection, seminal viscosity, and presence or absence of agglutination of sperm are considered.

2. Cervical mucus assessment
   a. At the height of estrogen stimulation, just before ovulation, cervical mucus is thin, has a low viscosity and cellularity, and appears in a large amount. It forms a fernlike pattern when allowed to dry on a glass slide. This pattern is observable under a microscope. At this point during the cycle, the cervical mucus also can be stretched into long strands.
   b. When progesterone levels rise, just after ovulation during the luteal phase, a fern pattern is no longer present.
   c. A **fern test** is done at midmenstrual cycle to confirm ferning. If there is no evidence of ferning, estrogen levels have not increased sufficiently. On the other hand, if a ferning pattern continues throughout the menstrual cycle, progesterone levels did not rise and the woman did not ovulate.
   d. A **spinnbarkeit test** can also be used to determine that high levels of estrogen are present. This test measures the "stretchability" of the cervical mucus and implies that ovulation is about to occur. In the presence of high levels of progesterone the mucus does not stretch and it is very thick. The woman can perform this test herself by stretching the sample between her thumb and forefinger.
3. Postcoital test
   a. The couple is instructed to have sexual intercourse at the presumed time of ovulation after a 48-hour period of abstinence.
   b. Immediately after intercourse, a sample of cervical mucus is examined microscopically to detect characteristics that enhance sperm survival and to assess adequacy of estrogen production.
4. Basal temperature recordings
   a. For several cycles, the woman takes and records oral temperatures daily when awakening.
   b. A biphasic pattern with persistent temperature elevation for 12 to 14 days before menstruation indicates that ovulation has occurred.
5. Hormonal assessment of ovulatory function
   a. **Gonadotropin levels** (follicle-stimulating hormone [FSH] and luteinizing hormone [LH]) provide valuable information concerning normal ovulatory function. The FSH level is drawn on cycle day 3 and is the most valuable test in assessing ovarian reserve and function; it should always be drawn on women over 35 years of age. LH levels are drawn early in the cycle to rule out disorders associated with androgen excess. Daily sampling of serum LH at midcycle can detect the LH surge. The day of the LH surge is believed to be the time of maximum fertility. Urine LH home testing kits are available to better time postcoital testing, insemination, and coitus.
   b. **Progesterone assays** furnish the best evidence of ovulation and corpus luteum function. Serum levels rise with the LH surge and peak 8 days later. A level of 5 ng/ml usually confirms ovulation. On day 21, a level of 10 ng/ml or higher indicates an adequate luteal phase.
   c. Elevated levels of **prolactin** (an anterior pituitary hormone) are a frequent cause of ovulatory dysfunction, which may include anovulation or amenorrhea.
   d. **Thyroid-stimulating hormone (TSH).** Thyroid hormone is necessary for most body functions. TSH stimulates prolactin secretion. Hypothyroidism may have a profound effect on ovulatory function, causing menstrual irregularities and bleeding problems.
   e. Excessive androgen levels usually result in such clinical symptoms as ovulatory dysfunction, which may include anovulation and amenorrhea.

6. Endometrial biopsy
   a. Endometrial biopsy provides direct histologic information about the endometrial tissue.
   b. If adequate secretory tissue is identified, secretion of progesterone and luteinizing hormone is normal, indicating that ovulation has occurred.
7. Hysterosalpingography
   a. Radiopaque dye is injected through the cervix into the uterus. Fluoroscopy shows whether the fallopian tubes fill with dye.
   b. A radiograph is taken 24 hours later to determine if the dye has dispersed in the pelvic cavity, an indication of fallopian tube patency.
   c. The study must be done after menstruation has ceased to prevent the possibility of old menstrual blood being pushed into the tubes and causing infection.
   d. The study also must be done before ovulation to prevent pushing a fertilized ovum out through the fimbrial end of the tubes.
8. Transvaginal ultrasound imaging
   a. Ultrasound waves can be used to determine the patency of the fallopian tubes and the depth and consistency of the lining of the uterus.
   b. Sonohysterography is a noninvasive ultrasound technique that can be carried out at any time during the menstrual cycle.
   c. Transvaginal ultrasound is the method of choice for monitoring women undergoing ovulation induction cycles, timing ovulation for insemination and intercourse, retrieving oocytes for in vitro fertilization, and monitoring early pregnancy.
9. Hysteroscopy
   a. Hysteroscopy is a visual inspection of the uterus through a hysteroscope.
   b. A thin hollow tube is inserted through the cervix.
   c. It is helpful in detecting uterine adhesions or other abnormalities.
10. Other tests
   a. **Immunoassays of semen and male or female serum** are done to determine if antibody formation against the partner's sperm is a factor in infertility.
   b. **Sperm penetration assay** is an in vitro test to determine the ability of the sperm to penetrate the zona pellucida of the ova from superovulated hamsters.

III. MEDICAL MANAGEMENT

A. Management of an underlying problem

1. General suggestions
   a. Alter acidic cervical mucus by having the woman douche with an alkaline solution 30 minutes before intercourse.
   b. Remove environmental hazards associated with oligospermia (for example, tight underclothes, hot tubs or saunas, and certain drugs, chemicals, and toxins).
2. Surgery
   a. Correct anatomic defects and remove obstructions in the female reproductive tract.
      - Remove uterine fibroid tumors.
      - Cerclage an incompetent cervix.
      - Perform microsurgery to open blocked fallopian tubes.
   b. Ligate varicocele in the man.

DRUG CHART 4-1
Medications used for infertility

Hormone classification	Uses	Selected interventions
Gonadotropins **Generic** Menotropins **Proprietary** Pergonal, Humegon	■ Management of infertility; production of ovarian follicular development and growth; followed by administration of human chorionic gonadotropin (HCG) to produce ovulation	■ Explain the importance of coordinating sexual relations with ovulation. ■ If injection is used, instruct the client appropriately. ■ Counsel the couple about the possibility of multiple births. ■ Assist the client to make a calendar for treatment schedule. ■ Observe for the following side effects and notify the primary care provider because treatment may need to be discontinued: ovarian enlargement, febrile reaction, multiple pregnancies, and ovarian hyperstimulation syndrome (abdominal and GI symptoms and peripheral edema).
Androgenic anabolic hormone **Generic** testosterone **Proprietary** Andro, Histerone, Testamone, Testoject	■ Possible increase of sperm count and motility	■ Measure and record I&O. ■ Monitor weekly weight gain (it should be no more than 5 lb). ■ Administer IM deep into the upper outer quadrant of gluteal muscle. ■ Monitor for side effects, including rash, dizziness, fatigue hirsutism, increased blood pressure, weight gain, and increased blood glucose.
Estrogen **Generic** estrogen **Proprietary** Depogen, Premarin CES	■ Restoration of hormone balance and maintenance of ovarian function	■ Advise the client to take the drug with food. ■ Measure weekly weight. ■ May cause increased triglycerides and cholesterol. ■ Monitor for side effects, including headache, dizziness, nausea, breast tenderness, thromboembolism, breakthrough bleeding, and leg cramps.
Estrogen agonist clomiphene citrate (Clomid)	■ Stimulation of the ovary. Binds with estrogen receptors and increases FSH and LH secretion from the hypothalamus	■ Obtain baseline hormonal studies and pelvic examination before starting therapy. ■ Use a calendar to plot treatment schedule and ovulation. ■ Warn clients to report any side effects, including abdominal distention, nausea, vomiting, breast tenderness, vasomotor flushing, and ovarian enlargement. ■ Warn clients that multiple births may occur with use of this drug.
Semisynthetic ergot derivative **Generic** bromocriptine **Proprietary** Parlodel	■ Hyperprolactinemia accompanying anovulation ■ High levels of prolactin may impair production of FSH and LH or block their action on the ovaries	■ Instruct client to: – Take drug with food. – Take first dose when lying down at bedtime. – Begin therapy during menses. ■ Use nonhormonal (mechanical) contraceptives while taking drug. ■ Discontinue at time of anticipated ovulation once normal ovulatory cycle is established. ■ Counsel the client that drug has teratogenic effects on fetal development if pregnancy occurs during therapy.

DRUG CHART 4-1
Medications used for infertility *(continued)*

Hormone classification	Uses	Selected interventions
Semisynthetic ergot derivative (continued)		▪ Tell the client to report nausea, vomiting, diarrhea, persistent watery nasal discharge, dizziness, headache, or fatigue. ▪ Inform the client that therapy should last no more than 6 to 12 months. ▪ Advise the client that intravaginal administration may decrease the occurrence of side effects.
Synthetic androgenic hormone **Generic** Danazol **Proprietary** Danocrine	▪ Treating infertility caused by endometriosis; suppresses ovulation and menstruation; to effect atrophy of the ectopic endometrial tissue; temporary suppression has been shown to result in healing of the endometriosis	▪ Ensure that the client is not pregnant before beginning therapy. ▪ Alert the client that weight gain, changes in hair distribution, and other androgenic effects may be irreversible. ▪ Arrange for periodic evaluation of hepatic function. ▪ Counsel the client to use barrier methods of contraception during therapy. ▪ Tell the client to report abnormal hair growth, bruising, bleeding, chills, fever, sore throat, and vaginal itching or irritation.

3. **Medications.** The following medications may be used to treat infertility (see *Drug Chart* 4-1).
   - *a.* Antibiotic therapy to treat infections
   - *b.* Testosterone to treat oligospermia
   - *c.* Estrogen therapy to increase the abundance of cervical mucus and enhance ferning and spinnbarkeit
   - *d.* Ovulation-induction medications to treat anovulation
4. Sexual therapy
   - *a.* This type of therapy for infertility involves treatment of sexual problems that may interfere with conception (such as vaginismus or dyspareunia without an identifiable organic, physical, or mechanical cause and psychogenic impotence).
   - *b.* One approach to sexual counseling involves gathering assessment data on a couple's sexual difficulties, then clarifying each member's perceptions of the other and of sexual activities in general.
   - *c.* The therapist facilitates communication between the two partners and their acceptance of each other's feelings and attitudes.
   - *d.* The couple may be taught specific exercises and different coital positions to assist in increasing control during sexual activity or enjoyment in the pleasure of sex.

B. Assisted reproductive techniques

1. Artificial insemination
   - *a.* This technique is used to instill the sperm into the cervix or uterus to aid in conception.

b. If the husband's sperm is used, the procedure is referred to as artificial insemination by husband.
c. If a donor sperm is used, the procedure is referred to as artificial insemination by donor.
d. If the man has an inadequate sperm count, a genetic defect, an irreversible vasectomy, or testicular cancer, he may choose to store sperm before therapy. The cryopreserved sperm will then be available for use if he desires children at a future time. This is referred to as therapeutic donor insemination (TDI).
e. TDI can also be used if the woman has no male partner, or has a vaginal or cervical factor that interferes with sperm motility.

2. In vitro fertilization (IVF)
   a. This technique is used when damaged or obstructed fallopian tubes impair transport of a fertilized egg to the uterus.
   b. Other reasons for use include oligospermia, absence of cervical mucus, presence of antisperm antibodies, when no cause has been determined, and when other options have been attempted and failed.
   c. The first recorded success was in 1978 in England.
   d. Following a course of menotropins (such as Pergonal and Humegon) to stimulate ovulation, the ovary is punctured during laparoscopy, and mature follicles are removed by suction.
   e. Each egg is incubated for several hours in a sugar, salt, and protein mixture designed to simulate maternal fluids found in the fallopian tubes.
   f. Semen is added, and the eggs and fluid are again incubated. If the egg is fertilized, it is incubated further until cell division begins. After cell division has begun, the fertilized egg is deposited in the woman's uterus using a thin plastic catheter.
3. Gamete intrafallopian transfer
   a. An ovum is surgically retrieved from the ovary and implanted into the fallopian tube.
   b. Sperm are then implanted into the fallopian tube.
   c. Fertilization may then occur naturally.
4. Zygote intrafallopian transfer
   a. The ovum is fertilized externally.
   b. The fertilized zygote is then returned to the fallopian tube by an instrument such as a laparoscope.
5. Surrogate embryo transfer (SET)
   a. This procedure is used when the woman does not ovulate and the male partner is fertile.
   b. The first child resulting from SET was born in 1984.
   c. Using hormonal therapy, the menstrual cycles of the donor woman and the recipient woman are synchronized.
   d. Sperm of the fertile partner is artificially inseminated in the fertile donor following her normal ovulation. Several days after fertilization occurs, the fertilized egg is washed from the donor's uterus and deposited in the recipient's uterus; if the procedure is successful, implantation occurs soon afterward.
   e. The embryo conceived in the donor woman is transplanted into the uterus of the infertile woman.
6. Intracytoplasmic sperm injection (ICSI)
   a. This procedure is a form of micromanipulation using a microscope with 200 to 400 times magnification and micromanipulators.

   b. ICSI enables injection of a sperm directly into an egg.
   c. The procedure has achieved fertilization when there is absence of sperm motility or extremely low sperm count, and when IVF therapy has failed.
7. Surrogate mothering
   a. This procedure is used when a woman not only is unable to conceive but also is unable to carry a fetus to viability.
   b. Semen from the infertile woman's partner is artificially inseminated into the host (surrogate mother).
   c. After birth, the newborn is given to the infertile couple.
   d. Legislation is pending in many states to regulate this practice.
8. Complementary and alternative therapy
   a. **Acupuncture** is used in traditional Chinese medicine and has become very popular in the United States. It involves inserting a needle into specific points on the body to control the flow of *chi* (life energy). For infertile couples, the acupuncturist would concentrate on the flow of chi in the kidneys and adrenal glands. Some clinical studies have shown acupuncture to be effective in treating infertility in both men and women.
   b. **Herbal therapies.** Herbs, especially ginseng and astragalus, are frequently recommended to treat infertility. Their success is attributed to their hormone-balancing effects. Historically, ginseng has been used in traditional Chinese medicine to improve male virility and fertility. Some studies indicate that ginseng and astragalus enhance in vitro sperm motility.
   c. The nurse should be alert for signs that the couple is pursuing these therapies out of desperation. They may not be using their best judgment.

NURSING PROCESS OVERVIEW

IV. CARE OF THE INFERTILE COUPLE

A. Assessment

1. Health history
   a. Evaluate the couple's sexual and reproductive history to rule out sexual dysfunction as a cause of infertility.
   b. Assess the couple's knowledge of sexuality, sexual techniques, and infertility.
   c. Assess the couple's general lifestyle, including use of medicines, drugs, and other substances; nutrition; exercise; rest patterns; and occupation.
   d. Evaluate the couple's usual strategies for coping with stress and anxiety.
   e. Assess the couple's psychosocial responses associated with infertility stage of emotional healing, cultural influences, belief systems, and effect on self-image.
   f. Assess the individual partner's general health, including illnesses, injuries, surgeries, and the woman's menstrual history.
   g. Determine fertility in other relationships, if applicable.
   h. Determine lifestyle choices, including use of alcohol and drugs, history of sexually transmitted diseases, and number of sex partners.
2. Physical examination
   a. Complete a general physical examination.
   b. Note distribution and condition of hair and fat.

c. Perform a careful examination of the genital tract. In women, assess for presence of infection, condition of cervix, and size, position, and mobility of uterus. In men, include presence of infection and size of the scrotum, testes, and prostate.

3. Laboratory and diagnostic studies
   a. Initially, the following studies are performed.
   - **Complete blood count**
   - **Triiodothyronine (T_3), thyroxine (T_4), and thyroid-stimulating hormone (TSH) (thyroid function studies)**
   - **Urinalysis and culture** represent normal kidney function and rule out the presence of infection.
   - **Serologic tests** for syphilis
   - **Rh factor and antibody titer**
   - **Sperm antibody tests** and **semen analysis**

   b. If these tests prove inconclusive, intensive infertility diagnostic studies will be performed on both partners (see section II).

B. Nursing diagnoses

1. Anxiety
2. Ineffective Family and Individual Coping
3. Decreased Self-esteem
4. Knowledge Deficit
5. Spiritual Distress
6. Fear
7. Grief
8. Health-Seeking Behavior

C. Planning and outcome identification

1. The couple will regain a sense of control.
2. The couple will receive advocacy and support during the decision-making process.
3. The couple will receive anticipatory guidance.
4. The couple will receive accurate information about infertility in general, and their case in particular.
5. The couple will resolve their feelings about infertility.

D. Implementation. The nurse must keep in mind that diagnosis and treatment of infertility typically occur over several months or years and represent a significant financial and emotional commitment on the part of the couple.

1. Assist the couple in regaining a sense of control.
   a. Use stress-reduction techniques.
   b. Point out successes and achievements in other areas of their lives.
   c. Suggest that the couple continue activities that they enjoy doing together.
   d. Suggest that they begin a new activity that is of interest to both partners.
2. Provide advocacy and support for decision-making.
   a. Listen and facilitate decision-making.
   b. Allot time to talk about ideas, concerns, and issues of conflict.
   c. Provide access to other sources and networks for information and support.
   d. Offer referral to appropriate agencies.
3. Provide anticipatory guidance.
   a. Explain the complex battery of diagnostic tests.
   b. Discuss protocols of fertility evaluation. (*Client and Family Teaching* 4-1)

CLIENT AND FAMILY TEACHING 4-1

How to collect a semen specimen

- Abstain from sexual activity for 2 to 4 days before collecting the specimen.
- Use a clean, dry container with a tight-fitting lid to collect the sample.
- Collect the specimen as close as possible to your usual schedule of sexual activity.
- Avoid using any lubricants when collecting the specimen.
- After the specimen is collected, close the container and write the time on the container.
- To keep the specimen at body temperature while you transport it, carry the container under your arm or next to your chest.
- The specimen must be analyzed within 1 hour of collection.

CLIENT AND FAMILY TEACHING 4-2

Activities to aid conception

- Determine the time of ovulation by using basal body temperature, analysis of cervical mucus, or a commercial kit to determine ovulation.
- Plan sexual relations for every other day at the time of ovulation. More frequent coitus may lower the sperm count.
- Men need sperm recovery time after ejaculation to maintain adequate sperm count. This is why coitus every other day during the fertile period may yield faster results.
- The male superior position is the ideal position because it places the sperm closest to the opening of the cervix.
- Elevating the woman's hips on a small pillow during coitus will help to collect sperm nearest to the cervical opening.
- The woman should stay on her back with her knees drawn up for at least 20 minutes after ejaculation to keep sperm near the cervical opening.
- Do not use douches or artificial lubricants before or after intercourse because they may interrupt sperm motility or change the pH of the vagina.

c. Point out responses to such procedures and the impact on sexual functioning and the couple's relationship.

4. Provide accurate information, and dispel myths associated with infertility that foster guilt, self-doubt, and feelings of inadequacy (*Client and Family Teaching* 4-2).
5. Help the couple resolve their feelings about infertility. For some couples, treatment for infertility will not be successful. These couples must be encouraged to consider other options, such as surrogate mothers, adoption, or child-free living.

F. Evaluation

1. The infertile couple exhibits evidence of healthy coping mechanisms when dealing with infertility.
2. The infertile couple makes decisions about their treatment with support from the nurse and other members of the health care team.
3. The infertile couple shows positive adjustment to the demands of the diagnostic and treatment regimens.
4. The infertile couple states that their questions are answered and they understand the treatment regimen. They acknowledge the possibility of failure.
5. The infertile couple verbalizes their individual and collective feelings related to infertility, diagnosis, and treatment.

Study questions

1. The medical record of a couple that has been trying to conceive for 2 years reveals no physiologic problem that would prevent conception. Which of the following statements by the couple would indicate that they need additional teaching about increasing the likelihood of conception by optimal timing of intercourse?
1. "Ovulation usually occurs 14 days before the onset of the menstrual cycle."
2. "An ovulated egg has a life span of 12 to 24 hours."
3. "Daily sexual intercourse increases the likelihood of conception."
4. "Ejaculated sperm have a life span of 24 to 48 hours."

2. A couple with one child has been trying, without success, for several years to have another child. Which of the following terms would describe their situation?
1. Primary infertility
2. Secondary infertility
3. Irreversible infertility
4. Sterility

3. When assessing the adequacy of sperm for conception to occur, which of the following is the most useful criterion?
1. Sperm count
2. Sperm motility
3. Sperm maturity
4. Semen volume

4. A client who is seeking help in becoming pregnant reveals that her mother took DES while pregnant with the client. The nurse's response would be based on the knowledge that maternal use of DES is associated with which of the following?
1. Pelvic inflammatory disease (PID) in female offspring.
2. Cervical incompetence in female offspring.
3. No specific problems in either male or female offspring.
4. Reproductive problems in male offspring.

5. Which of the following best explains why data about a client's medical history, which includes a ruptured appendix and resulting peritonitis, would be pertinent to the client's infertility problems?
1. Scarring and adhesions may have created anatomic deformities or tubal blocking.
2. The infection may have caused sterility.
3. The appendix is important to tubal functioning.
4. Surgical removal of the appendix is likely to sever the fallopian tubes.

6. A couple who wants to conceive but has been unsuccessful during the last 3 years has undergone many diagnostic procedures. When discussing the situation with the nurse, one partner states, "All the couples we know in our age-group are having their second or third child, yet we are so inadequate that we can't even produce one. With our luck, we'd probably have a defective baby anyway." Which of the following would be the most pertinent nursing diagnosis for this couple?
1. Fear related to the unknown.
2. Pain related to numerous procedures.
3. Ineffective family coping related to infertility.
4. Self-esteem disturbance related to infertility.

7. A couple who is infertile has never used contraception and engages in intercourse usually three to four times a week. Both independently express a high degree of sexual satisfaction. They practice some sexual experimentation with position, time, and location, and they use petroleum jelly for additional lubrication. The man's sperm count is lower than normal, but other assessment data appear to be well within normal limits. Based on these data, the nurse's recommendation for potentially increasing the likelihood of conception would include which of the following?

1. Advise the couple to reduce frequency of intercourse to once a week.
2. Advise them to be more consistent in how they have intercourse.
3. Instruct them to stop using the additional lubrication.
4. Clarify the validity of their sexual satisfaction.

8. Introduction of radiopaque material into the uterus and fallopian tubes to assess tubal patency is known as which of the following?

1. Spinnbarkeit test
2. Hysteroscopy
3. Ferning test
4. Hysterosalpingography

9. The results of various diagnostic procedures indicate serious problems for a man with a low sperm count and a woman with fibroid tumors blocking the fallopian tubes. Both partners begin to laugh when one says, "Oh, we were so worried nothing could be done to help us begin a family. We'll just take care of these two things, and then we'll have a baby." The couple's reaction to the seriousness of their fertility problem most likely indicates which of the following?

1. Denial of the seriousness of the problem.
2. Concealed anger with each other.
3. Joyful relief toward the seriousness of the problem.
4. Coping with a positive attitude.

10. Desperately desiring children, a couple has spent 10 years undergoing numerous procedures, including corrective surgery and marital therapy, to help them cope with anger and disappointment. Today they reveal that they have decided to adopt a child. While discussing their decision with the nurse, they are smiling and holding hands. The man says, "I'm glad I'll never have to see this place [the fertility clinic] again." Based on this information, the nurse would most accurately evaluate their behavior as an indication of which of the following?

1. Denial of their chance to have their own child.
2. Anger at the nurse for wasting their time.
3. Apathy concerning their state of infertility.
4. Acceptance of their state of infertility.

11. The nurse working with a young woman in the infertility clinic explains how to take and record a daily basal body temperature. The young woman states that she works nights in a box factory, goes to bed at 6 a.m., and gets up to take her husband to work at 8 a.m.. She gets home and goes back to bed at 9 a.m., and sleeps about 5 or 6 hours before getting up to cook dinner and get ready for work. When during the day should she record her basal body temperature?

1. at 6 a.m.
2. at 9 a.m.
3. at 2 p.m.
4. at 8 a.m.
5. at 10 p.m.

Answer key

1. The answer is **3.**
Daily sexual intercourse may actually lower the sperm count, or the daily schedule may become a source of added stress on the relationship, possibly impairing conception. Thus, the couple would need more teaching. Ovulation on the average occurs approximately 14 days before the onset of the menstrual cycle. An ovulated egg's life span is approximately 12 to 24 hours, whereas that of ejaculated sperm ranges from 24 to 48 hours.

2. The answer is **2.**
Because the couple successfully conceived previously, their situation would be accurately described as secondary infertility. Primary infertility would apply if the couple had never conceived a child. This scenario does not suggest irreversible infertility, also called sterility.

3. The answer is **2.**
Although all of the factors listed are important, sperm motility is the most significant criterion when assessing male infertility. Sperm count, sperm maturity, and semen volume are all significant, but they are not as significant as sperm motility.

4. The answer is **2.**
Maternal use of DES during pregnancy has been linked to problems involving cervical incompetence in female offspring, contributing to possible problems with infertility. PID and male reproductive problems are not associated with maternal use of DES.

5. The answer is **1.**
A history involving a ruptured appendix and resultant peritonitis is significant because scarring and adhesions are possible. These may result in anatomic deformities or blockage of the client's fallopian tubes, possibly causing infertility problems. Sterility from the infection or severing of the tubes during surgery is not likely. The appendix plays no role in tubal functioning.

6. The answer is **4.**
Based on the partner's statement, the couple is verbalizing feelings of inadequacy and negative feelings about themselves and their capabilities. Thus, the nursing diagnosis of self-esteem disturbance is most appropriate. Fear, pain, and ineffective family coping also may be present but as secondary nursing diagnoses.

7. The answer is **3.**
Petroleum jelly and some water-soluble lubricants have been shown to be spermicidal. Reducing the frequency of intercourse will not increase the probability of conception. No information is presented in the scenario to indicate that consistency in how the couple has intercourse or the validity of their statements about their sexual satisfaction are factors involved with the couple's ability to conceive.

8. The answer is **4.**
The injection of radiopaque dye through the cervix into the uterus followed by fluoroscopy to show whether the fallopian tubes fill with dye is a hysterosalpingography. With this test, a radiograph is taken 24 hours later to determine if the dye has dispersed in the pelvic cavity, an indication of fallopian tube patency. Spinnbarkeit tests and ferning tests assess cervical mucus. A hysteroscopy is a visual inspection of the uterus through a hysteroscope. A thin hollow tube is inserted through the cervix to detect uterine adhesions or other abnormalities.

9. The answer is **1.**
The couple's statement indicates denial, a typical initial reaction to "bad news" that allows time for adjusting to a threatening situation. Although the couple may be angry

with each other, no data are provided in this scenario to support this analysis. The couple's statement and situation involves neither joy nor positive feelings.

10. The answer is 4.
The couple's statement reveals feelings of acceptance and moving on by taking steps to obtain children despite their infertility. This couple's history of 10 years of therapeutic assistance indicates that they have moved through anger and denial. Through their continued pursuit and involvement to conceive, they have not demonstrated apathy and resignation but have made every effort to achieve conception.

11. The answer is 3, 4.
This is often a problem because many women work outside the home on a variety of shifts, frequently going without a long period of sustained aleep. In order to determine a pattern and establish a baseline, this young woman should take her temperature twice a day—on awakening in the morning (8 a.m.) and on awakening after her longest period of sleep during the day (2 p.m.). Whichever of these times shows the most constant temperature would be her baseline basal body temperature.

5 Biopsychosocial Aspects of Pregnancy

I. BIOLOGICAL ASPECTS OF PREGNANCY

A. Overview

1. All maternal body systems are altered by pregnancy. These changes are normal, inevitable, and temporary.
2. Pregnancy represents a state of wellness; it is not an illness.

B. Signs and symptoms of pregnancy

1. Presumptive (subjective) changes
   a. Amenorrhea
   b. Nausea and vomiting
   c. Urinary frequency
   d. Breast tenderness and changes
   e. Excessive fatigue
   f. Uterine enlargement
   g. Quickening
2. Probable (objective) changes
   a. Changes in pelvic organs
      - Goodell sign is softening of the cervix.
      - Hegar sign is softening of the lower uterine segment.
      - Piskacek sign is enlargement and softening of the uterus.
      - McDonald's sign is an ease in flexing the body of the uterus against the cervix.
      - Chadwick's sign is a blue-purple discoloration of the cervix.

   b. Serum laboratory tests for pregnancy based on detection of the presence of human chorionic gonadotropin (HCG)
      - The serum test for HCG is 95% to 98% accurate. For this reason, a positive HCG is considered a probable sign of pregnancy.
      - HCG is a hormone produced by the chorionic villi of the placenta. It is measurable in both the serum and urine of pregnant women. However, urine tests are not usually used today because serum levels of HCG can be measured earlier in the pregnancy.
      - HCG appears in trace amounts in the serum as early as 24 to 48 hours after implantation. It reaches measurable levels at 7 to 9 days after conception (50 mIU). The level peaks at 100 mIU between 60 and 80 days of gestation. The level then declines throughout pregnancy until at term only trace amounts remain.

   c. Uterine souffle, which is a soft, blowing sound at the rate of the maternal pulse
   d. Changes in skin pigmentation
   e. Ultrasonographic evidence of a gestational sac
3. Positive (diagnostic) changes
   a. Fetal heartbeat is audible at 10 to 12 weeks' gestation by Doppler ultrasound and at 16 to 20 weeks' gestation with a fetoscope. The normal fetal heart rate is 120 to 160 beats per minute.
   b. Fetal movements palpable by examiner are a positive finding.
   c. Ultrasonography confirms the presence of a fetus.

C. Reproductive system changes of pregnancy involve the uterus, cervix, ovaries, vagina, and breasts.

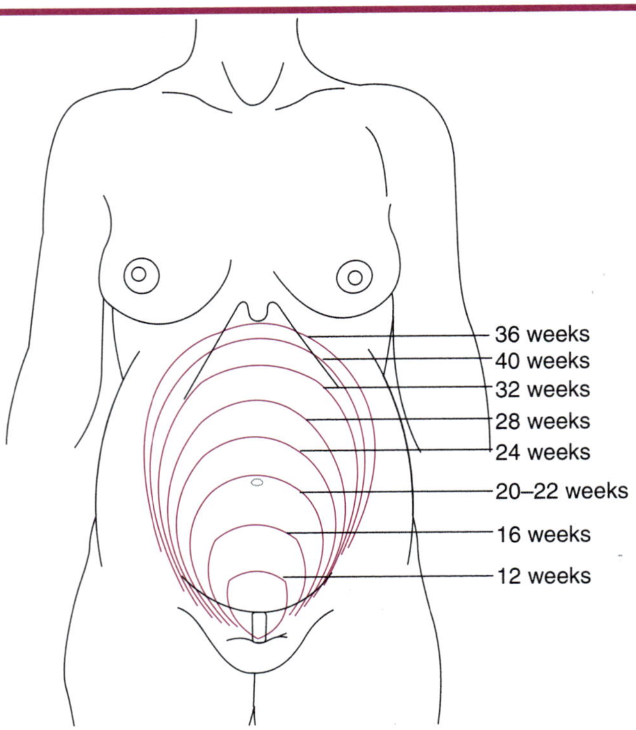

FIGURE 5–1

Fundal height at various weeks of pregnancy.

1. Uterus
   a. Uterine growth occurs as follows:
   - Length increases from 6.5 to 32 cm.
   - Width increases from 4 to 24 cm.
   - Depth increases from 2.5 to 22 cm.
   - Weight increases from 60 to 1,100 g.
   - Capacity increases from 1 to 10 ml to 5,000 ml.

   b. Uterine enlargement results from growth of new myometrial muscle cells and stretching of existing myometrial cells.

   c. Increased formation of fibroelastic tissue adds strength and elasticity to the uterine muscle wall by binding the muscle fibers together.

   d. Uterine circulatory requirements increase; accordingly, so do the size and number of blood vessels and lymphatics.

   e. Braxton Hicks contractions (painless contractions) occur intermittently throughout pregnancy and can be felt by the woman by the fourth month.

   f. Normal uterine growth, measured in terms of fundal height, is evaluated in relation to other anatomic structures.
   - Uterine growth is steady, constant, and predictable throughout pregnancy.
   - After 20 weeks' gestation, fundal height in centimeters approximates the weeks of pregnancy up to 36 weeks (*Figure* 5-1).

2. Cervix
   a. Stimulated by estrogen, the cervix becomes vascular and edematous.
   b. Endocervical glands secrete thick mucus that forms a mucus plug.
      - The mucus plug seals the endocervical canal and prevents contamination of the uterus by bacteria and other substances.
      - The mucus plug is expelled just before the onset of labor.
   c. Goodell sign, softening of the cervix, results from increased cervical vascularization.
3. Ovaries
   a. The ovaries do not produce ova during pregnancy.
   b. The corpus luteum, which develops from the ruptured follicle, produces hormones (estrogen and progesterone) for the first 16 weeks of pregnancy; it then regresses in size and becomes indistinct.
4. Vagina and external genitalia
   a. Increased vascularization causes tissues to thicken and soften.
   b. Increased vascularization of the vagina causes a blue-purple coloration. This is called Chadwick sign.
   c. Vaginal discharge tends to be thick, white, and acidic (pH 4 to 5) during pregnancy.
5. Breasts
   a. Breast size increases, and breasts become more nodular owing to glandular hyperplasia and hypertrophy.
   b. The nipple and areola darken; superficial veins become more prominent.
   c. Striae may develop in late pregnancy.
   d. Colostrum may leak or be expressed from the breast during the last 3 months of pregnancy.

D. Respiratory system changes

1. The diaphragm elevates and the substernal angle increases owing to an enlarging uterus.
2. Displacement of the diaphragm causes shortness of breath.
3. Nasal stuffiness and epistaxis are common owing to edema and vascular congestion, which is caused by increased estrogen levels.
4. Respiratory function is affected in the following ways:
   a. Respiratory rate increases by about two breaths per minute.
   b. Vital capacity may remain unchanged or increase slightly.
   c. Breathing more deeply increases the efficiency of gas exchange.
   d. Functional residual capacity and residual volume are decreased owing to elevation of the diaphragm.
   e. Plasma Po_2 increases to between 104 and 108 mm Hg.
   f. Tidal volume increases by 30% to 40%.
   g. Plasma Pco_2 decreases to between 27 and 32 mm Hg.
   h. Plasma pH increases to between 7.40 and 7.45.

E. Cardiovascular system changes

1. The heart is displaced upward, to the left, and forward.
2. As the uterus enlarges, pressure on blood vessels increases and slows circulation. This process can lead to edema and varicosities of the legs, vulva, and rectum.
3. The pressure of the enlarged uterus on the vena cava causes supine hypotensive syndrome during the second trimester (when the woman lies supine).

4. Cardiovascular function is affected in the following ways:
   a. Blood volume increases 30% to 50% during pregnancy.
   b. Red blood cell volume increases 20% to 30%.
   c. Hematocrit decreases 7%, causing physiologic anemia of pregnancy.
   d. Fibrinogen level may increase by as much as 40%.
   e. Leukocytes increase to 20,500.
   f. Pulse rate increases 10 to 15 beats per minute.
   g. Blood pressure decreases slightly, then returns to prepregnant level during the third trimester.
   h. Cardiac output increases by 25% to 50%.
   i. Heart rate increases by 10 to 15 beats per minute.
   j. Plasma volume increases from 2,600 ml to 3,600 ml.
   k. Total protein decreases from 7.0 g/dl to 5.5 to 6.0 g/dl.

F. Gastrointestinal system changes

1. Nausea and vomiting, especially in the morning, are common during the first trimester.
2. Gum tissue may become soft and bleed when the teeth are brushed.
3. Secretion of saliva may increase.
4. Gastric acidity decreases. Heartburn and flatulence may result owing to the reduction in gastric acidity, a growing uterus, and smooth-muscle relaxation.
5. Bloating and constipation may occur owing to delayed gastric emptying time and decreased intestinal motility.

G. Urinary system changes

1. Urine output increases; urine-specific gravity decreases.
2. Dilation of the kidneys and urethra may occur, especially on the right side, owing to the pressure of the enlarged uterus.
3. Urinary stasis and urinary tract infections may occur as a result of pressure on the ureter and urethra from the growing uterus.
4. Bladder capacity increases to 1,500 ml.
5. There is an increased risk of glycosuria because reabsorption of glucose by the renal tubules occurs at a fixed rate. During pregnancy, there is an increased glomerular filtration rate, which leads to increased filtration of glucose into the tubules. This creates an opportunity for spillage of glucose into the urine.
6. Urinary frequency occurs in the first and third trimesters owing to pressure from the enlarged uterus.

H. Integumentary system changes

1. Pigmentation changes occur in the areola, nipple, abdomen, thighs, and vulva.
2. Facial chloasma (mask of pregnancy) and vascular spider nevi may develop.
3. Striae (stretch marks) commonly appear on the abdomen, breasts, and thighs.
4. Activity of sebaceous and sweat glands may increase.

I. Skeletal system changes

1. Sacroiliac, sacrococcygeal, and pubic joints relax during pregnancy.
2. The symphysis pubis may separate slightly.
3. Lumbodorsal spinal curve is increased during the third trimester, commonly producing low back pain.

TABLE 5-1
Recommended total weight gain ranges for pregnant women

Pregnancy weight-for-height category	Recommended total gain lb	kg
Low (BMI < 19.8)	28–40	12.5–18
Normal (BMI 19.8–26)	25–35	11.5–16
High (BMI > 26.0–29.0)	15–25	7.0–11.5
Obese (BMI > 29.0)	≥15	≥7

Note: For singleton pregnancies. The range for women carrying twins is 16–20 kg (35–45 lb). Young adolescents (< 2 years after menarche) and African-American women should strive for gains at the upper end of the range. Short women (< 57 cm or < 62 in) should strive for gains at the lower end of the range.

From Institute of Medicine Subcommittee for a Clinical Application Guide (1992). *Nutrition During Pregnancy and Lactation: An Implementation Guide.* Washington, D.C.: National Academy Press, p. 44.

From Olds, S., London, M., Laderwig, P., et al. (2004). *Maternal-Newborn Nursing and Women's Health Care.* 7 ed. Upple Saddle River, New Jersey: Pearson Prentice Hall.

J. Metabolic changes

1. Metabolism accelerates 20% during pregnancy.
2. Average weight gain during pregnancy is 25 to 35 lb, which is composed of:
   a. Fetus — 7.5 lb
   b. Placenta and membrane — 1.5 lb
   c. Amniotic fluid — 2 lb
   d. Uterus — 2.5 lb
   e. Breasts — 3 lb
   f. Increased blood volume — 2 to 4 lb
   g. Extravascular fluid and fat — 5 to 10 lb (*Table* 5-1)
3. Increased water retention is a basic chemical alteration of pregnancy.
   a. Water is retained during pregnancy to support the increase in blood volume and to serve as a ready source of nutrients for the fetus. Normal increase results in a total body-water level of about 7.5 L.
      - The fetus, placenta, and amniotic fluid account for 3.5 L of the increased amount of fluid.
      - Increased blood volume, interstitial fluid, and hypertrophied maternal organs account for 3.5 L of the increased amount of fluid.
   b. Factors contributing to water retention include:
      - Increased level of steroid sex hormones
      - Lowered serum protein
      - Increased intracapillary pressure and permeability

K. Endocrine system changes

1. Thyroid gland
   a. There is an increase in vascularity and hyperplasia.
   b. A rise in thyroxine (T_4) occurs.
   c. Basal metabolic rate increases by 25%.
2. Parathyroid gland
   a. There is increased parathyroid hormone production.
   b. There is an increase in the size of the gland.
3. Pituitary gland
   a. The gland becomes slightly hypertrophic during pregnancy.
   b. The anterior pituitary gland increases secretion of prolactin, which is responsible for beginning lactation after delivery.
   c. The posterior pituitary gland releases oxytocin, to produce uterine contractions, and vasopressin, to promote vasoconstriction and an antidiuretic effect.
4. Adrenal glands
   a. The adrenal glands undergo little structural change.
   b. Cortisol levels regulate metabolism of carbohydrates and proteins.
   c. Increased levels of aldosterone and corticosteroids suppress an inflammatory response.
5. **Pancreas.** The pancreas increases production of insulin.
6. Placenta
   a. The placenta is the endocrine gland of pregnancy.
   b. It secretes the hormones of pregnancy—human chorionic gonadotropin (HCG), estrogen, progesterone, human placental lactogen (HPL), and relaxin.
      - HCG is originally produced by the trophoblast cells of the blastocyst. At about the 8th gestational week, the placenta takes over production of this hormone. HCG stimulates the corpus luteum to produce estrogen and progesterone early in the pregnancy before the placenta takes over production of these hormones.
      - Estrogen stimulates the development of a uterine environment suitable for the fetus (that is, it increases the uterus's size and weight and augments the blood supply).
      - Progesterone maintains the endometrium and decreases contractility of the uterus.
      - HPL increases circulating free fatty acids for maternal metabolism.
      - Relaxin decreases uterine activity and softens the cervix.

L. Nutrition during pregnancy

1. The total energy cost of pregnancy is 85,000 calories. This breaks down to about 300 extra calories each day averaged over the entire pregnancy. Specific dietary increases are recommended by the National Academy of Sciences (*Table* 5-2) and are discussed in section III.
   a. Protein requirements increase to provide sufficient amino acids for fetal development, increased blood volume, and breast and uterine tissue growth; the recommended daily allowance is 30 g/day more than nonpregnant needs.
   b. Pregnancy increases requirements for all vitamins. However, vitamin oversupplementation may lead to vitamin toxicity.
   c. Commonly recommended prenatal nutritional supplements contain vitamins B_6, C, D, and E; folic acid; pantothenic acid; iron; calcium; magnesium; zinc; and copper.

TABLE 5-2

Average recommended nutritional requirements for nonpregnant, pregnant, and breast-feeding women

Nutrients	Nonpregnant women Age 11 – 14	Age 15 – 18	Age 19 – 30	Age 31 – 50	Pregnant	Breast-feeding
Calories	2200	2200	2200	1800	2100–2500	2300–2700
Protein (g)	46	44	46	46	60	60
Fats (g)	(Unchanged during pregnancy and lactation; should account for 30% of total caloric intake)					
Fat soluble vitamins						
Vitamin A (μg)	700	700	700	700	750–770	1200–1300
Vitamin D (μg)	5	5	5	5	5	5
Vitamin E (mg)	15	15	15	15	15	19
Vitamin K (μg)	60	75	90	90	90	90
Water soluble vitamins						
Vitamin C (mg)	45	65	75	75	80–85	115–120
Thiamine (mg)	1.1	1.1	1.1	1.1	1.4	1.4
Riboflavin (mg)	1.1	1.1	1.1	1.1	1.4	1.6
Niacin (mg)	14	14	14	14	18	17
Vitamin B_6 (mg)	1.0	1.2	1.3	1.5	1.9	2.0
Vitamin B_{12} (μg)	1.8	2.4	2.4	2.4	2.6	2.8
Minerals						
Folate (μg)	400	400	400	400	600	500
Calcium (mg)	1300	1300	1000	1000	1300	1300
Phosphorus (mg)	1250	1250	700	700	700–1250	700–1250
Iron (mg)	8	15	18	18	27	9–10
Zinc (mg)	8	9	8	8	11–13	12–13
Iodine (μg)	120	150	150	150	220	290
Selenium (μg)	40	55	55	55	60	70
Magnesium (mg)	240	360	310	320	350-360	310–360

From Institute of Medicine (1997-2001). *Dietary Reference Intakes.* Washington, D.C.: National Academy Press. Also available at http://www.nap.edu

d. Dietary calcium is the best way to increase calcium intake to support the growing fetus (for example, dairy products, beans, and leafy, green vegetables [collard, mustard, kale, turnip, and broccoli]).
e. Because of the mixed effects of calcium on iron and zinc absorption, daily calcium supplements exceeding 100 g are not recommended during pregnancy.

2. Some **hormonal effects** of pregnancy are the basis for the increased nutritional requirements and dietary allowances.
   a. Progesterone causes relaxation of the smooth muscle, including the GI tract, and reduced motility, allowing more nutrients to be absorbed. Progesterone also increases maternal fat deposition and increases renal sodium excretion.
   b. Estrogen increases water retention.
   c. HCG is implicated in nausea.
3. Some metabolic adjustments during pregnancy are the basis for the increased nutritional requirements and dietary allowances. These include:
   a. A 50% greater plasma volume by 34 weeks' gestation, creating an increased need to carry oxygen and nutrients
   b. Increased serum lipid levels (such as triglycerides, cholesterol, free fatty acids, and vitamin A), which are probably due to increased circulating steroids (cholesterol is a precursor for the synthesis of progesterone and estrogen in the placenta)
   c. Increased blood flow through the kidneys and an increased glomerular filtration rate to facilitate the clearance of waste products from the woman and fetus

II. PSYCHOSOCIAL ASPECTS OF PREGNANCY

A. Overview

1. Pregnant women may become more dependent and may need increased nurturing so that they can nurture their developing offspring.
2. Pregnant women may need varied social service programs to help meet their health care needs.
3. Family-centered care has helped involve the family as well as the mother in childbirth.
4. Cultural background may determine activities that are acceptable or not acceptable during pregnancy (*Box* 5-1).

B. Psychosocial stages of pregnancy

1. **Anticipatory stage**. Women train for the role of expectant parent and interact with babies and children.
2. **Honeymoon stage.** Women fully assume the pregnancy role and initially may seek help from family members.
3. **Plateau stage.** The pregnancy role is fully exercised; the expectant parent validates the adequacy of the current role.
4. **Disengagement.** The termination stage precedes and includes termination of the pregnancy role (that is, labor and birth of the infant [although the pregnancy role may terminate in other ways]).

C. Meaning and effect of pregnancy on the couple

1. The coming child represents the synthesis of three distinct role relationships.
   a. Relationship of the woman and her partner
   b. Relationship of the woman and her developing fetus
   c. Relationship of the woman and her newborn

BOX 5-1
Developing cultural competence

Nurses who are interacting with expectant families from a different culture or ethnic group can provide more effective, culturally sensitive nursing care by:

- Critically examining their own cultural beliefs
- Identifying personal biases, attitudes, stereotypes, and prejudices
- Making a conscious commitment to respect the values and beliefs of others
- Using sensitive, current language when describing others' cultures
- Learning the rituals, customs, and practices of the major cultural and ethnic groups with whom they have contact
- Including cultural assessment of the family's expectations of the health care system as a routine part of prenatal nursing care
- Incorporating the family's cultural practices into prenatal care as much as possible
- Fostering an attitude of respect for and cooperation with alternative healers and caregivers whenever possible
- Providing for services of an interpreter if language barriers exist
- Learning the language (or at least several key phrases) of at least one of the cultural groups with whom they interact
- Recogizing tha ultimately it is the woman's right to make her own health care choices
- Evaluating whether the client's health care beliefs have any potential negative consequences for her health

From Olds, S., London, M., Laderwig, P., et al. (2004). *Maternal-Newborn Nursing and Women's Health Care.* 7 ed. Upple Saddle River, New Jersey: Pearson Prentice Hall, p. 319.

2. The mother can never again be a single unit.
3. Men may experience physical and psychological changes during their partner's pregnancy. This common experience is referred to as couvade syndrome.
4. The male partner may feel left out or jealous of the growing baby, or he may be unable to express his feelings.
5. Necessary tasks of pregnancy for a woman or the couple include the following:
   a. Belief that she is pregnant and incorporation of the fetus into her body image
   b. Preparation for physical separation with the birth of the newborn
   c. Resolution and identification of conflicts that accompany role transition; this will prepare for smooth functioning of the family.
   d. Resolution of previous life experiences; the pregnant woman will examine her relationship with her own mother.
   e. Fantasizing about what it will be like to be a parent and what the baby will be like
6. Common emotional reactions of the woman or the couple to pregnancy include the following:
   a. **First trimester.** Ambivalence, fear, fantasies, or anxiety
   b. **Second trimester.** Well-being, increased need to learn about fetal growth and development, narcissism, passivity, or introversion (may seem egocentric and self-centered)
   c. **Third trimester.** Feels awkward, clumsy, unattractive; becomes more introverted; or reflects on own childhood

NURSING PROCESS OVERVIEW

III. THE BIOPSYCHOSOCIAL ASPECTS OF PREGNANCY

(see also Chapter 8: Antepartum Care)

A. Assessment

1. Overview
   - *a.* Begin a biopsychosocial assessment at the initial prenatal visit and perform ongoing data collection at each subsequent visit.
   - *b.* Make every effort to include the expectant father in prenatal visits.
2. Obtain detailed family, menstrual, and obstetric histories.
3. Elicit a description of the **cardinal signs and symptoms** of pregnancy, including onset, duration, location, and precipitation (see section I, B).
4. Evaluate the expectant parents for **risk factors** associated with poor adaptation to pregnancy.
   - *a.* Prior negative childbearing or childrearing experiences
   - *b.* Inadequate preparation for childbearing or childrearing
   - *c.* Significant health concerns
   - *d.* Negative response to the pregnancy
   - *e.* Conflicts or problems in support system

B. Nursing diagnoses

1. Anxiety
2. Knowledge Deficit
3. Altered Nutrition: Less Than Body Requirements
4. Body Image Disturbance

C. Planning and outcome identification

1. The couple will experience decreased anxiety.
2. The couple will acquire knowledge about what to expect during pregnancy.
3. The expectant mother will increase her intake of calories and nutrients to meet the demands of pregnancy.
4. The expectant mother will maintain a healthy body image.

D. Implementation

1. Alleviate anxiety.
   - *a.* Reassure the woman that episodes of nausea and vomiting typically cease by the end of the first trimester.
   - *b.* Explain to expectant fathers that many men do not feel involved in the pregnancy until the last few weeks, but offer assistance in adapting to the pregnancy (*Client and Family Teaching* 5-1).
   - *c.* Plan time to address questions and concerns of both expectant parents. This approach will help alleviate anxiety and increase the couple's understanding of their roles.
   - *d.* Encourage communication between the couple.
   - *e.* Encourage the woman to continue her usual social and physical activities as long as she is comfortable.

CLIENT AND FAMILY TEACHING 5-1

Assisting the expectant father to adapt to pregnancy

The nurse should explain that paternal responses change throughout the pregnancy. They depend on the man's ability to view the infant as real, to internalize the role of parent, and to create a role as an involved father. Be an advocate for the man by remembering to include the following points in your care:

- Some expectant fathers develop a cluster of signs and symptoms of pregnancy similar to the mother. This is called *couvade syndrome*. Assure the man that this is normal and temporary.
- Encourage the expectant father to come to prenatal visits if possible; schedule the prenatal visits at a time when he will be able to attend.
- Allow the expectant father to listen to the fetal heart rate.
- Provide an opportunity for the expectant father to ask questions and discuss concerns.
- Show the expectant parents the sonogram and explain the "picture."

CLIENT AND FAMILY TEACHING 5-2

Alleviating backache during pregnancy

The nurse should explain that backache is a common problem during pregnancy as a result of strain on the lower vertebrae from carrying extra weight, a shift in the body's center of gravity, and a forward curving of the lumbar spine to accommodate the pregnancy. The following suggestions may help alleviate backache:

- Maintain correct posture; avoid wearing high-heeled shoes.
- Squat rather than bend from the waist to pick up objects.
- When sitting, use arm rests, foot supports, and pillows placed behind your back.
- Taylor sitting, pelvic rocking, and shoulder-circling exercises strengthen your back.
- Report backache if urinary frequency and pain accompany it, localized pain in the back, back pain that comes and goes frequently, or backache not relieved by rest.

2. Provide family teaching.
   a. Explain what biophysical and psychosocial changes to expect next month.
   b. Teach the woman how to cope with backache during pregnancy (*Client and Family Teaching* 5-2).
3. Encourage the woman to increase her intake of calories and nutrients to meet the demands of pregnancy.
   a. Offer tips on alleviating nausea and vomiting (*Client and Family Teaching* 5-3, page 72).
   b. Provide sample diets.
   c. Refer the expectant mother to a nutritionist.
   d. Provide information on government nutrition programs for expectant mothers with limited incomes (such as Women, Infant, Children [WIC] food program).
4. Promote a positive body image.
   a. Explain that the physical changes are normal and temporary.
   b. Encourage the woman to continue her exercise routine, with appropriate modifications for pregnancy.
   c. Encourage the woman to wear clothes that flatter her changing figure.
   d. Compliment good grooming and personal hygiene.
   e. Allow time for the woman to express her feelings. It is OK for the woman to have times when her pregnancy does not produce euphoria.

CLIENT AND FAMILY TEACHING 5-3

Alleviating nausea and vomiting of pregnancy

The nurse should explain that nausea and vomiting are a common occurrence during the first trimester of pregnancy but that these symptoms will disappear as the woman enters the second trimester. The following remedies may be helpful in alleviating nausea and vomiting:

- Eat dry crackers or toast *before* getting out of bed in the morning. Get up slowly.
- Eat dry crackers every 2 hours throughout the day to avoid having an empty stomach.
- Eat five or six small meals rather than three big ones.
- Drink fluids separately rather than with your meals.
- Avoid fried, greasy, gas-producing, or spicy foods, and foods with strong odors.

E. Outcome evaluation

1. The couple states their anxiety level is decreased.
2. The couple exhibits progress toward healthy adaptation to childbearing.
3. The couple reports increased knowledge concerning all aspects of pregnancy.
4. The expectant mother's caloric intake is sufficient to support expected weight gain.
5. The expectant mother makes positive statements about her changing body.

Study questions

1. Which of the following urinary symptoms does the pregnant woman most frequently experience during the first trimester?
1. Dysuria
2. Frequency
3. Incontinence
4. Burning

2. Heartburn and flatulence, common in the second trimester, are most likely the result of which of the following?
1. Increased plasma HCG levels
2. Decreased intestinal motility
3. Decreased gastric acidity
4. Elevated estrogen levels

3. On which of the following areas would the nurse expect to observe chloasma?
1. Breasts, areola, and nipples
2. Chest, neck, arms, and legs
3. Abdomen, breast, and thighs
4. Cheeks, forehead, and nose

4. A pregnant client states that she "waddles" when she walks. The nurse's explanation is based on which of the following as the cause?
1. The large size of the newborn
2. Pressure on the pelvic muscles
3. Relaxation of the pelvic joints
4. Excessive weight gain

5. Which of the following represents the average amount of weight gained during pregnancy?
1. 12 to 22 lb
2. 15 to 25 lb
3. 20 to 30 lb
4. 25 to 35 lb

6. Which of the following would be the nurse's best response to a woman who, at 5 months' gestation, reports that she has felt intermittent, painless, irregular contractions of her uterus?
1. "It is important to time these contractions because it may be the beginning of labor."
2. "If these contractions occur again, call your physician immediately."

3. "The contractions help stimulate the movement of blood through the placenta."
4. "They are called Braxton Hicks contractions. They may occur throughout pregnancy."

7. When talking with a pregnant client who is experiencing aching, swollen leg veins, the nurse would explain that this is most probably the result of which of the following?
1. Thrombophlebitis
2. Pregnancy-induced hypertension
3. Pressure on blood vessels from the enlarging uterus
4. The force of gravity pulling down on the uterus

8. Cervical softening and uterine souffle are classified as which of the following?
1. Diagnostic signs
2. Presumptive signs
3. Probable signs
4. Positive signs

9. Which of the following would the nurse identify as a presumptive sign of pregnancy?
1. Hegar sign
2. Nausea and vomiting
3. Skin pigmentation changes
4. Positive serum pregnancy test

10. Which of the following common emotional reactions to pregnancy would the nurse expect to occur during the first trimester?
1. Introversion, egocentrism, narcissism
2. Awkwardness, clumsiness and unattractiveness
3. Anxiety, passivity, extroversion
4. Ambivalence, fear, fantasies

11. The nurse is palpating the uterus of a client who is 20 weeks pregnant to measure fundal height. Identify the area on the abdomen where the nurse should expect to feel the uterine fundus.

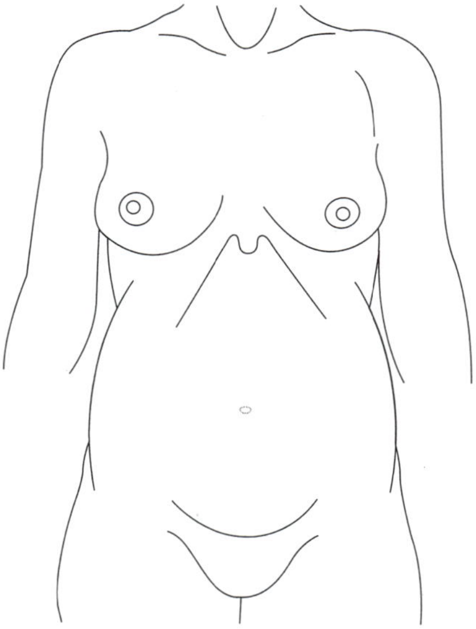

Answer key

1. The answer is 2.
Pressure and irritation of the bladder by the growing uterus during the first trimester is responsible for causing urinary frequency. Dysuria, incontinence, and burning are symptoms associated with urinary tract infections.

2. The answer is 3.
During the second trimester, the reduction in gastric acidity, in conjunction with pressure from the growing uterus and smooth-muscle relaxation, can cause heartburn and flatulence. HCG levels increase in the first, not the second, trimester. Decreased intestinal motility would most likely be the cause of constipation and bloating. Estrogen levels decrease in the second trimester.

3. The answer is 4.
Chloasma, also called the mask of pregnancy, is an irregular hyperpigmented area found on the face. It is not seen on the breasts, areola, nipples, chest, neck, arms, legs, abdomen, or thighs.

4. The answer is 3.
During pregnancy, hormonal changes cause relaxation of the pelvic joints, resulting in the typical "waddling" gait. Changes in posture are related to the growing fetus. Pressure on the surrounding muscles causing discomfort is due to the growing uterus. Weight gain has no effect on gait.

5. The answer is 3.
The average amount of weight gained during pregnancy is 24 to 30 lb. This weight gain consists of the following: fetus — 7.5 lb; placenta and membrane — 1.5 lb; amniotic fluid — 2 lb; uterus — 2.5 lb; breasts — 3 lb; increased blood volume — 2 to 4 lb; and extravascular fluid and fat — 4 to 9 lb. A gain of 12 to 22 lb is insufficient, whereas a weight gain of 15 to 25 lb is marginal. A weight gain of 25 to 40 lb is considered excessive.

6. The answer is 4.
Braxton Hicks contractions are a normal antepartum phenomenon that probably result from stretching of the uterine muscles. Braxton Hicks contractions are not a sign of labor. Because these contractions are normal, their occurrence does not warrant notifying the physician. Additionally, these contractions have no effect on placental perfusion.

7. The answer is 3.
Pressure of the growing uterus on blood vessels results in an increased risk of venous stasis in the lower extremities. Subsequently, edema and varicose vein formation may occur. Thrombophlebitis is an inflammation of the veins due to thrombus formation. Pregnancy-induced hypertension is not associated with these symptoms. Gravity plays only a minor role with these symptoms.

8. The answer is 3.
Cervical softening (Goodell sign) and uterine souffle are two probable signs of pregnancy. Probable signs are objective findings that strongly suggest pregnancy. Other probable signs include Hegar sign, which is softening of the lower uterine segment; Piskacek sign, which is enlargement and softening of the uterus; serum laboratory tests; changes in skin pigmentation; and ultrasonic evidence of a gestational sac. Presumptive signs are subjective signs and include amenorrhea, nausea and vomiting, urinary frequency, breast tenderness and changes, excessive fatigue, uterine enlargement, and quickening.

9. The answer is 2.
Presumptive signs of pregnancy are subjective signs. Of the signs listed, only nausea and vomiting are presumptive signs. Hegar sign, skin pigmentation changes, and a positive serum pregnancy test are considered probable signs, which are strongly suggestive of pregnancy.

10. The answer is 4.
During the first trimester, common emotional reactions include ambivalence, fear, fantasies, and anxiety. The second trimester is a period of well-being accompanied by the increased need to learn about fetal growth and development. Common emotional reactions during this trimester include narcissism, passivity, and introversion. At times the woman may seem egocentric and self-centered. During the third trimester, the woman typically feels awkward, clumsy, and unattractive, often becoming more introverted or reflective of her own childhood.

11. At 20 weeks' gestation, fundal height should be at the level of the umbilicus (see *Figure* 5-1, page 62). Fundal height should be measured from the symphysis pubis to the top of the uterus. Serial measurements assess fetal growth over the duration of the pregnancy. Between 18 and 34 weeks, the centimeters measured are approximately equal to the week of gestation.

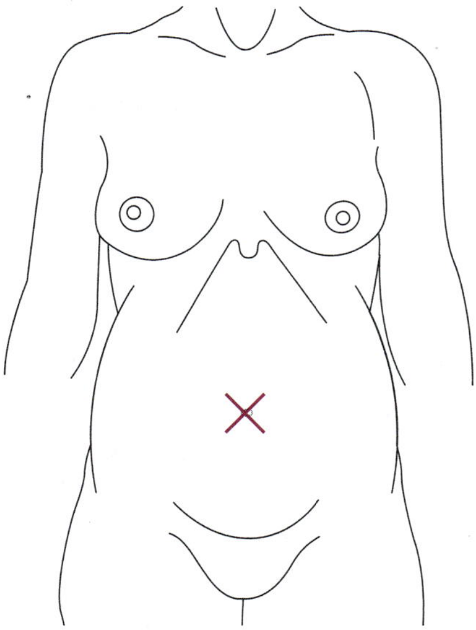

6 Fetal Growth and Development and Genetic Principles

I. FETAL GROWTH AND DEVELOPMENT

Growth and development of the fetus begins with fertilization. After fertilization, fetal development occurs in three stages — preembryonic, embryonic, and fetal.

A. Fertilization

1. Following ejaculation into the vagina, sperm live about 48 to 72 hours but are believed to be healthy and highly fertile for only about 24 hours. Ova are considered fertile for about 12 to 24 hours after ovulation. Thus, for fertilization to occur, coitus must be accomplished no more than 24 hours before or after ovulation.
2. Fertilization refers to the union of an ovum (egg) and a spermatozoan (sperm), which results in a zygote. Fertilization occurs in the ampulla (outer one-third) of the fallopian tube following ovulation.

B. Preembryonic stage

1. This stage encompasses the first 14 days after conception.
2. When the zygote implants in the decidua, about 8 to 10 days after fertilization, the structure is referred to as an embryo.
3. After implantation, the embryo undergoes rapid growth and differentiation. Establishment of embryonic membranes and development of tissues and organs from the three primary germ layers of the embryo occur as follows:
   a. **Ectoderm.** The tissues and organs that develop from the ectoderm include the central nervous system; peripheral nervous system; sensory epithelium of ear, nose, eye, sinus, mouth, and anal canal; skin (epidermis), hair, nails, sebaceous glands, sweat glands, hair follicles; and mammary glands, pituitary gland, enamel of teeth, and oral glands.
   b. **Mesoderm.** The tissues and organs that develop from the mesoderm include bone, cartilage, skeleton; connective tissue, smooth and striated muscles; cardiovascular and lymphatic systems; blood and lymph cells; kidneys and reproductive organs; subcutaneous tissues of the skin; serous membrane lining of the pericardial, pleural, and peritoneal cavities; and spleen.
   c. **Endoderm.** The tissues and organs that develop from the endoderm include respiratory tract epithelium, epithelial lining of GI tract (pharynx, tongue, tonsils, thyroid, parathyroid, thymus), epithelial lining of urinary bladder and urethra, liver, and pancreas.

C. Embryonic stage

1. This stage begins during the third week after conception and continues until the embryo reaches a crown-to-rump length of 3 cm (1.2 in) at about the eighth week. At this time, the embryo is referred to as a **fetus.**
2. During this stage, differentiation of tissues into organs and development of main external features occur.

D. Fetal stage

1. The fetal stage begins 8 to 10 weeks after conception and continues until the end of the pregnancy.
2. At this time, the fetus is fully developed structurally. The remainder of the gestational period is devoted to refinement of structures and organization and perfection of function. *Box* 6-1, page 78 shows fetal development by gestational month.
3. Fetal circulation differs from extrauterine blood flow. The fetus receives oxygen and excretes carbon dioxide through the placenta. Fetal lungs are fluid filled and do not func-

BOX 6-1

Milestones of fetal development

Four weeks

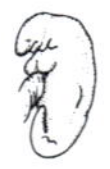
4 weeks

- The embryo is 4 to 5 mm in length.
- Trophoblasts embed in decidua.
- Chorionic villi form.
- Foundations for nervous system, genitourinary system, skin, bones, and lungs are formed.
- Buds of arms and legs begin to form.
- Rudiments of eyes, ears, and nose appear.

Five to eight weeks

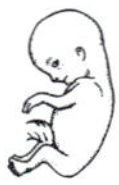
8 weeks

- The fetus is 27 to 31 mm in length and weighs 2 to 4 g.
- Fetus is markedly bent.
- Head is disproportionately large as a result of brain development.
- Sex differentiation begins.
- Centers of bone begin to ossify.

Nine to twelve weeks

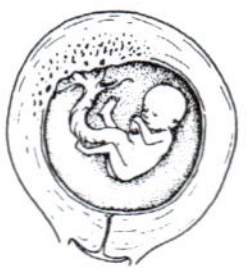
12 weeks

- The fetus average length is 50 to 87 mm and weight is 45 g.
- Fingers and toes are distinct.
- Placenta is complete.
- Rudimentary kidneys secrete urine.
- Fetal circulation is complete.
- External genitalia show definite characteristics.

Thirteen to sixteen weeks

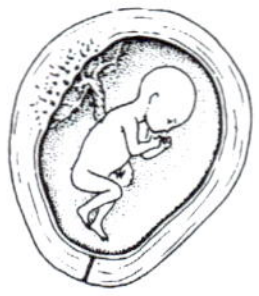
16 weeks

- The fetus is 94 to 140 mm in length and weighs 97 to 200 g.
- Head is erect.
- Lower limbs are well developed.
- Coordinated limb movements are present.
- Heartbeat is present.
- Lanugo develops.
- Nasal septum and palate close.
- Fingerprints are set.

Seventeen to twenty weeks

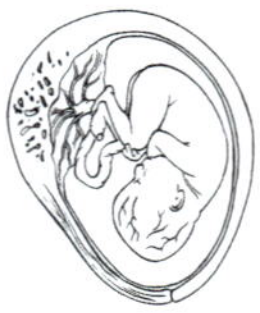
20 weeks

- The fetus is 150 to 190 mm in length and weighs approximately 260 to 460 g.
- Lanugo covers entire body.
- Fetal movements are felt by woman.
- Eyebrows and scalp hair are present.
- Heart sounds are perceptible by auscultation.
- Vernix caseosa covers skin.

All lengths are given crown to rump

Twenty-one to twenty-five weeks

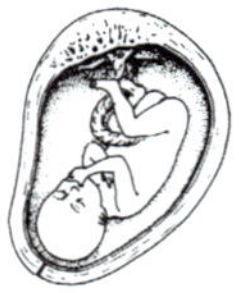
25 weeks

- The fetus is about 200 to 240 mm in length and weighs 495 to 910 g.
- Skin appears wrinkled and pink to red.
- REM begins.
- Eyebrows and fingernails develop.
- Sustained weight gain occurs.

Twenty-six to twenty-nine weeks

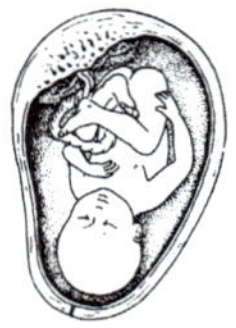
29 weeks

- The fetus is 250 to 275 mm in length and weighs about 910 to 1,500 g.
- Skin is red.
- Rhythmic breathing movements occur.
- Pupillary membrane disappears from eyes.
- The fetus often survives if born prematurely.

Thirty to thirty-four weeks

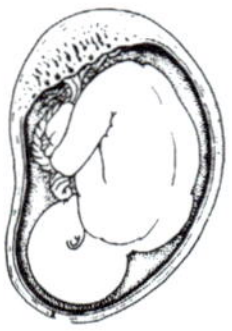
34 weeks

- The fetus is 280 to 320 mm in length and weighs 1,700 to 2,500 g.
- Toenails become visible.
- Eyelids open.
- Steady weight gain occurs.
- Vigorous fetal movement occurs.

Thirty-five to thirty-seven weeks

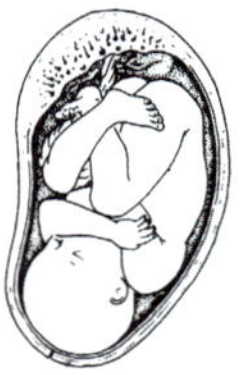
37 weeks

- The fetus average length is 330 to 360 mm: weight is about 2,700 to 3,400 g.
- Face and body have a loose wrinkled appearance because of subcutaneous fat deposit.
- Body is usually plump.
- Lanugo disappears.
- Nails reach fingertip edge.
- Amniotic fluid decreases.

Thirty-eight weeks (full term)

- The average fetus is 360 mm in length and weighs 3,400 to 3,600 g.
- Skin is smooth.
- Chest is prominent.
- Eyes are uniformly slate colored.
- Bones of skull are ossified and nearly together at sutures.
- Testes are in scrotum.

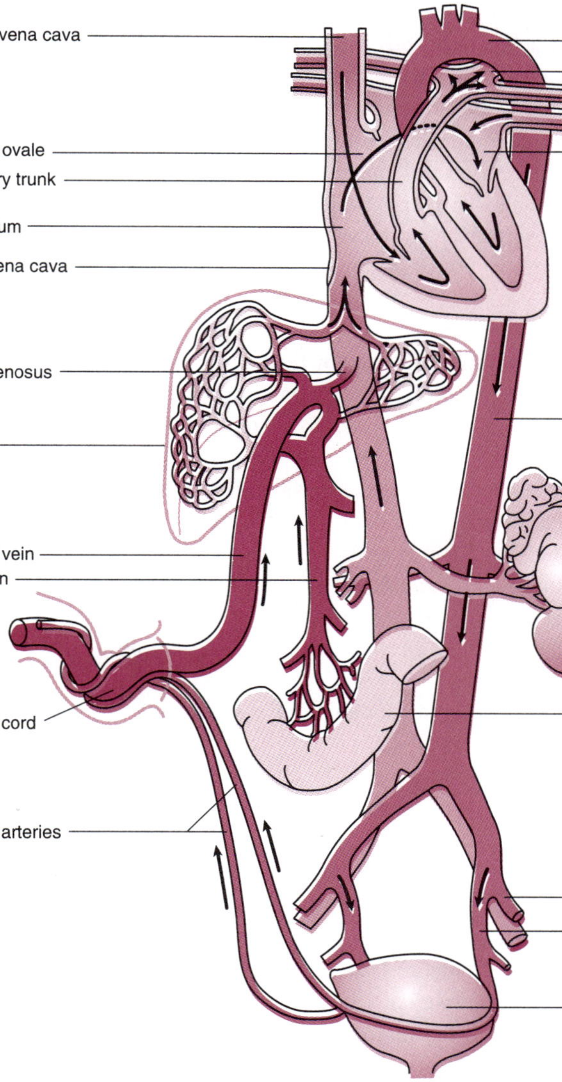

FIGURE 6-1
Fetal circulation shortly before birth. Arrows indicate the direction of blood flow.

tion for gas exchange. There are three shunts in fetal circulation that must close at birth — ductus arteriosus, ductus venosus, and the foramen ovale. There are two umbilical arteries and one vein (*Figure* 6-1).

4. Usually by the 12th week of gestation, external genitalia are developed enough to be distinguishable with ultrasonography.
5. In a female fetus, the ovary has many primitive follicles and produces small amounts of estrogen.
6. In a male fetus, the gonads play a critical role in forming the genital tract. The testes produce androgenic hormones that promote growth and differentiation of male genitalia.

E. Embryonic and fetal support structures

1. The **corpus luteum** supplies most of the estrogen and progesterone in the first two gestational months before the placenta is fully developed. The persistence of the corpus luteum in supplying these hormones is essential for sustaining the uterine endometrium and preventing menstruation.
2. **Decidua**. The endometrium (the lining of the inside of the uterus) becomes the decidua following conception and implantation. The portion directly under the blastocyst, where the chorionic villa intersect with the maternal blood vessels, is the decidua basalis. The portion covering the blastocyst is called the decidua capsularis, and the portion lining the rest of the uterus is the decidua vera. It will protect and nourish the developing embryo.
3. **Placenta**
   a. The placenta begins to function by the fourth week of gestation; by the 14th week, it is a complete, independently functioning organ.
   b. It transmits nutrients and oxygen to the fetus and removes waste and carbon dioxide by diffusion.
   c. The **endocrine** organ of pregnancy, the placenta, produces the following hormones:
   - **Estrogen** (primarily estriol)
     - It stimulates the growth of uterine muscle (myometrium) and glandular epithelium (endometrium), and induces the synthesis of receptors for progesterone.
     - Estrogen stimulates uterine growth and uteroplacental blood flow.
     - Estrogen enhances growth of all organs and ensures nourishment of developing tissue.
     - It indicates placental function, fetal maturity, and fetal well-being (levels of maternal serum estriol).
   - **Progesterone**
     - Progesterone promotes thickening and increased viscosity of cervical mucus (the mucus plug) to protect the fetus against invading bacteria.
     - Progesterone decreases motility of oviducts and uterus.
     - It stimulates growth of glandular breast tissue (acini cells) in preparation for lactation.
     - Progesterone maintains uterine lining for implantation.
     - It relaxes uterine smooth muscle.
   - **Human chorionic gonadotropin (HCG)**
     - HCG is secreted by trophoblast cells of the blastocyst (the early product of conception) and the placenta (after the second gestational month). It is partly responsible for maintaining the corpus luteum.
     - HCG is detected in the urine and plasma (by day 8), and is the first indicator of a positive pregnancy.
     - HCG levels may also be monitored later in the pregnancy to determine fetal well-being.
   - **Human placental lactogen,** or human chorionic somatomammotropin, levels increase after 20 weeks of gestation.
     - It is a growthlike substance that stimulates maternal metabolism.
     - It facilitates glucose transport across the placenta.
     - It also stimulates breast development to prepare for lactation.

4. **Membranes and amniotic fluid**
   a. Two membranes form to protect and support the embryo.
   - **Chorion,** the outside embryonic membrane
   - **Amnion,** the innermost membrane

   b. **Amniotic fluid** is contained within the amnion. Fluid volume normally ranges from 500 to 1,000 ml. The functions of the amniotic fluid are as follows:
   - Protects the embryo and fetus
   - Controls temperature
   - Supports symmetrical growth
   - Prevents adherence to amnion
   - Allows the embryo or fetus to move within the amniotic cavity

5. **Umbilical cord**
   a. At term, it is 30 to 90 cm long and 2 cm in diameter.
   b. It contains two arteries and one vein.
   c. Two arteries carry blood from the fetus to the placenta.
   d. One vein returns blood and nutrients to the fetus.
   e. The umbilical cord is normally inserted at the center of the placenta.
   f. The cord also contains a clear, jellylike substance called Wharton jelly, which is a connective tissue that prevents compression of the blood vessels.

F. Multiple pregnancy

1. About 2% of births in the United States are multiple. Twins occur in about 1 in 80 pregnancies; triplets in 1 in 8,000. Multiple births greater than triplets are rare, but the incidence is rising because of the increasing use of gonadotropins to treat women with ovulatory failure.
2. **Dizygotic** (fraternal) multiple pregnancy involves two or more ova fertilized by separate sperm. Fetuses have separate placentas, amnions, and chorions (although the placenta may fuse to resemble a single one) and may be the same or different sexes.
3. **Monozygotic** (identical) multiple pregnancy develops from a single fertilized ovum. Fetuses share a common placenta and chorion but have separate amnions; they are the same sex and have the same genotype (*Figure* 6-2, page 82).

G. Factors influencing embryonic and fetal development

1. **Environment**
   a. Poverty
   b. Malnutrition
   c. Maternal alcohol, nicotine, or illicit drug use
   d. Maternal prescription drug use (for example, anticoagulants, aspirin, anticonvulsants, antibiotics)
2. **Anatomic problems**
   a. Maternal problems include ectopic pregnancy, uterine abnormality, retroversion of the uterus, and incompetent cervical os.
   b. Fetal problems include chromosomal defects (see section II) and poor implantation.
3. **Maternal complications** (such as infection, Rh incompatibility, cyanotic heart disease, renal diseases, hypertension, and urinary tract infection)
4. **Fetal complications** (such as premature rupture of membranes, preterm labor, and postmaturity)
5. **Physiologic problems** (such as folate deficiency, endocrine deficiency, and defective sperm)

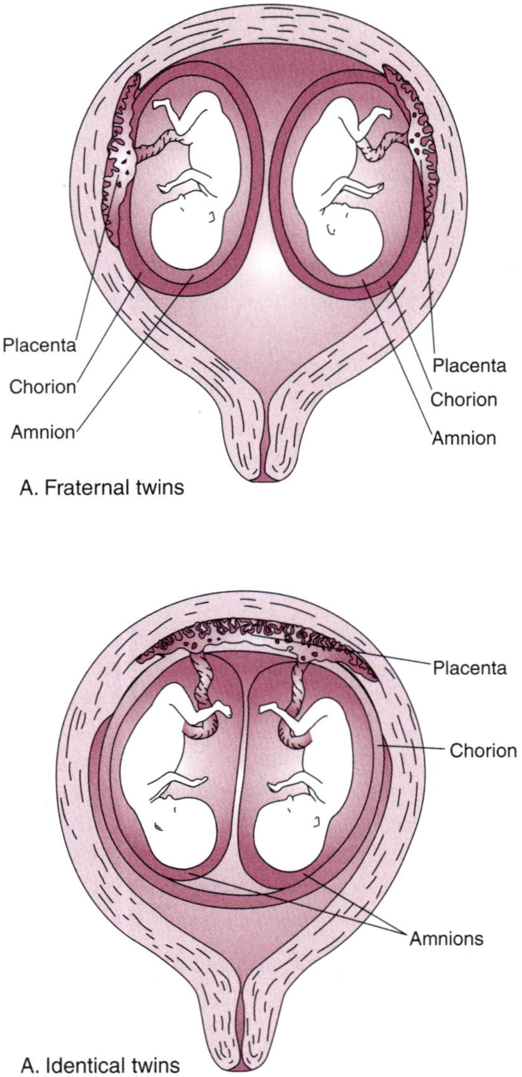

FIGURE 6-2
Multiple gestations. (A) Dizygotic (fraternal) twins showing two placentas, two chorions, and two amnions. (B) Monozygotic (identical) twins with one placenta, one chorion, and two amnions. (Courtesy of Pillitteri, A [2003]. *Maternal and Child Health*, 4th ed. Philadelphia: Lippincott Williams & Wilkins, p. 412.)

II. GENETIC PRINCIPLES INFLUENCING FETAL GROWTH AND DEVELOPMENT

A. Chromosomal structure

1. **Chromosomes,** in the nucleus of the cell, carry the hereditary material that determines the individual's physical characteristics. They are threadlike strands of DNA.
2. **Genes** are small segments of DNA contained in the chromosomes. Some are dominant, some are recessive, and some may be sex linked.
3. **Alleles** are pairs of genes. There are two genes for every human trait. One gene comes from the ovum and one comes from the sperm.
4. **Phenotype** is an individual's physical appearance determined by the alleles.
5. **Genotype** refers to the individual's actual gene composition.
6. Normal embryonic cell tissue contains 46 chromosomes (23 pairs): 44 homologous (22 pairs) and two sex (one pair) chromosomes.
7. Each chromosome contains 22 autosomes and one sex chromosome (Y) from the male and 22 autosomes and one sex chromosome (X) from the female.
8. Fetal cells and organs develop from chromosomes. Human life begins as a single cell, a zygote, that reproduces itself (as does each new cell).
9. The sex of the fetus is determined at the time of fertilization by the combination of the sex chromosomes of the sperm (X or Y) and the ovum (X or X). The resulting pair of sex chromosomes is either XX (female) or XY (male) (*Figure* 6-3).

B. Inheritance patterns

1. The science of genetic disorders seeks to explain the underlying causes of disorders present at birth. It also explores the patterns in which inherited disorders pass from one generation to the next.
2. A person who has two genes for a trait is homozygous for that trait.
3. A person who has two genes that differ (one is dominant, one is recessive) is heterozygous for that trait.
4. The dominant gene will be expressed for any trait.
5. Recessive genes will be expressed only if both genes in the allele carry them.
6. Mendelian laws allow us to predict inheritance of characteristics such as eye and hair color. We can also predict whether the child will be born with a genetic disorder.

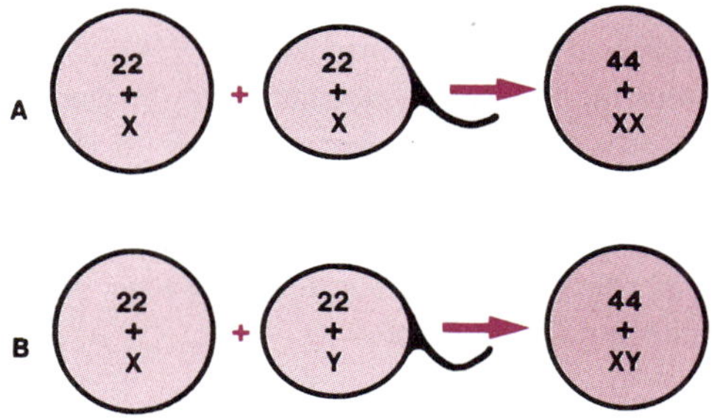

FIGURE 6-3
Fetal sex is determined genetically at fertilization. (A) Ovum fertilized by sperm bearing X chromosome will form a female zygote. (B) Ovum fertilized by sperm bearing Y chromosome will form a male zygote.

C. Chromosomal inheritance disorders

1. **Autosomal dominant disorder.** The clinical expression of a gene when one allele at a given chromosome locus is mutant (heterozygous). An example of an autosomal dominant disorder is achondroplastic dwarfism.
2. **Autosomal recessive disorder.** The clinical expression of a gene when both alleles at a given chromosome locus are mutant (homozygous). An example of an autosomal recessive disorders is cystic fibrosis.
3. **X-linked dominant disorder.** The terms dominant and recessive in X-linked traits refer only to women. Men, having only one X chromosome and one Y chromosome, will always be affected if they inherit an X-linked mutant gene.
   - *a.* X-linked dominant disorders are rare but appear in every generation of an affected family.
   - *b.* Women, having two X chromosomes, will be affected if heterozygous or homozygous for an X-linked dominant trait.
   - *c.* Examples of an X-linked dominant disorder are fragile X syndrome and vitamin D–resistant rickets.
4. **X-linked recessive disorder**
   - *a.* Women will be asymptomatic for a trait if heterozygous for an X-linked recessive trait.
   - *b.* Women will be affected if homozygous for an X-linked recessive disorder.
   - *c.* Examples of X-linked recessive disorders are hemophilia A, color blindness, and muscular dystrophy.
5. **Multifactorial inheritance** involves traits and disorders resulting from the interaction of many genetic factors (polygenetic inheritance) or the interaction of genetic and environmental factors. Examples of multifactorial disorders include:
   - *a.* Congenital heart defects
   - *b.* Clubfoot
   - *c.* Neural tube defects
   - *d.* Pyloric stenosis
   - *e.* Cleft lip and cleft palate
   - *f.* Congenital hip dysplasia

D. Chromosomal abnormality disorders

1. Causes may be hereditary or nonhereditary. Contributing factors include:
   - *a.* Exposure to teratogens, such as radiation, certain drugs, viruses, toxins, and chemicals
   - *b.* Advanced maternal age at conception
2. Types of chromosomal abnormalities include:
   - *a.* **Numeric abnormalities** (usually too many; too few chromosomes usually results in miscarriage) in sex chromosomes and autosomes (for example, Klinefelter and Turner syndromes, and trisomy 13, 18, or 21)
   - *b.* **Structural disorders,** such as deletions (for example, cri du chat syndrome) and translocations, which are aberrations that result when part of a chromosome is transferred to a different chromosome.

III. GENETIC COUNSELING

A. Goals

1. Enables individuals or couples to make informed reproductive decisions
2. Provides psychological support for decision-making
3. Provides clients with information about the defect in question
4. Communicates to clients the risk of transmitting the defect in question to future children

B. Indications for prenatal genetic screening

1. Parent is a carrier of, or is affected by, a chromosomal or metabolic disorder.
2. Family history of genetic disorders, including family with an ethnic background that is highly susceptible to certain inherited disorders (such as Tay-Sachs disease in Jews of Eastern European [Ashkenazi] descent, sickle cell disease in people of African descent, and beta-thalassemia [Cooley anemia] in people of Mediterranean descent)
3. Previous birth of child with a congenital abnormality or with multiple anomalies who has had no chromosomal studies done
4. Advanced maternal age (35 years of age and older)
5. History of spontaneous abortion
6. Willingness to interrupt pregnancy if an abnormal fetus is detected

C. Screening for genetic traits and disease

1. The goal of screening is to prevent tragic genetic diseases and offer various reproductive options to at-risk couples (*Box* 6-2, page 86).
2. Accurate screening hinges on the education and advocacy of physicians and nurses caring for people of reproductive age.
3. Specific diagnostic tests include:
   a. **Karyotyping** — a visual display of the individual's actual chromosome pattern
   b. **Heterozygote screening** — directed at detecting clinically normal carriers of a disease-causing mutant gene, particularly in people of ethnic groups with high frequency of the mutant gene under investigation
   c. **Maternal serum alpha-fetoprotein** (MSAFP) screen — selectively done when an open neural tube defect, anencephaly, omphalocele, or gastroschisis is suspected (MSAFP is not diagnostic; there is, however, a 5% to 10% risk of the defect when MSAFP level is elevated at 16 to 18 weeks' gestation.) Low MSAFP level has been associated with Down syndrome.
   d. **Triple screening** — analysis of three indicators from maternal serum alpha-fetoprotein, estriol, and human chorionic gonadotropin; yields more reliable results than MSAFP
   e. **Chorionic villi sampling** — the retrieval of chorionic villi for chromosomal analysis
   - It may be done as early as the fifth week of pregnancy.
   - It is more often done between the 8th and 10th week of pregnancy.
   - Results of this analysis are extremely accurate.
   - This test cannot detect all inherited diseases.

   f. **Amniocentesis** — the withdrawal of a sample of amniotic fluid (2 to 5 ml) transabdominally for genetic analysis
   - It is usually done with ultrasound visualization between 14 and 16 weeks.

BOX 6-2

Genetic screening recommendations for various ethnic and age groups

Population at Risk	Abnormality	Screening Test	Definitive Test
Ashkenazic Jewish, French-Canadians, Cajuns	Tay-Sachs disease	Decreased serum hexosaminidase-A	Chorionic villi sampling (CVS) or amniocentesis for hexosaminidase-A assay
African-Hispanic (from the Caribbean, Central America or South America), Arabs, Egyptians, Asian-Indians	Sickle cell anemia	Presence of sickle cell hemoglobin; confirmatory hemoglobin electrophoresis	CVS or amniocentesis for genotype determination, direct molecular studies
Southeast Asians (Vietnamese, Laotian, Cambodian), Filipino	Alpha-thalassemia	Mean corpuscular volume < 80%; confirmatory hemoglobin electrophoresis	CVS or amniocentesis for genotype determination (direct molecular studies)
Greek, Italian	Beta-thalassemia	Mean corpuscular volume < 80%; confirmatory hemoglobin electrophoresis	CVS or amniocentesis for genotype determination (direct molecular studies or indirect restriction fragment length polymorphism analysis)
Women over age 35 (all ethnic groups)	Chromosomal trisomies	None	CVS or amniocentesis for cytogenic analysis
Women of any age (all ethnic groups; particularly suggested for women from British Isles, Ireland)	Neural tube defects and selected other anomalies	Maternal serum alpha-fetoprotein (MSAFP)	Amniocentesis for amniotic fluid, alpha-fetoprotein, and acetylcholinesterase assays
Ashkenazic Jewish	Gaucher disease	Decreased glucocerebrosidase	CVS
Caucasians (Northern Europeans, Celtic population), Ashkenazic Jewish	Cystic fibrosis	Delta F508 amino acid mutation	CVS or amniocentesis for genotype; definitive diagnosis for all fetuses not possible

(From Olds, S., London, M., Ladewig, P., and Davidson, M. [2004]. *Maternal-Newborn Nursing & Women's Health Care,* 7th ed. Upper Saddle River, New Jersey: Pearson Education, Inc. p. 276.)

- It may be used to analyze skin cells, alpha-fetoprotein, or acetylcholinesterase (a breakdown product of blood). Acetylcholinesterase helps decrease false-positive results.
- Amniocentesis carries only a 0.5% risk of spontaneous abortion.

g. **Percutaneous umbilical blood sampling** — removal of blood from the umbilical vein

- Blood studies include karyotyping, complete blood count, direct Coombs' test, and measurement of blood gases.

- It uses a technique similar to amniocentesis to obtain the blood sample.
- An Rh-negative mother should be given RhoGAM because blood may enter maternal circulation after the procedure as a result of oozing at the puncture site.

h. **Sonography** — a diagnostic tool used to assess a fetus for general size. It can also be used to examine structural disorders of the internal organs, spine, and limbs. It uses sound waves to create a "picture."

i. **Fetoscopy** — the insertion into the mother's uterus of a fiberoptic fetoscope through a small incision in her abdomen
- It is used to inspect for fetal anomalies or confirm an ultrasound finding.
- It can be used to remove fetal skin cells for DNA analysis.
- It also may be used to perform corrective surgery for congenital anomalies.

NURSING PROCESS OVERVIEW

IV. GENETIC PRINCIPLES INFLUENCING FETAL GROWTH AND DEVELOPMENT

(Note: Nursing process overview for fetal growth and development is covered in Chapter 8, Antepartum Care.)

A. Assessment

1. **Health history** should focus on determining the couple's risk for having a baby with an inherited disorder. In the next section are general areas that the nurse should focus on for assessing risk. *Box* 6-3, page 88, contains a more complete list of topics related to risk.
   a. A relevant preliminary **genetic history,** being alert to information indicating the need for referral to genetic counseling, is important. Note if genetic disorders are present in family members of both the mother and father. It may be necessary to assess other members of the family as well as the couple.
   b. **Ethnic background** is important because certain disorders occur more frequently in some ethnic groups compared to others.
   c. Assessment of the **general medical history** of the couple and of the couple's family members (including those who are deceased) is important.
   d. Asking the **mother's age** is also important because risk commonly increases with age.
2. **Laboratory and diagnostic studies.** Arrange for specific genetic screening tests (see section III).

B. Nursing diagnoses

1. Knowledge Deficit
2. Decisional Conflict
3. Anticipatory Grieving
4. Health-Seeking Behavior

C. Planning and outcome identification

1. **Provide education.**
   a. Describe the couple's risk for having a child with an inherited disorder.
   b. Provide sufficient and correct information about the genetic problem in question.
   c. Explain the genetic testing required.
   d. Provide information about possible treatments for the disorder (if any).
   e. Provide information about available resources.

BOX 6-3
Assessment of risk factors

Obstetric History
- History of infertility
- Grand multiparity
- Incompetent cervix
- Uterine/cervical anomaly
- Previous preterm labor/preterm birth
- Previous macrosomic infant
- Previous ectopic pregnancy
- Previous stillborn or neonatal death
- Previous multiple gestation
- Previous prolonged labor
- Previous low-birth-weight infant
- DES exposure in utero

Medical History
- Cardiac disease
- Metabolic disease
- Seizure disorders
- Emotional disorders
- Family history of inherited disorders
- Pulmonary disease
- Endocrine disorders
- Sexually transmitted diseases
- Mental retardation
- Surgery during pregnancy

Current OB Status
- Inadequate prenatal care
- Intrauterine growth-restricted infant
- Large-for-gestational-age infant
- Rh sensitization
- Gravida
- Stillbirths
- Fetal manipulation
- Polyhydramnios
- Fetal/placental malformation
- Abnormal fetal surveillance tests
- Para
- Abnormal presentation

Psychosocial Factors
- Inadequate finances
- Social problems
- Adolescent
- Poor nutrition
- Inadequate support systems
- Lack of acceptance of pregnancy
- Inadequate housing
- Unwed
- Minority status
- Parental occupation
- No help at home
- Psychiatric history

Demographic Factors
- Maternal age < 16 or > 35
- Education < 11 years
- Ethnic background

Lifestyle
- Smokes > 10 cigarettes/day
- Substance use/abuse
- Number of sex partners
- Alcohol intake
- Unusual stress
- Father of infant not involved

2. **Provide emotional support.**
   a. Identify the counseling needs of families with a history of inherited disorders.
   b. Provide risk-appropriate health care and counseling.
   c. Assist the couple in coping with the results of genetic testing.
   d. Refer the couple to appropriate health care providers, support groups, and community resources for help in managing the crisis in their lives.
   e. Serve as a liaison between the genetic counselor and the family.
3. **The couple will verbalize possible risk of a genetic disorder based on the results of testing.**

D. Outcome evaluation

1. The couple states that they received adequate information about patterns of inheritance, their risk in having a child with an inherited disorder, the disorder itself, and treatments and available resources.
2. The couple demonstrates positive coping skills and states that they are able to make a reasonable choice about the outcome of genetic testing and counseling.
3. The couple identifies factors associated with the risk of the genetic disorder.
4. The couple voices understanding of genetic testing.
5. The couple states the chances that their offspring will have the genetic disorder.

Study questions

1. Which of the following terms refers to the thickened endometrium in which the fertilized embryo implants?
1. Endoderm
2. Decidua
3. Amnion
4. Chorion

2. The fetal nervous system is formed by the germ layer known as which of the following?
1. Ectoderm
2. Mesoderm
3. Endoderm
4. Entoderm

3. The corpus luteum acts as the placenta for the implanted ovum until the end of which of the following gestational months?
1. First
2. Second
3. Fourth
4. Fifth

4. An expectant mother in the prenatal clinic states, "I'm sure I'm going to have a boy because my husband says he knows it's a boy." Which of the following would be the nurse's best response?
1. "You could be right that it's a boy."
2. "The woman determines the sex of the newborn."
3. "There are more girls born than boys."
4. "The man determines the sex of the newborn."

5. Which of the following would the nurse estimate as the approximate gestational age for a 19-cm fetus expelled by a client?
1. 2 months
2. 3 months
3. 4 months
4. 5 months

6. Which of the following substances is measured in the maternal serum when a neural tube defect is suspected?
1. Estrogen
2. Progesterone
3. Alpha-fetoprotein (AFP)
4. Luteinizing hormone (LH)

7. By which of the following does the placenta transport nutrients and oxygen to the fetus?
1. Capacitation
2. Diffusion
3. Fertilization
4. Ustulation

8. An expectant mother asks the nurse in the prenatal clinic, "When can I expect to feel my baby move?" Which of the following would be the nurse's best response?
1. At about 2 months
2. At about 3 months
3. At about 4 months
4. At about 5 months

9. An expectant mother in the prenatal clinic informs the nurse that she smokes and asks if she could continue to do so. Which of the following responses best demonstrates the nurse's understanding of smoking's effect on a pregnancy?
1. "How much do you smoke?"
2. "You should decrease the number of cigarettes used."
3. "Smoking may adversely affect your baby's development."
4. "That is something you should ask the physician."

10. Which of the following responses by the nurse would be most appropriate for an expectant mother in the prenatal clinic who confides that she has frequent headaches and has always taken aspirin?
1. "Did you take aspirin in the first 4 weeks of your pregnancy?"
2. "The physician may recommend another medication for your headaches."
3. "Could you tell me more about these headaches and when you get them?"
4. "We do not recommend using any medication during pregnancy."

11. The number of chromosomes found in each sperm is ______________________.

Answer key

1. The answer is 2.
The decidua is the thickened endometrium into which the fertilized ovum implants. The endoderm is a germ layer. The amnion and chorion form the placenta.

2. The answer is 1.
The ectoderm forms the fetal nervous system. The mesoderm forms muscles, bone, cartilage, teeth dentin, ligaments, tendons, kidneys, heart, and other structures. The endoderm, also called the entoderm, forms the epithelium of the digestive tract and respiratory tract.

3. The answer is 2.
The corpus luteum supplies most of the estrogen and progesterone in the first two gestational months before the placenta is fully developed. By the end of the second gestational month, the placenta is functional and becomes active. The placenta is not yet developed enough by the end of the first gestational month. By the fourth and fifth gestational months, the placenta has been actively functioning.

4. The answer is 4.
The sex of the fetus is determined at the time of fertilization by the combination of the sex chromosomes of the sperm (X or Y) and the ovum (X or X). The resulting pair of sex chromosomes is either XX (female) or XY (male). Because the sperm contains either X or Y chromosomes, the man, not the woman, determines the sex of the fetus. Telling the client that she could be right is a nonprofessional response that offers no instruction. Stating that more girls are born than boys, although correct, is not the most appropriate response to the client's statement.

5. The answer is 4.
The average fetal length at 5 months' gestation is 19 cm. At 2 months, the fetus is about 2.5 cm; at 3 months, 6 to 9 cm, and at 4 months, 12 to 17 cm in length.

6. The answer is 3.
Maternal serum alpha-fetoprotein (MSAFP) screening is selectively done when an open neural tube defect is suspected. Estrogen and progesterone work together to maintain pregnancy and promote fetal well-being. Luteinizing hormone (LH) stimulates follicular growth.

7. The answer is 2.
Most nutrients and oxygen move across the placenta by diffusion. Capacitation refers to changes in the ovum that facilitate penetration by the sperm. Fertilization refers to impregnation by the union of an ovum and a sperm. Ustulation refers to drying of a moist drug by heat.

8. The answer is 3.
At about five gestational months, the mother usually feels fetal movements. At this time, the average fetus is about 19 cm long and weighs about 300 g. On average, 2, 3, or 4 months' gestation are all too early for the mother to sense defined movement.

9. The answer is 3.

Smoking during pregnancy has been proven to increase the risk of a developmental problem, especially small-for-gestational age newborn. The nurse's statement about smoking adversely affecting the baby's development demonstrates the nurse's understanding of this effect. Asking how much the client smokes and telling her that she should decrease the number of cigarettes smoked per day may be appropriate but only after acknowledging the effect of nicotine on the baby. Because the nurse can intervene independently of the physician in this situation, telling the client to ask the physician is inappropriate.

10. The answer is 3.

By asking the client to tell the nurse more about the headaches, the nurse keeps in mind the possible developmental complications associated with medication use while also seeking additional information about the characteristics and frequency of the headaches. Asking the client about taking aspirin during the first 4 weeks of pregnancy is inappropriate because it would alarm the client. Telling the client that the physician may recommend another headache medication may be true. However, it does not yield information about the headaches, which may impact on the quality of care given to the mother and newborn. Telling the client about recommendations for not using any medication during pregnancy is too restrictive.

11. The answer is 23.

Each sperm contains 22 autosomes and 1 sex chromosome from the male. The same is true for the female. At conception normal embryonic cell tissue contains 46 chromosomes — 23 chromosomes from each parent.

7 Childbirth Education

I. OVERVIEW

A. Essentials of childbirth education

1. The childbirth education movement began in the 1950s and grew until prepared childbirth education is now recommended for all expectant parents by most care providers and by *Healthy People 2010.*
2. Preconception care and education are designed to assist a couple in making conscious conception choices, foster health maintenance, promote healthy behaviors for the woman and her potential fetus, and provide risk management as needed.
3. The term *natural childbirth* initially described a particular approach to childbirth—labor and birth without analgesia or anesthesia. However, it has come to mean being prepared for the birth experience through information, instruction, exercises, and techniques developed to deal with the discomforts of pregnancy, labor, and birth. As a result, childbirth education has become a standard part of prenatal care in the United States.
4. Regardless of the approach, childbirth education classes provide the following information:
   a. Preconception education
   b. Prenatal care and planning for the birth
   c. Fetal growth and development
   d. Preparation for labor and delivery
   e. Preparation of grandparents and siblings for the birth
   f. Postpartum care of the mother and newborn
5. Inclusion of fathers and other family members in the birthing process is an important aspect of childbirth education.
6. Childbirth educators see themselves as expectant parents' advocates. Childbirth education has grown from a small consumer movement to a significant force in maternity care in the United States.
7. Among the most important choices the couple will make are the choice of a primary birthing attendant and the setting in which the birth will take place.

B. Goals of childbirth education

1. Provide expectant parents with knowledge and skills necessary to cope with the stresses of pregnancy, labor, and birth.
2. Prepare expectant parents to be informed health care consumers.
3. Assist the mother in managing pain using a variety of pain management techniques and minimal pharmacologic intervention.
4. Assist parents in achieving a positive, safe, and rewarding labor and birth experience.

C. Effectiveness of childbirth education

1. Research demonstrates that childbirth preparation courses can increase satisfaction, reduce the amount of reported pain, and increase feelings of control for the pregnant woman and her partner.
2. Whether a woman wants to, or is able to, take a childbirth preparation course depends on cultural and socioeconomic factors and individual choice.
3. Learning stress reduction and relaxation techniques enables the woman to cope more effectively with the rigors of labor.
4. Women and their partners enjoy the opportunity to share their fears and hopes about their pregnancy with others.
5. Neonatal health is improved with minimal or no medication during labor and birth.

6. Parent-newborn bonding is facilitated when the mother and newborn are awake and aware at the time of birth.

D. Creating a birth plan

1. A birth plan can help prepare the woman and her partner to establish realistic goals, which relate to the concern for the safety of the mother and the infant. A birth plan usually includes information regarding the couple's preferences for labor, birth, and the immediate care of the newborn. Plans also are included for complications that may arise. The ultimate goal of any birth plan is a healthy infant born to healthy parents.
2. Childbirth education assists couples in making important choices, which will go into their written birth plan. The most important choices include:
   a. Selecting a primary birth attendant (such as obstetrician, pediatrician, family practice physician, nurse practitioner, or certified nurse midwife)
      - Some expectant couples select their primary birthing attendant (for example, obstetrician) and allow the attendant to make decisions on their behalf.
      - Other couples decide what they want in the childbearing experience and choose their primary birthing attendant accordingly.
      - Some couples decide to use the services of a **doula**. A doula is professionally trained to provide physical, emotional, and informational support to women and their partners during labor and birth. The doula does not become involved in clinical tasks. The doula's primary goal is assisting the woman in achieving her personal goals.

   b. Determining where they prefer the birth to occur (for example, hospital with traditional maternity center or birthing center, community agency, private hospital, freestanding birthing center, or at home)
   c. Selecting a preferred birthing approach for managing labor (such as Lamaze or Bradley)
   d. Deciding whether or not to use medications and what type (for example, narcotics or regional anesthesia) to manage pain during labor and delivery
   e. Deciding what medical interventions are acceptable or not during labor and delivery (such as use of forceps or vacuum, or episiotomy)
   f. Deciding what types of activities to implement during labor and birth (such as music, walking, and use of videotape or photography to document the birth)
   g. Deciding the direction of postpartum events, such as:
      - Immediate contact with newborn
      - A chance to breast-feed immediately after birth
      - Allowing the support person to cut the cord
      - Rooming-in of mother and baby
      - Use of pacifiers and supplemental feedings for the newborn
      - Delaying newborn eye treatment
      - Early discharge
3. Couples must understand that birth plans may need to be modified to meet the specific demands and challenges of their individual birth experience.

II. PRENATAL AND POSTPARTUM EDUCATION PROGRAMS

A. Teaching methods. The following teaching methods can be used for all types of prenatal and postpartum education courses.

1. Individual teaching and counseling

2. Groups and classes structured as informational classes, counseling groups, or discussion groups
3. Tours of available facilities and the options offered (such as birthing rooms, medications frequently used, visitors during labor, midwives on staff)

B. Prenatal childbirth education programs

1. Overview
   a. Prenatal childbirth education programs vary widely in length, goals, content, and cost. Typically, each class covers 4 to 8 hours of content and classes are spaced over a 4- to 8-week period.
   b. First-trimester classes commonly focus on such issues as early physiologic changes, fetal development, sexuality during pregnancy, and nutrition; some early sessions may include prepregnant couples.
   c. Second- and third-trimester classes may focus on preparation for birth, parenting, and newborn care.
2. Content of prenatal education programs (*Table* 7-1, page 96)
   a. Prenatal care and planning
      - Nutrition, exercise, and rest
      - Discomforts and self-care measures
      - Choosing a birth setting, primary birthing attendant, and birth approach (such as Lamaze or Bradley)
      - **Recognition of danger signals during pregnancy, which include vaginal bleeding, headaches, persistent vomiting, abdominal pain, edema, increased temperature, rapid weight gain, painful urination, visual disturbances, signs of preterm labor, and rupture of membranes (leaking of amniotic fluid)**
   b. Fetal development
      - Maternal use of drugs, alcohol, and smoking
      - Maternal nutrition
      - Medications used to treat an existing medical condition
      - Environmental hazards
      - Developmental milestones
   c. Preparation for labor and delivery
      - The birth process
      - Breathing techniques and relaxation exercises
      - Creating a birth plan, which includes plans for getting to the birthplace and child-care arrangements
      - Understanding fetal monitoring
      - Hydration during labor
      - Analgesia and anesthesia (Because individuals vary in their response to stress and because the characteristics of individual labor vary, the carefully considered use of pain medication along with breathing and relaxation techniques may enhance the woman's ability to maintain control during the labor process.)
      - Preparation for possible cesarean birth, including indications, advantages and disadvantages, risks, partner's involvement, and anesthesia
   d. Postpartum care
      - Self-care
      - Newborn care (for example, sleeping and waking patterns, newborn safety, bathing and feeding techniques, cord care, and circumcision)
      - Evaluation of feeding methods
      - Maternal nutrition, exercise, and rest needs

TABLE 7-1
Sample content for childbirth preparation education program

Lesson I: Physiologic changes of pregnancy and fetal growth

Lesson II: Personal care during pregnancy
1. Nutrition
2. Hygiene
3. Exercise
4. Rest
5. Sexuality
6. Discomforts
7. Danger signals
8. Feeding choices

Lesson III: Emotional changes associated with pregnancy

Lesson IV: Labor and birth
1. The birth process
2. Breathing techniques and exercises
3. Pharmacologic agents
4. View a video on birth

Lesson V: Postpartum concerns

Lesson VI: Infant care and feeding
1. Hygiene
2. Safety
3. Immunizations
4. Infant stimulation

Lesson VII: Creating a birth plan
1. Types of birth settings available to the couple
2. What to take to the birth setting
3. Child care and transportation
4. Tour of facility

Lesson VIII: Reproductive life planning

(Adapted from Pillitteri, A. [2003]. *Maternal and Child Health Nursing,* 4th ed. Philadelphia: Lippincott WIlliams & Wilkins, p. 310.)

- Recognition of danger signs and symptoms, which include heavy vaginal bleeding after lochia has become dark red-brown or pale; fever; increased vaginal discharge (especially foul smelling); swollen, tender, red, or hot area on one leg; area of swelling or tender, red, hot, area on a breast; painful urination; and perineal or pelvic pain

3. **Approaches to childbirth education**
   a. Contemporary childbirth education methods tend to be eclectic, combining features of many approaches, particularly Dick-Read, Lamaze, and Bradley.
   b. Grantly Dick-Read method
   - This method is based on the premise that education decreases fear, tension, and pain.
   - Teaches exercises to improve muscle tone and increase relaxation.
   - Stresses slow breathing, muscle relaxation, and pushing techniques.

c. The **Lamaze,** or psychoprophylactic, **method** combines relaxation, concentration, focusing, and complex, well-paced breathing patterns to reduce the perception of pain through a conditioned response to labor contractions.

d. The **Bradley technique** is very similar to Dick-Read's approach with the addition of a labor coach.
- Focuses on slow breathing and deep relaxation for labor
- Focuses on reduced responsiveness to external stimuli
- Focuses on the role of the male partner as coach

e. The **Wright,** or "new childbirth," **method** involves slower but more complex breathing patterns than the Lamaze method.

f. The **Kitzinger** (psychosexual) **method**
- Uses sensory memory as an aid to understanding and working with the body in preparation for childbirth
- Pregnancy, labor, and birth are considered continuing points in the woman's life cycle.

g. **Yoga** teaches relaxation, concentration, and "complete breathing" (combination of chest and abdominal breathing).

h. **Hypnosis** may be of benefit for some clients.

C. Breast-feeding programs

1. The American Academy of Pediatrics recommends that infants be breast-fed exclusively for the first 6 months of life and that breast-feeding should continue for at least 12 months (American Academy of Pediatrics Work Group on Breast Feeding, 1997).
2. Healthy People 2010 goals state that 75% of women will breast-feed at birth; 50% will continue for 6 months, and 25% will breast-feed for 1 year (Department of Health and Human Services, 2000).
3. Content of breast-feeding programs includes preparation of breasts, techniques for breast-feeding, and the advantages versus disadvantages of breast-feeding (*Table* 7-2, page 98).
4. These classes are offered by hospitals, birthing centers, clinics, individuals, and the La Leche League.
5. Fathers are included more frequently because these programs provide an opportunity to express their feelings (both positive and negative) about breast-feeding. These classes also provide fathers with knowledge they can use to support the mother as she learns to breast-feed the newborn.
6. Nurses often work in collaboration with lactation consultants in hospitals, physician's offices, and community agencies. Lactation consultants have had specialized education, training, and clinical experience related to breast-feeding. Most are certified by the International Board of Lactation Consultant Examiners and have met specific criteria for academic and clinical experience and have passed the certifying examination. Lactation consultants provide information, assistance, and support for breast-feeding mothers.

D. Sibling preparation classes

1. Purposes of these classes include:

a. Preparing children for what to expect when they visit mother and newborn in the hospital

b. Reducing the problems associated with separation when mother goes to the hospital

TABLE 7-2
Comparing breast-feeding with bottle-feeding

Feeding method	Advantages	Disadvantages
Breast-feeding	▪ Breast milk is considered ideal food source for newborn. ▪ Breast milk is always the perfect temperature ▪ No special preparations or supplies are needed. ▪ Breast-feeding speeds involution (return of uterus to normal size) for the mother. ▪ Maternal antibodies transferred in breast milk decrease incidence of allergies.	▪ It takes about 3 weeks for milk supply in the breast to become fully established, during which time a large newborn may be unsatisfied. ▪ It may be inconvenient or difficult for the mother who is employed outside of home. ▪ Physical and psychological preparations for breast-feeding may be too demanding or inconvenient for some women. ▪ Father cannot participate in feeding newborn.
Bottle-feeding	▪ Feeding preparation replicates mother's milk as much as possible. ▪ Formula containers are marked, making it easy to measure the newborn's intake. ▪ Father can participate in feeding and bonding. ▪ Immediately replenishable supply of formula helps satisfy appetite of larger newborns	▪ Some feeding formulas may contribute to colic. ▪ Feeding formula does not contain immune antibodies from the mother. ▪ Feeding formula may require extensive preparation (for example, supplies, measuring, mixing, and storage). ▪ Formula requires refrigeration and must be warmed before feedings. ▪ Method requires planning; parents must pack and carry feeding supplies when away from home. ▪ Bottle-feeding costs more than breast-feeding. ▪ Preparation of formula increases chance for feeding error.

c. Facilitating the parents' preparation of children for the introduction of the newborn in the home. This involves coping with sibling rivalry by:
- Providing extra attention
- Giving siblings undivided attention before introducing the newborn to them

2. Few programs prepare children for attendance at the birth; a sibling support person is expected to accompany the child to reduce distraction of the mother during labor.

E. Grandparent preparation classes

1. Classes are frequently offered in maternity centers that encourage grandparent visits and direct contact with the newborn, and that have extended visiting hours.

2. Purposes of these classes include:

a. Increasing grandparents' awareness of changes that have occurred in childbearing and childrearing

b. Increasing grandparents' awareness of their own feelings

3. Some grandparents are an integral part of the birthing experience and need information about being a "coach."

4. The need for knowledgeable extended family support systems becomes increasingly important with shorter hospital stays.

F. Postpartum education programs

1. With the emergence of shorter hospital stays, classes following delivery are being offered through hospitals, clinics, private agencies, and health professionals in private practice.
2. Although these programs vary widely in length, goals, and content, they all provide support for parents.
3. These programs often are extensions of the prenatal classes and deal with issues as they emerge from parents' concerns (such as mother's body image concerns, newborn care and safety, and birth control).

NURSING PROCESS OVERVIEW

III. CHILDBIRTH EDUCATION

A. Assessment

1. Determine the woman's or couple's expectations about instruction and about childbirth.
2. Identify cultural expectations and influences on the mother's behavior during pregnancy, labor, and birth.
3. Assess the couple's readiness for decision-making.
4. Assess their learning needs as a couple and as individuals.
5. Evaluate the clients' knowledge of:
   a. Physical and physiologic changes of pregnancy
   b. Fetal development
   c. What to expect during prenatal visits
   d. Preparation for labor and delivery
   e. Newborn care
   f. Self-care

B. Nursing diagnoses

1. Anxiety
2. Fear
3. Knowledge Deficit
4. Ineffective Management of Therapeutic Regimen: Noncompliance
5. Powerlessness
6. Decisional Conflict

C. Planning and outcome identification

1. The couple's anxiety and fear related to pregnancy and childbirth will be reduced
2. The couple plans to attend childbirth education classes and other prenatal and postpartum education programs as appropriate.
3. The couple will keep all prenatal appointments.
4. The couple will plan for pregnancy, childbirth, and newborn care by making informed decisions.
5. The expectant mother's partner will play an integral role in preparation for childbirth.

D. Implementation

1. Reduce the couple's anxiety and fears related to pregnancy and childbirth.
   a. Maintain an open nonjudgmental atmosphere.
   b. Promote realistic goals and expectations regarding the entire childbirth experience.

CLIENT AND FAMILY TEACHING 7-1

Sample birth plan

Birth attendant	■ James Fishburn, MD (obstetrician)
Birth setting, hospital	■ Labor, delivery, recovery, and postpartum (LDRP) room #2 at Valley General Hospital
Support person	■ Alice Bloom, my mother
Activities during labor	■ Walk, watch TV, rock in the rocking chair ■ Visit with family as long as possible ■ Listen to soft music ■ Discuss medications that may be needed
Birth	■ I do not want an episiotomy. ■ My mother wants to cut the cord. ■ We want to videotape the birth.
Postpartum	■ I want to breast-feed immediately. ■ I want to keep my baby with me. ■ I want to room in with my baby. ■ I want the infant's eye treatment delayed until after first feeding. ■ I want to go home as soon as possible after the birth.

2. Provide family teaching.
   a. Refer the couple to a childbirth preparation course.
   b. Determine the couple's needs and refer them to additional appropriate prenatal and postpartum education programs (such as sibling preparation class or breast-feeding class)
   c. Explain what to include in a birth plan and review the birth plan with the couple (*Client and Family Teaching* 7-1).
3. Promote prenatal care compliance in the pregnant woman and her partner.
   a. Stress the importance of prenatal care to the woman and her partner.
   b. Advise the couple to make arrangements for transportation and childcare, if needed, in order to keep prenatal appointments.
   c. Address the couple's questions and concerns honestly and promptly.
   d. Encourage attendance at childbirth education programs.
4. Encourage the couple to take charge of their planning for pregnancy and birth, and to make informed decisions.
   a. Provide the woman and her partner with accurate information about available options for birth settings (*Client and Family Teaching* 7-2).
   b. Explain the differences between the types of primary birthing attendants (for example, obstetrician versus certified nurse midwife).
   c. Stress the importance of creating a birth plan.
5. Integrate the partner into preparation for childbirth. Provide such information as:
   a. How to coach the mother during labor and delivery
   b. The importance of helping the mother keep antepartum appointments
   c. The significance of fetal heart tones (FHTs) and the sonogram; listening to FHTs and viewing the sonogram
   d. How to participate in preparing the home for the newborn
   e. Preparing siblings for the newborn

CLIENT AND FAMILY TEACHING 7-2

Choosing a birth setting

Selecting a birth setting for yourself, your partner, and the baby is a matter of personal choice and depends on the type of care available in your area. Some questions to consider are:

- What type of caregiver do I want to supervise my care during pregnancy, labor, and birth? What type of caregiver do I want to supervise my baby's care?
- Will the same person I see at prenatal visits be available for the birth?
- Does the agency offer childbirth education classes?
- What types of birth settings are available to me?
- Is the amount and kind of pharmacologic agents to be used during labor negotiable?
- Can I choose my support person and can he or she participate in the labor and birth?
- Can I breast-feed immediately and keep the baby with me for an extended time following birth? Is rooming-in available?
- Does the birth setting have an early discharge policy? Do they have follow-up visits or phone calls?
- Can I record the birth on video or in photographs?
- What if an emergency occurs; is the setting prepared for swift transfer of my baby or me?

E. Outcome evaluation

1. The couple's anxieties and fears are reduced.
   a. Their expectations of themselves and each other are realistic.
   b. The couple's goals for labor are realistic and flexible.
2. The couple verbalizes an understanding of the major concepts and content of childbirth education, other prenatal and postpartum programs, and what to include in a birth plan.
3. The couple attends all prenatal care appointments and participates in childbirth education classes.
4. The expectant parents voice a feeling of control in planning for childbirth.
   a. The couple makes an informed decision about a delivery setting and a primary birthing attendant.
   b. The birth plan is prepared by the beginning of the third trimester and includes information regarding the woman's preferences for labor, birth, and newborn care; it also delineates preferences should complications arise.
5. The partner verbalizes an understanding of the role and responsibilities of the support person in the childbirth process.

Study questions

1. Which of the following best defines childbirth education?

1. The minimal level of teaching requirements for prenatal care in this country, as advocated by health care professionals
2. Approach to childbirth involving the use of a coach and advocation of "natural childbirth" without analgesia
3. Achievement of a positive, safe, and rewarding labor and birth experience for parents and family members.
4. Information, exercises, and techniques to deal with the discomforts of pregnancy, labor, and birth.

2. During which of the following would the focus of classes be mainly on physiologic changes, fetal development, sexuality during pregnancy, and nutrition?

1. Prepregnant period
2. First trimester
3. Second trimester
4. Third trimester

3. Which of the following approaches to childbirth education advocates slow breathing, deep relaxation, and a person to act as coach?
1. Dick-Read method
2. "New childbirth" method
3. Bradley method
4. Lamaze method

4. Which of the following would the nurse identify as the best purpose for sibling preparation classes?
1. They prepare the child for what to expect when visiting mother during labor and delivery.
2. They prepare the child to visit mother and newborn in the hospital and for babysitting when at home.
3. They prepare the child for what to expect when visiting mother and newborn in the hospital.
4. They prepare the child to understand the reasons why mother cannot give the child all of her attention.

5. Which of the following best identifies the reason for grandparent preparation classes?
1. Prepare the grandparents for hospital visits during labor and delivery
2. Increase the grandparents' awareness of changes in childbearing
3. Prepare the grandparents to be more up to date in babysitting situations
4. Prepare the grandparents for the emotional problems of aging and grandparenting

6. Which of the following would be a disadvantage of breast-feeding?
1. Involution occurs more rapidly but with greater blood loss.
2. The incidence of allergies increases due to maternal antibodies.
3. The father may resent the infant's demands on the mother's body.
4. There is a greater chance for error during preparation.

7. Which of the following identifies the best reason for a father to be included in breast-feeding programs?
1. He will be able to understand why his wife has to spend so much time with the newborn.
2. He will be prepared to explain the procedure of breast-feeding to the children at home.
3. He will be able to help his wife with problems of self-esteem, body image, and frustration.
4. He will have an opportunity to express his positive and negative feelings about the process.

8. Which of the following best describes the effectiveness of childbirth education?
1. It provides expectant parents with knowledge and skills necessary to cope with pregnancy.
2. It prepares expectant parents to be informed consumers of birthing attendants and facilities.
3. It provides a long time for expectant parents to express their concerns and fears.
4. It improves newborn health, parent-newborn bonding, and ability to cope with labor.

9. Which of the following topics should be included in childbirth education for pregnant adolescents?
Select all that apply:
1. interpersonal relationships
2. sexuality issues
3. weight gain
4. sibling preparation classes
5. physical changes during pregnancy
6. availability of community resources

Answer key

1. The answer is 4.
Childbirth education is defined as being prepared for the birth experience through information, instruction, exercises, and techniques developed to deal with the discomforts of pregnancy, labor, and birth. As a result, childbirth education has become a standard part of prenatal care in the United States. It does involve teaching but not at the minimal level. The term *natural childbirth* initially described a particular approach to childbirth — labor and birth without analgesia or anesthesia. Achieving a positive, safe, and rewarding labor and birth experience is one of the goals of childbirth education.

2. The answer is 2.
First-trimester classes commonly focus on such issues as early physiologic changes, fetal development, sexuality during pregnancy, and nutrition. Some early classes may include prepregnant couples. Second- and third-trimester classes may focus on preparation for birth, parenting, and newborn care.

3. The answer is 3.
The Bradley technique focuses on slow breathing and deep relaxation for labor, reduced responsiveness to external stimuli, and the role for an individual as a coach. It is basically Dick-Read's approach with the addition of a labor coach. The Grantly Dick-Read approach suggests that education decreases fear, tension, and pain. This method teaches exercises to improve muscle tone and increase relaxation, and stresses slow breathing, muscle relaxation, and pushing techniques. The Wright, or "new childbirth," method involves slower but more complex breathing patterns than the Lamaze method. The Lamaze, or psychoprophylactic, method combines relaxation, concentration, focusing, and complex, well-paced breathing patterns to reduce the perception of pain through a conditioned response to labor contractions.

4. The answer is 3.
Sibling preparation classes typically prepare the child for what to expect when visiting mother and newborn in the hospital. Few programs exist to prepare the child for attendance at the birth. A sibling support person is usually expected to accompany the child to reduce distraction of mother during labor. Sibling preparation classes do not prepare the child for babysitting, nor do they help the child understand the reasons for not receiving attention during this time.

5. The answer is 2.
Grandparent preparation classes help increase the grandparents' awareness of changes that have occurred in childbearing and childrearing, and increase grandparents' awareness of their own feelings. Some grandparents are an integral part of the birthing experience and need information about being a "coach." Preparing them for hospital visits, up-to-date babysitting situations, or the emotional problems of aging and grandparenting are not addressed with grandparent preparation classes.

6. The answer is 3.
The father knows that his body is not capable of providing the milk for the newborn, and he may fear that breast-feeding will interfere with his feeding the newborn, providing fewer chances for bonding. He may also be jealous of the infant's demands on his wife's time and body. Breast-feeding is advantageous because uterine involution occurs more rapidly, thus minimizing blood loss. The presence of maternal antibodies in breast milk helps decrease the incidence of allergies in the newborn. A greater chance for error is associated with bottle-feeding. No preparation is required for breast-feeding.

7. The answer is **4.**
Breast-feeding programs typically include content such as preparation of breasts, techniques for breast-feeding, and advantages versus disadvantages of breast-feeding. Fathers are included more frequently because these programs provide an opportunity for expression of their feelings — both positive and negative — about breast-feeding. Understanding the amount of time spent with the newborn, being able to explain the procedure to children at home, and helping his wife with problems with self-esteem and body image are not associated with breast-feeding programs.

8. The answer is **4.**
The effectiveness of childbirth education is demonstrated by improved newborn health, parent-newborn bonding, and the parents' ability to cope with labor. Providing expectant parents with necessary knowledge and skills and preparing them to be informed consumers are goals of childbirth education. Childbirth education does not provide a long time for expectant parents to express their concerns and fears.

9. The answer is **1, 2, 3, 5, 6.**
Adolescents have special learning needs during pregnancy. Areas of special interest are peer relationships, altered body image, weight gain issues, and sexuality issues. The pregnant adolescent is often without adequate support from parents or a partner. The nurse should assist her in identifying and accessing community resources for herself and her baby. Sibling preparation classes are not usually a concern.

8 Antepartum Care

I. OVERVIEW

A. Essential concepts

1. Antepartum care refers to the medical and nursing care given to the pregnant woman between conception and the onset of labor.
2. Consideration is given to the physical, emotional, and social needs of the woman, the unborn child, her partner, and other family members.
3. Pregnancy is viewed as a normal physiologic process, not a disease process. Nevertheless, at no other time in life does a woman need such intense, regular care as during pregnancy.
4. With the advent of highly sophisticated instrumentation and monitoring, the nurse must be particularly alert that these techniques are used to augment practice and should never replace the therapeutic process.
5. Although the value of prenatal care in terms of maternal-fetal outcome is well documented, prenatal care, even of the highest quality, does not guarantee a positive outcome.
6. The process of data gathering and analysis is ongoing; the nurse cannot expect to cover all areas during the initial antepartum visit and, therefore, should focus on trimester-specific issues.
7. Every woman who has been menstruating and then misses a menstrual period is usually considered pregnant until proven otherwise. Pregnancy must be ruled out in any instance of amenorrhea, even though the woman insists that she is not pregnant.
8. The following methods are commonly used to determine pregnancy:
   a. Pregnancy tests (urine or serum) at home or in the health care facility
      - Pregnancy tests are not infallible.
      - A negative result may occur when pregnancy exists or there may be a positive result when there is no pregnancy (*Table* 8-1).

   b. Presumptive evidence of pregnancy (for example, amenorrhea, nausea, and breast tenderness)
   c. Probable evidence of pregnancy (for example, enlarged abdomen and quickening)
   d. Positive evidence of pregnancy (for example, fetal heartbeat and ultrasound visualization)

B. Goals of antepartum care

1. The expectant mother's and family's knowledge of pregnancy increases.
2. The expectant mother and other family members learn about actions they can take to facilitate a positive birth outcome.
3. Family members experience pregnancy in a positive way.
4. The newborn is successfully integrated into the family.

C. Factors affecting the antepartum experience

1. Previous experience with pregnancy
2. Cultural and personal expectations
3. Prepregnant health and biophysical preparedness for childbearing
4. Motivation for childbearing
5. Socioeconomic status
6. Mother's age and partnered versus unpartnered status
7. Accessibility of prenatal care
8. Level of education
9. Availability of resources

TABLE 8-1
Causes of false pregnancy test results

Causes	False-positive results	False-negative results
Human	▪ Error in reading ▪ Error in recording	▪ Error in reading ▪ Error in recording
Poor test sample or condition	▪ Recent pregnancy (for example, test done fewer than 10 days after abortion) ▪ Proteinuria ▪ Hematuria ▪ Test performed during ovulation	▪ Test performed too early or too late in pregnancy ▪ Urine too dilute ▪ Urine stored too long at room temperature
Substance	▪ Luteinizing hormone cross-reaction interference ▪ Aspirin in large doses, phenothiazines (antipsychotic medications), marijuana, methyldopa (Aldomet) ▪ Treatment with human chorionic gonadotropin (HCG) for infertility (affects blood tests only) ▪ HCG secreted by tumor	▪ N/A (as in menopause)
Other	▪ Pregnancy recently terminated (within 10 days of test) ▪ Trophoblastic disease (molar pregnancy or choriocarcinoma)	▪ Missed abortion ▪ Ectopic pregnancy ▪ Impending spontaneous abortion

II. EVALUATION OF FETAL WELL-BEING

A. Fetal heart rate (FHR)

1. FHR usually is auscultated at the midline suprapubic region with a Doppler ultrasound transducer at 10 to 12 weeks' gestation.
2. FHR can be auscultated with a fetoscope, a specially designed stethoscope, at about 20 weeks' gestation.
3. An FHR of 120 to 160 beats per minute can be distinguished from the slower maternal heart rate by palpating the mother's pulse while auscultating the FHR.
4. A regular heartbeat is normal; irregularity is abnormal.
5. The heartbeat will be muffled when the mother's abdominal wall is thick, if she is obese, or if there is a large volume of amniotic fluid.
6. Fundic souffle, caused by blood rushing through the umbilical arteries, is synchronous with the FHR; uterine souffle, the sound of blood passing through the uterine blood vessels, is synchronous with the maternal pulse.
7. Failure to hear FHR may result from one or more of the following:
   a. Inexperience with the Doppler ultrasound transducer or fetoscope
   b. Defective Doppler ultrasound transducer or fetoscope, or a noisy environment
   c. Early pregnancy or miscalculation of gestational age
   d. Obesity
   e. Loud placental souffle obscuring the FHR
   f. Posterior position of the fetus
   g. Hydramnios
   h. Small-for-gestational-age fetus
   i. Fetal death

B. Ultrasonography (sonograms)

1. Serial sonograms provide useful information when assessing fetal growth and well-being.
2. Ultrasonography provides direct information about the fetus during each trimester.
   a. **First trimester**
   - Assessment of gestational age
   - Evaluation for congenital anomalies
   - Diagnostic evaluation of vaginal bleeding
   - Confirmation of suspected multiple gestation
   - Evaluation of fetal growth
   - Adjunct to prenatal testing, such as amniocentesis or chorionic villus sampling (CVS)

   b. **Second trimester**
   - Assessment of gestational age
   - Evaluation for congenital anomalies (such as hydrocephaly)
   - Assessment of fetal growth
   - Guidance of procedures, such as amniocentesis and fetoscopy
   - Assessment of placental location
   - Diagnosis of multiple gestation

   c. **Third trimester**
   - Determination of fetal position
   - Estimation of fetal size
3. A second-trimester sonogram is recommended as a baseline for all clients considered to be at risk for complications.
4. A full bladder may improve ultrasonic resolution before 20 weeks' gestation. Clients may be instructed to drink a quart or more of fluid 1 to 2 hours before the procedure.
5. When used as an adjunct to prenatal diagnoses, ultrasonic visualization of the fetus may support the difficult decision of whether or not to terminate the pregnancy.
6. Depending on the skill of the technician, it may be possible to visualize the sex of the fetus in addition to other structures. The parents should be asked whether they want to know the sex of the child before the information is provided.

C. Measurement of fundal height (McDonald rule)

1. Assessment begins during the second trimester, when the fundus is palpable at the level of the umbilicus (at 20 weeks), and continues until it reaches the xyphoid process (at 36 weeks).
2. Measurement involves using a nonelastic, flexible measuring tape, placing the zero point on the superior border of the symphysis pubis, and stretching the tape across the abdomen at the midline to the top of the fundus.
3. After 20 to 22 weeks' gestation, the fundal height in centimeters normally approximates the gestational age in weeks until the 36th week. After this time, the fetus is gaining weight rather than height and near the onset of labor settles into the mother's pelvis in preparation for birth. For these reasons, a fundus that is truly at 40 weeks may be the same height as it was at 36 weeks.
4. Possible causes of greater-than-expected fundal height include multiple gestation, polyhydramnios, and fetal macrosomia.
5. Possible causes for less-than-expected fundal height include abnormal fetal presentation, fetal growth restriction, congenital anomalies, and oligohydramnios.

D. Fetal movement (quickening)

1. In primigravidas (first-time mothers), quickening normally is detected between 18 and 20 weeks' gestation.
2. In multigravidas, quickening may occur as early as 16 weeks.
3. Quickening is typically described as a light fluttering feeling; it may be mistaken for flatus.

E. Electronic fetal heart monitoring (EFHM)

1. EFHM may be used during the antepartum period to evaluate fetal status. It can demonstrate fetal heart rate changes in response to fetal movement and spontaneous or induced uterine contractions.
2. An increase in fetal heart rate with fetal movement indicates adequate oxygenation, a functioning neural pathway to the heart, and the ability of the fetal heart to respond to stimuli.
3. Contractions stress the fetus by decreasing uterine perfusion. In a fetus already compromised by disease, cord compression, or other factors, contractions may alter the heart rate, which is detectable on EFHM.
4. Common EFHM studies are the nonstress test (NST) and the contraction stress test (CST).

   a. **NST**

   - This is the least invasive test of fetal well-being involving the use of an electronic fetal monitor. The baseline FHR and the presence of periodic patterns are identified and correlated to contractions observed on the uterine activity tracing.
   - Adequate perfusion is necessary to maintain fetal central nervous system integrity and reflex responses.
   - In a healthy fetus, fetal movement causes an accelerated heart rate; in this case, the test is reactive.
   - Among the various assessment protocols, the most common involves two FHR accelerations within a 10-minute period, with each acceleration increasing the heart rate by at least 15 beats per minute and lasting at least 15 seconds.
   - The fetus typically is monitored for at least 40 minutes (to account for a normal sleep period); the entire tracing is then evaluated.
   - Abnormal or nonreactive NST results require further evaluation that same day.
   - Even with a reactive NST, follow-up is indicated if the FHR falls outside the range of 120 to 160 beats per minute or if decelerations (early, late, or variable) are detected.

   b. **CST.** This test would not be performed until about 38+ weeks and only if there were other indications of a problem such as may be detected in the biophysical profile or maternal serum alpha-fetoprotein (MSAFP). Delivery of the compromised fetus would be the goal of such testing to protect its welfare. There are two ways to do this–nipple stimulation and intravenous oxytocin drip.

   - Perfusion through the spinal arteries of the uterus decreases during contractions. Recordings of the heart rate of the fetus with limited reserve show late decelerations in response to the stress of contractions (a positive CST finding). The healthy fetus responds to the stress of contractions with a normal heart rate and no decelerations apparent on the fetal monitoring strip (a negative CST result).
   - During fetal testing, contractions may occur spontaneously; most commonly, however, stimulation will be necessary. This is done either by breast stimulation (such as nipple rolling or application of moist hot pads) to trigger prolactin release or by low-dose intravenous oxytocin infusion (oxytocin challenge test [OCT]).

- Three contractions within 10 minutes, ideally lasting 40 to 60 seconds each, must be evaluated to assess fetal response to stress.
- During an OCT, oxytocin may precipitate labor.

F. Other procedures

1. **Fetal activity determination,** also referred to as "kick counts," is assessed by the mother, and a marker is placed on the monitor strip. FHR in relation to fetal movement is evaluated. There should be a slight rise in FHR immediately before movement. The heart rate should remain within normal limits. The determination is usually done when the mother reports a decrease, or absence, of fetal movement.
2. Routine **maternal urinalysis** and **serum assays** help monitor fetal status. For example, serum human chorionic gonadotropin indicates a viable fetus, and serum estriol and human placental lactogen reflect fetal homeostasis.
3. **Triple screening** includes MSAFP, human chorionic gonadotropin, and unconjugated estriol. Together they increase the detection of trisomy 18 and trisomy 21. They are performed between 15 and 22 weeks and are considered positive if all three markers are low. Further testing for karyotyping is usually offered.
4. **CVS** is a first-trimester (10 to 12 weeks) alternative to amniocentesis for prenatal diagnosis of genetic abnormalities. This procedure is accomplished by needle aspiration of a sample of chorionic villi, either by the transcervical or transabdominal route.
5. **Amniocentesis** can determine fetal maturity and detect certain birth defects (such as Down syndrome or spina bifida), hemolytic disease of the newborn, and sex and chromosomal abnormalities.
6. **Percutaneous umbilical blood sampling** (PUBS; *Figure* 8-1), also called cordocentesis, may be performed in the second or third trimester to investigate or treat conditions requiring direct access to the fetal vascular system. PUBS is being used with less frequency because newer tests have replaced the need for a direct fetal sample.
7. **Fetoscopy** enables direct fetal visualization through a fetoscope, a fiberoptic optical instrument, inserted through the abdominal and uterine walls to identify fetal developmental abnormalities. The fetoscope can retrieve tissue and blood samples to detect hemophilia or other disorders and may be used for some types of fetal surgery. This procedure has been replaced by amniocentesis, PUBS, ultrasound, and biochemical marker identification.
8. **Fetal fibronectin (fFN)** is a glycoprotein produced by the trophoblast and other fetal tissues. The presence of cervicovaginal fetal fibronectin between 20 and 34 weeks' gestation is a strong predictor of preterm birth caused by spontaneous preterm labor or premature rupture of membranes. Fetal fibronectin levels can be measured with an enzyme immunoassay.
9. **Phosphatidylglycerol (PG)** is the second most abundant phospholipid in surfactant. PG appears at about 36 weeks' gestation and increases in amount until term. PG is not present in blood or vaginal fluid; therefore, its presence is reliable for indicating lung maturity. It is not measured in specific concentration; instead, the presence of PG is associated with very low development of respiratory distress syndrome (RDS). The absence of PG is associated with development of RDS. Lung maturity can be confirmed in most pregnancies if PG is present with a lecithin-to-sphingomyelin (L/S) ratio of 2:1.
10. **Biophysical profile (BPP)** represents an assessment of five fetal biophysical variables: FHR acceleration, fetal breathing, fetal movements, fetal tone, and amniotic fluid volume. FHR acceleration is assessed with NST (See Section II, E, 4, a). The other four variables are assessed by ultrasound scan. BPP helps to identify the compromised fetus and

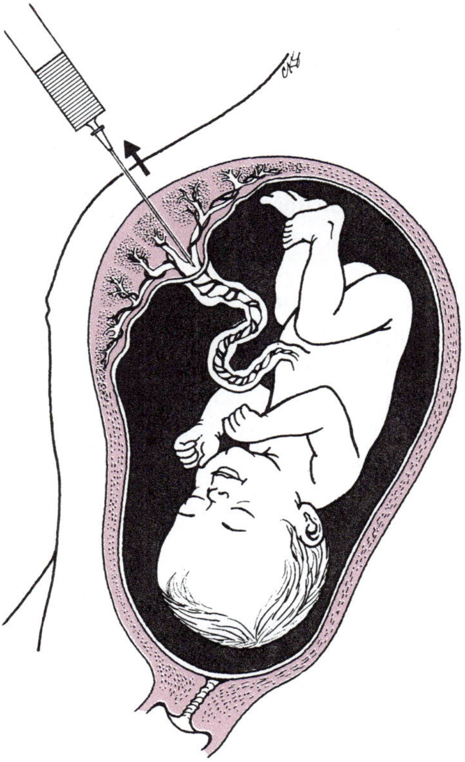

FIGURE 8-1
Percutaneous umbilical blood sampling involves inserting a needle into the fetal umbilical cord and aspirating blood for analysis. The procedure is guided by ultrasonography and is used to screen karyotypes (chromosomes), examine antibodies for teratogenic viruses, and provide access for fetal blood transfusions.

confirms the healthy fetus. Normal variables are assigned a score of 2 each. Abnormal variables are assigned a score of zero (0). The highest score possible for a normal fetus is 10.

11. **Alpha-fetoprotein (AFP)** is a fetal protein produced in the yolk sac during the first 6 weeks of gestation and later by the fetal liver. AFP is found in the amniotic fluid and maternal serum. If the fetus has a neural tube defect, AFP levels are elevated.
12. **Doppler blood flow studies** use ultrasound technology to study blood flow changes that occur in maternal and fetal circulation and to assess placental function. They are most useful when intrauterine growth restriction occurs no matter the cause. These studies have no demonstrated value in postterm pregnancy, diabetes, or systemic lupus erythematosus, and in detecting fetal compromise in the general obstetric population.

NURSING PROCESS OVERVIEW

III. CARE OF THE WOMAN DURING THE ANTEPARTUM PERIOD

A. Initial prenatal assessment

1. Health history
    a. **Current pregnancy history** should include first day of the last menstrual period, cramping or bleeding, results of the pregnancy test, and discomfort (for example, nausea, vomiting, headache, urinary frequency, and fatigue).
    b. **History of previous pregnancies** should include gravida, para, number of abortions, number of living children, prenatal education, cesarean births, length of labor, stillbirths, preterm labors, gestational age, and birth weight.
    c. **Gynecologic history** should include previous infections, previous surgery, age of menarche and menstrual cycle, and sexual, menstrual, and contraception history.
    d. **Current medical history** should include weight, blood type and Rh, medications presently taking (prescription and over the counter), habits (such as smoking, alcohol, caffeine, or drugs), allergies, potential teratogenic effects on this pregnancy (such as infections, medications, radiographs, or toxins in home or workplace), medical conditions (such as diabetes, hypertension or cardiovascular, renal, or congenital disorders), and immunizations.
    e. **Medical history** should include childhood diseases, medical diseases and treatment, sexually transmitted diseases, surgeries, bleeding disorders or previous blood transfusions, emotional problems, and accidents.
    f. **Family medical history** should include medical disorders (such as cancer, heart disease, or diabetes), multiple births, and genetic or congenital disorders.
    g. **Occupational history** should include type of work and health hazards (*Client and Family Teaching* 8-1).
    h. **History of the baby's father** should include age, health problems, habits, blood type and Rh, genetic or congenital disorders, occupation, and attitude toward the pregnancy.
    i. **Personal information** should include racial, cultural, and religious practices; exercise (*Client and Family Teaching* 8-2); housing and living conditions; income; support system; use of health care system; and work.

CLIENT AND FAMILY TEACHING 8-1

Tips for pregnant working women

- Know your work environment, such as what toxins are present in the work you do.
- Use your break and lunch periods to rest with your legs elevated to decrease edema.
- When resting, lie on your left side to promote circulation to the uterus.
- Wear support hosiery to promote circulation in your lower extremities.
- If you must stand for long periods of time, think of ways to walk around your workplace.
- Empty your bladder every 2 hours to prevent infection.
- Avoid excessive overtime to lessen fatigue.
- Avoid activities that require balance, climbing, or reaching.
- Wear your seat belt properly positioned for pregnancy.
- Get extra rest on days off or on weekends.
- Stop working 2 to 4 weeks before your expected date of birth.
- Stop smoking or decrease the amount you smoke.

CLIENT AND FAMILY TEACHING 8-2
Exercise during pregnancy

- Consult your primary care provider before you exercise. Do not exceed target heart rates.
- Exercise at least three times per week rather than sporadically.
- Avoid jerky or bouncy movements, jumping and jarring, or fast changes of direction.
- Do not do strenuous exercise (for example, tennis or running) in hot, humid weather.
- Always start your exercise with a warm-up and end with a cool-down.
- Do not overstretch your joints.
- When lying on the floor, get up slowly. Do not lay on your back or point your toes when exercising after the fourth month.
- Drink liquids liberally.
- Maintain a caloric intake adequate to your needs and the additional requirements of pregnancy.
- Stop exercising and contact your primary care provider if unusual symptoms occur.

2. Determination of the estimated date of delivery (EDD) or estimated date of confinement
   a. The average length of pregnancy is 280 days (40 weeks, 10 lunar months, or 9 calendar months), as calculated from the first day of the last menstrual period (LMP).
   b. To calculate the EDD by Nägele rule, count backward 3 calendar months from the month in which the last menstrual period occurred. Using the date of the first day of this menses, add 7 days. Change the year, if necessary. For example, an LMP of May 15, 2003 would yield an EDD of February 22, 2004.
   c. The following are ways to date the pregnancy when LMP is unknown.
      - Uterine size is reported in terms of weeks of gestation at the first prenatal visit.
      - Presence of the uterus in the abdomen (fundal height) indicates at least 12 weeks' gestation.
      - Uterus in the pelvis (fundal height) indicates less than 12 weeks' gestation.
      - Quickening indicates about 20 weeks' gestation in primigravidas; it may occur earlier in multigravidas.
      - Fetal heart tones can be detected at 10 to 12 weeks' gestation with a Doppler ultrasound transducer and at 16 to 20 weeks with a fetoscope.
      - Ultrasound can detect pregnancy 5 to 6 weeks after the LMP.

3. Assessment of risk factors
   a. Early identification of potential risk factors may provide opportunities for appropriate interventions.
   b. Risk factors that could have a negative effect on the pregnancy may be characterized as demographic, obstetric, medical, and miscellaneous (*Table* 8-2, page 114).

4. Physical examination. Perform a complete physical examination, including vital signs, height, and weight (current and prepregnant), and a pelvic examination. Two additional parts of the physical examination include assessment of the pelvic size for adequacy and a breast examination.
   a. **Assessment of pelvic size for adequacy** (see Chapter 2 for discussion of pelvic measurements.)
      - This assessment consists of measurement of the dimensions and proportion of the bony pelvis.
      - Measurements are obtained during the bimanual portion of the pelvic examination by moving the fingers over the landmarks of the bony pelvis and estimating their size.

TABLE 8-2
Perinatal risk assessment

Areas to be assessed	Conditions associated with increased risk
Antepartum course	
General prenatal information	■ Lack of prenatal care ■ Weight gain ($\leq$ 5 lb or $\geq$ 35 lb)
Maternal health	■ Medical conditions – Insulin-dependent diabetes* – Heart disease – Chronic hypertension ■ Habits – Smoking – Substance abuse ■ Infections during pregnancy – Rubella – Venereal disease ■ Complications of pregnancy – Pregnancy-induced hypertension – Third-trimester bleeding* – Rh sensitization; severe sensitization* – Multiple fetuses*
Results of antepartum tests	■ Estriol levels: decreased or no increase after 36 wk ■ Ultrasound: growth retardation $\geq$ 2 wk ■ Amniocentesis: – Bilirubin or meconium present – L/S ratio < 2:1 ■ Nonstress test: nonreactive ■ Stress test: positive

Areas to be assessed	Conditions associated with increased risk
Intrapartum course	
Length of pregnancy	■ < 34 wk, $\leq$ 37 wk, $\geq$ 42 wk
Duration and character of labor	■ Prolonged first or second stage* ■ Precipitous labor or delivery ■ Premature rupture of membrane > 24 hr ■ Difficult labor ■ Cephalopelvic disproportion
Maternal conditions	■ Preexisting problems (see antepartum course) ■ Progressive hypotension ■ Progressive hypertension ■ Excessive bleeding* ■ Signs of infection
Fetal presentation and position	■ Breech* ■ Transverse lie*
Events indicating possible fetal distress	■ Fetal monitoring findings ■ Persistent late decelerations* ■ Severe variable decelerations* ■ Heart rate < 120 or >160 for > 30 min ■ Poor beat-to-beat (short-term and long-term) variability ■ Scalp pH $\leq$ 7.25* ■ Meconium-stained fluid* ■ Prolapsed cord*
Analgesia	■ Large or repeated doses of analgesia (for example, meperidine may cause neonatal respiratory depression for up to 4 hr after administration) ■ I.M. analgesia between 1 and 4 hr of delivery ■ I.V. analgesia within 30 min of delivery
Anesthesia	■ General anesthesia ■ Conduction anesthesia with maternal hypotension
Method of delivery	■ Cesarean birth* ■ Midforceps or high-forceps delivery* ■ Failed vacuum extraction

*Conditions usually requiring presence at delivery of someone skilled in resuscitation.

- This assessment may be delayed until later in pregnancy, when the procedure may be more comfortable for the mother; it is not crucial to determine pelvic adequacy at the initial assessment.

b. Inspection and palpation of the breasts for normal and questionable changes of pregnancy
- Normal changes associated with pregnancy include increased size, tenderness, darkening and enlargement of areola; erection of nipples; leaking of colostrum late in the first trimester;and the appearance of a venous pattern and striae formation.
- Questionable changes include recent lumps or masses that feel hard or fixed, dimpling, redness, edema, ulceration, and nipple retraction or elevation.

5. **Laboratory and diagnostic studies.** During the initial assessment of physical status, which typically occurs during the first prenatal visit, baseline data are obtained (*Table* 8-3, page 116). These data provide a measure against which subsequent data are evaluated.

a. **Urinalysis** includes tests for protein, glucose, ketones, bilirubin, red blood cells, white blood cells, and bacteria.

b. **Blood tests**
- **CBC** to determine hemoglobin and hematocrit levels
- **Blood group and type test** to determine blood type, Rh factor, and presence of antibodies to blood group antigens.
- **Blood glucose tests** to screen for diabetes; usually done between the 24th and 28th week of gestation because of hormonal effects that block insulin usage.
- **Rubella antibody titer** to screen for rubella.
- **Blood culture** to detect specific infectious microorganisms.
- **VDRL, ART, and RPR** are blood tests to detect the presence of certain sexually transmitted diseases.
- **Hemoglobin and hematocrit** determination
- **Hepatitis B test**
- **Human immunodeficiency virus test**
- **Sickle cell test** to screen for sickle cell trait and disease

c. **Papanicolaou smear** and **cytologic study** to screen for cervical dysplasia and assess hormone cytology and inflammatory disease of the female genital tract.

6. Evaluation of fetal well-being. See section II.

7. **Psychosocial assessment** during the initial visits should include:

a. Expectations for the pregnancy; emotional and financial impact on the family; and the partner's attitude toward the pregnancy (for example, excitement or apprehension)

b. Whether or not the pregnancy was planned

c. Educational needs and resources

d. Support systems

e. Religious beliefs and cultural practices related to childbirth and parenting

f. Family functioning, living situation, and sexual activity

g. Preparation for childbirth and parenthood

B. Subsequent prenatal assessments. In a low-risk pregnancy, prenatal visits are scheduled every 4 weeks for the first 28 weeks; every 2 weeks from 28 to 36 weeks; and then weekly until delivery.

1. History and physical assessment with each prenatal visit should include:

a. Data concerning the course of the pregnancy (such as common discomforts and how they are alleviated)

TABLE 8-3
Common prenatal laboratory tests

Test	Timing	Significant value
HCG	Initial visit	Positive
CBC		
Hct	Initial visit, 28 and 36 wks	< 32%
Hgb	Initial visit, 28 and 36 wks	< 11 g/dl
WCT	Initial visit, 28 and 36 wks	>15,000 mm^3
Blood type and Rh	Initial visit	Mother Rh– Father Rh+
Antibody screen	Initial visit, 28 and 36 wks	Positive
Serology	Initial visit and 36 wks	Positive
Rubella titer	Initial visit	≤1.8
1-hr serum glucose	24 to 28 wks	>140 g/dl
HBsAg	Initial visit, if indicated	Positive
Urinalysis	Initial visit	Positive
Urine C&S	Initial visit	Positive for infection
Urine		
Glucose	Each visit	Positive
Protein	Each visit	Greater than 2+
Pap smear	Initial visit	Abnormal cytology
PPD	Initial visit	Positive
HIV	Offer at initial visit	Positive
Sickle cell screen	Offer at initial visit	Positive for trait or anemia
Tay-Sachs screen	Offer at initial visit	Carrier
GC culture	Initial visit and 36 wks	Positive
Rh antibody	Initial visit, 28 and 36 wks	Negative
MSAFP	15 to 20 weeks	≥2.0
Biophysical profile	Third trimester	≤8–10

(From Simpson, KR and Creehan, PA. (1996). *AWHONN's Perinatal Nursing.* Philadelphia: Lippincott Williams & Wilkins, p. 86.)

b. Maternal vital signs, including temperature, pulse, respiration, and blood pressure
c. Weight gain (distribution per trimester)
d. Presence of edema
e. Uterine size (fundal height)
f. FHR
g. Urine for protein and glucose
h. **Danger signals, including vaginal bleeding, visual disturbances, leaking of amniotic fluid, rapid weight gain, elevated blood pressure, headaches, persistent vomiting, abdominal pain, edema, increased temperature, painful urination, signs of preterm labor, and gross rupture of membranes.**
i. Signs of impending labor (after 38 weeks), including lightening, engagement, cervical changes, and presence of contractions.

2. **Psychosocial assessment** should focus on any specific concerns of the woman or her partner, which may include sexual activity, preparation for parenting, preparation for childbirth, and signs of labor.
3. Nutritional assessment should include:
   a. Review of dietary intake of iron, nutritional supplements, and herbs (*Box* 8-1, page 119)
   b. 24-hour diet recall
   c. Comparison of prepregnancy weight with weight gained during the pregnancy
      - During the course of the pregnancy, a total weight gain of 24 to 30 lb is recommended.
      - A normal pattern of weight gain is 1.5 lb in the first 10 weeks; 9 lb at 20 weeks; 19 lb by 30 weeks; and 27.5 lb by 40 weeks.
      - Nondietary factors affecting weight gain include increased blood pressure and excess fluid retention.

C. Assessment of common minor discomforts of pregnancy

1. First trimester
   a. Nausea and vomiting (morning sickness) generally occur early in pregnancy and subside by the fourth month of pregnancy. This is most likely a systemic reaction to increased estrogen or decreased glucose levels in the blood (*Client and Family Teaching* 8-3, page 118).
   b. Nasal stuffiness and epistaxis occur owing to nasal edema from elevated estrogen levels.
   c. Urinary frequency, caused by the growing uterus pressing on bladder, is seen in the first trimester and again in the later part of the third trimester.
   d. Breast tenderness occurs early in pregnancy and continues throughout the pregnancy owing to hormonal changes.
   e. Ptyalism (excessive salvation) occurs, probably as a local reaction to the influence of estrogen.
   f. Leukorrhea (increased vaginal discharge that is white) results from the increased activity of vaginal epithelial cells as they prepare for distention during the birth process.
   g. Headaches are due to emotional tension, eye strain, vascular engorgement, and congestion of sinuses from hormonal stimulation.
2. Second and third trimesters
   a. Heartburn, owing to regurgitation of acidic gastric contents into the esophagus, may be associated with tension and vomiting in the third trimester.
   b. Ankle edema is due to decreased venous return in the lower extremities.
   c. Varicose veins are due to poor circulation and weakened vessel walls.

CLIENT AND FAMILY TEACHING 8-3

Relieving the common discomforts of pregnancy

Discomfort	Solution
Ankle edema	Rest with your feet elevated. Avoid standing for long periods. Avoid restrictive garments on the lower half of your body.
Backache	Apply local heat. Avoid long periods of standing. Stoop to pick up objects. Tylenol in usual adult dose may help. Wear low-heeled shoes.
Breast tenderness	Wear a supportive bra. Decrease the amount of caffeine and carbonated beverages ingested.
Constipation	Increase fiber in your diet. Drink additional fluids. Have a regular time for bowel movements.
Difficulty sleeping	Drink a warm, caffeine-free drink before bed and practice relaxation techniques.
Fatigue	Schedule a rest period daily. Have a regular bedtime routine. Use extra pillows for comfort.
Faintness	Move slowly. Avoid crowds. Remain in a cool environment. Lie on your left side when at rest.
Headache	Avoid eye strain. Visit your eye doctor. Rest with a cool cloth on your forehead. Take Tylenol in regular adult dose, as needed. Report frequent or persistent headaches to your primary care provider.
Heartburn	Eat small, frequent meals each day. Avoid overeating, as well as spicy, fatty, and fried foods.
Hemorrhoids	Avoid constipation and straining with a bowel movement. Take a sitz bath. Apply a witch hazel compress.
Leg cramps	Avoid pointing your toes. Straighten your leg and dorsiflex your ankle.
Nausea	Eat six small meals per day rather than three. Eat a piece of dry toast or some crackers before getting out of bed. Avoid foods or situations that worsen the nausea. If it persists, report this problem to your primary care provider.
Nasal stuffiness	Use cool air vaporizer or humidifier, increase fluid intake, place moist towel on the sinuses, and massage the sinuses.
Ptyalism	Use mouthwash as needed. Chew gum or suck on hard candy.
Round ligament pain	Avoid twisting motions. Rise to a standing position slowly and use your hands to support the abdomen. Bend forward to relieve discomfort.
Shortness of breath	Use proper posture. Use pillows behind head and shoulders at night.
Urinary frequency	Void as necessary, at least every 2 hours. Increase fluid intake. Avoid caffeine. Practice Kegel exercises.
Vaginal discharge	Wear cotton underwear. Bathe daily. Avoid tight pantyhose.
Varicose veins	Walk regularly. Rest with feet elevated. Avoid long periods of standing. Do not cross your legs when sitting. Avoid knee-high stockings. Wear support hosiery.

(Adapted from Pillitteri, A. (1999). *Maternal and Child Health Nursing, 3rd ed.* Philadelphia: Lippincott Williams & Wilkins, p. 263.)

BOX 8-1

Complementary and alternative therapies

Herbs used to prevent miscarriage

Three herbs are used for the prevention of miscarriage—black haw, cramp bark, and false unicorn root. Black haw and cramp bark are part of the same family and are sometimes considered to be synonymous. These herbs may be given in combination and should only be dispensed by a qualified herbalist.

Pregnant women should avoid licorice in any form because it has a hypertensive effect.

Black haw

This is usually administered as a tincture, tea, or capsule; it has a uterine relaxant effect.

Cramp bark

This also may have a relaxing effect on the uterine muscles.

False unicorn root

This is administered as a tincture or in dried root form. It is considered a uterine tonic.

Herbs used to prevent hypertension

Burdock

Burdock seeds are used for their hypotensive and diuretic effects. Burdock is administered as an extract, tincture, or tea. Burdock root should not be used by pregnant women because its effect is stronger and it may be a uterine stimulant.

Dandelion

The dandelion root is used as an antihypertensive. It is also used as a diuretic, thus reducing the effects of hypertension. It is administered as an extract, tincture, capsule, or tea.

Hawthorne

Hawthorne is used to treat cardiac disorders and hypertension. Its leaves and flowers are used, and it is administered as an extract, tincture, capsule, or tea. Pregnant women should not use the berries because they may stimulate uterine activity.

Coenzyme Q10

Coenzyme Q10, also known as ubiquinone, is a fat-soluble vitamin-like compound. It is used to treat a variety of cardiac disorders, including hypertension.

Ginger and acupuncture for morning sickness

Ginger and acupuncture are among the most frequently used alternative therapies for the nausea and vomiting caused by morning sickness.

Ginger

Many clinical trials have confirmed the effectiveness and safety of ginger. However, when used in large doses it can act as an abortion-inducing agent. It should be used with caution in pregnant women, and the dosage should not exceed 1 g of dried root daily. It is available in capsules, candied, or as tea.

Acupuncture

Acupuncture is a therapy based on the ancient philosophy of traditional Chinese medicine. It involves the application of pressure to stimulate and balance the body's healing energy. A specific pressure point for nausea is located on the forearm, three fingerwidths above the wrist closest to the palm, toward the elbow. The point is pressed firmly for 10 seconds every few minutes. Pressure can also be applied through the use of a commercially prepared wristband used for motion sickness.

(Adapted from Olds, S., London, M., and Davidsson, M. [2004]. *Maternal-Newborn Nursing and Women's Health Care*, 7th ed. Upper Saddle River, NJ: Pearson/Prentice Hall, pp. 363, 471, 495.)

d. Hemorrhoids may occur from pressure of the gravid uterus on the spine, which interferes with venous circulation.

e. Constipation is caused by decreased intestinal peristalsis and displacement of the intestines from a gravid uterus, insufficient fluid intake, or use of iron supplements.

f. Backache results from altered posture due to increased curvature of the lumbosacral vertebrae from the enlarging uterus.

g. Leg cramps may be caused by spasms of the gastrocnemius muscle, possibly from insufficient calcium.

h. Faintness is due to changes in blood volume and postural hypotension.

i. Shortness of breath occurs owing to pressure exerted on the diaphragm by an enlarging uterus.

j. The enlarged uterus causes difficulty sleeping.

k. Round ligament pain results from stretching and hypertrophy of the ligaments; this should not to be mistaken for labor.

D. Nursing diagnoses

1. Health-Seeking Behaviors
2. Noncompliance
3. Altered Nutrition: Less Than Body Requirements
4. Altered Nutrition: More Than Body Requirements
5. Knowledge Deficit
6. Altered Role Performance

E. Planning and outcome identification

1. The woman will have a complication-free pregnancy.
2. The woman will achieve adequate nutritional status and fluid intake.
3. The woman will learn how to relieve common discomforts of pregnancy.
4. The woman and her partner will achieve a positive psychosocial adjustment toward the pregnancy.

F. Implementation

1. Stress the importance of regular prenatal appointments throughout the pregnancy to detect prenatal complications and to assess fetal growth and development.
   a. Explain prenatal testing to the woman and her partner.
   b. Prepare the woman and her partner for prenatal testing.
   c. Teach the woman about the danger signals of pregnancy (see section IV, B, 1, h).
2. Promote an adequate nutritional status and fluid intake.
   a. Stress well-balanced meals; review the United States Department of Agriculture's food pyramid, and discuss vitamin and mineral supplementation (*Figure* 8-2 and *Drug Chart* 8-1).

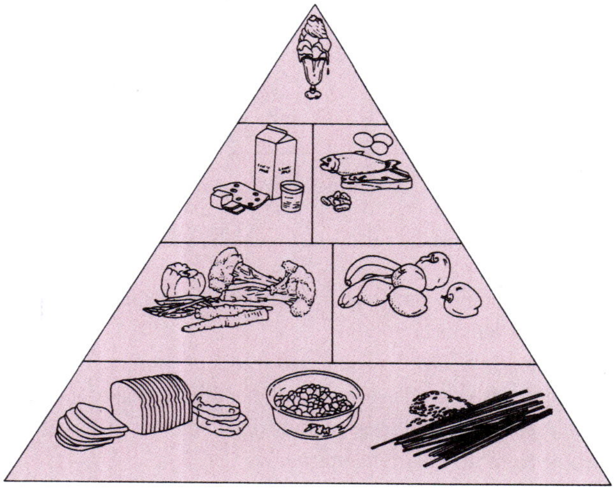

FIGURE 8-2
Food pyramid. In 1992, the United States Department of Agriculture (USDA) published recommended dietary guidelines. The USDA recommended daily servings from the basic food group of bread, cereal, rice, and pasta (10 or more servings); vegetables (3 to 5 servings); fruits (3 to 4 servings); milk, yogurt, and cheese (4 or more servings); meat poultry, fish, dry beans, eggs, and nuts (6 servings); and fats and sweets (sparingly). Some single-serving equivalents are 1 oz of breakfast cereal, 4 oz of cooked green beans, 2 oz of meat, 1 banana, and 8 oz of milk. During pregnancy, recommended daily servings may increase.

DRUG CHART 8-1

Prenatal vitamins

Classifications	Used to	Selected interventions
Prenatal multiple vitamins (contain both fat- and water-soluble vitamins, and an increased amount of folic acid and iron)	▪ Combat vitamin deficiency or supplement nutrition ▪ Prevent certain gestational defects (for example, a link has been found between neural tube defects and folic acid deficiency) ▪ Prevent maternal megaloblastic anemia	▪ Assess client for signs of a nutritional deficiency. ▪ Provide the client with information related to a nutritional diet. ▪ Explain the need for added vitamins during pregnancy and lactation. ▪ Help the client comply by identifying a routine time for taking the vitamin. ▪ Teach the client that side effects are rare. ▪ Caution client to keep medication out of reach of small children. Excessive folic acid and iron can cause poisoning in small children. ▪ Maternal overdose of vitamin C may cause withdrawal scurvy in the infant at birth.

(From Pilitteri, A. [2003]. *Maternal & Child Health Nursing*, 4th ed. Philadelphia: Lippincott Williams & Wilkins, pp. 288-289.)

b. Explain the importance of increasing fluid intake to prevent urinary tract infection and improve kidney function.

3. Provide client teaching about ways to relieve the common discomforts of pregnancy (see *Client and Family Teaching* 8-3, page 118).
4. Promote a positive psychosocial adjustment to pregnancy.
   a. Discuss sexual concerns with the client and partner, as appropriate; include reasons for altered libido (increased or decreased).
   b. Provide information concerning parenting, sibling, and grandparent classes.

G. Outcome evaluation

1. The woman exhibits no signs of complications, and fetal growth and development are normal.
2. Maternal weight gain, nutritional status, and fluid intake are within normal limits.
3. The woman reports increased comfort.
4. The woman and her partner demonstrate a positive psychosocial adjustment to pregnancy.

Study questions

1. Which of the following is an expected outcome of antepartum care?
1. Trimester-specific physiologic and psychosocial assessment
2. Increased expectant mother's and family's knowledge of pregnancy
3. Education and counseling for the pregnant woman and her family
4. Assessment of the client's previous experiences and cultural expectations

2. Which of the following would cause a false-positive result on a pregnancy test?
1. The test was performed less than 10 days after an abortion.
2. The test was performed too early or too late in the pregnancy.
3. The urine sample was stored too long at room temperature.
4. A spontaneous abortion or a missed abortion is impending.

3. Fetal heart rate (FHR) can be auscultated with a fetoscope as early as which of the following?
   1. 5 weeks' gestation
   2. 10 weeks' gestation
   3. 15 weeks' gestation
   4. 20 weeks' gestation

4. An ultrasound is typically performed during the third trimester for which of the following reasons?
   1. To evaluate the fetus for possible congenital anomalies
   2. To determine the fetal position and estimate fetal size
   3. To confirm the suspicion of possible multiple gestation
   4. To enhance prenatal testing and evaluation of pelvic mass

5. Quickening in primagravidas usually can be detected during which of the following weeks of gestation?
   1. 10 to 14 weeks
   2. 15 to 17 weeks
   3. 18 to 20 weeks
   4. 20 to 22 weeks

6. Which of the following best characterizes the contraction stress test (CST)?
   1. The fetus typically is monitored for at least 40 minutes; then the entire monitoring strip (or tracing) is analyzed.
   2. Any abnormal or nonreactive stress test results require further evaluation that same day.
   3. It is the least invasive test of fetal well-being that involves using an electronic fetal monitor.
   4. Three contractions within 10 minutes must be evaluated. Ideally, each contraction should last from 40 to 60 seconds.

7. A client's last menstrual period (LMP) began July 5. Her estimated date of delivery (EDD) should be which of the following?
   1. January 2
   2. March 28
   3. April 12
   4. October 12

8. Which of the following fundal heights indicates less than 12 weeks' gestation when the date of the last menstrual period (LMP) is unknown?
   1. Uterus in the pelvis
   2. Uterus at the xiphoid
   3. Uterus in the abdomen
   4. Uterus at the umbilicus

9. Which of the following danger signs should be reported promptly during the antepartum period?
   1. Constipation
   2. Breast tenderness
   3. Nasal stuffiness
   4. Leaking amniotic fluid

10. Which of the following prenatal laboratory test values would the nurse consider as significant?
    1. Hematocrit 33.5%
    2. Rubella titer less than 1:8
    3. White blood cells 8,000/mm^3
    4. One-hour glucose tolerance test 110 g/dl

11. A pregnant client at 26 weeks' gestation took a 1-hour glucose tolerance test as part of the recommended screening for gestational diabetes. The need for further testing is indicated by a result greater than or equal to how many mg/dl ?

Answer key

1. The answer is 2.
One of the expected outcomes of antepartum care is increased parental knowledge about pregnancy. Trimester-specific assessments, education, counseling, and assessment of previous experiences and cultural expectation are interventions associated with pregnancy.

2. The answer is 1.
A false-positive reaction can occur if the pregnancy test is performed less than 10 days after an abortion. Performing the tests too early or too late in the pregnancy, storing the urine sample too long at room temperature, or having a spontaneous or missed abortion impending can all produce false-negative results.

3. The answer is 4.
The FHR can be auscultated with a fetoscope at about 20 weeks' gestation. FHR usually is auscultated at the midline suprapubic region with a Doppler ultrasound transducer at 10 to 12 weeks' gestation. FHR cannot be heard any earlier than 10 weeks' gestation.

4. The answer is 2.
Ultrasound is typically performed during the third trimester to determine fetal position and estimate fetal size. During the second trimester, an ultrasound is performed to evaluate for congenital anomalies (such as hydrocephaly), assess fetal growth, guide procedures (such as amniocentesis and fetoscopy), assess placental location, and diagnose multiple gestation. During the first trimester, ultrasound may be done to assess gestational age, evaluate for congenital anomalies, obtain diagnostic evaluation of vaginal bleeding, confirm suspected multiple gestation, evaluate fetal growth, provide an adjunct to prenatal testing, such as amniocentesis or chorionic villus sampling, and provide diagnostic evaluation of pelvic mass or pain.

5. The answer is 3.
Quickening, typically described as a light fluttering feeling, can usually be detected between 18 and 20 weeks' gestation in primigravidas. However, in multigravidas, fetal movement can be detected as early as 16 weeks' gestation.

6. The answer is 4.
During the CST, three contractions within 10 minutes — ideally, each lasting 40 to 60 seconds — must be evaluated to assess fetal response to stress. A nonstress test, the least invasive test of fetal well-being using an electronic fetal monitor, is characterized by monitoring the fetus for at least 40 minutes, with the entire monitoring strip analyzed afterward and with any abnormal or nonreactive stress test results requiring further evaluation the same day.

7. The answer is 3.
To determine the EDD when the date of the client's LMP is known, use Nägele rule. To the first day of the LMP, add 7 days, subtract 3 months, and add 1 year (if applicable) to arrive at the EDD as follows: $5 + 7 = 12$; 7 (July) minus $3 = 4$ (April). Therefore, the client's EDD is April 12.

8. The answer is 1.
When the LMP is unknown, the gestational age of the fetus is estimated by uterine size or position (fundal height). The presence of the uterus in the pelvis indicates less than 12 weeks' gestation. At about 12 to 14 weeks, the fundus is out of the pelvis above the symphysis pubis. The fundus is at the level of the umbilicus at about 20 weeks' gestation and reaches the xiphoid at term, or 40 weeks.

9. The answer is 4.
Danger signs that require prompt reporting include leaking of amniotic fluid, vaginal bleeding, blurred vision, rapid weight gain, and elevated blood pressure. Constipation,

breast tenderness, and nasal stuffiness are common discomforts associated with pregnancy.

10. The answer is **2.**
A rubella titer should be 1:8 or greater. Thus, a finding of a titer less than 1:8 is significant, indicating that the client may not possess immunity to rubella. A hematocrit of 33.5%, a white blood cell count of 8,000/mm^3, and a 1-hour glucose tolerance test of 110 g/dl are within normal parameters.

11. The answer is **140.**
Screening for gestational diabetes using a 1-hour glucose tolerance test is recommended for all pregnant women between 24 and 28 weeks' gestation. An abnormal 1-hour glucose tolerance test is defined as a level of 140 mg/dl or greater. A 3-hour standard glucose tolerance test should be performed if results of the 1-hour test are abnormal.

9 Intrapartum Care

I. OVERVIEW

A. Intrapartum care

1. The intrapartum period extends from the beginning of contractions that cause cervical dilation to the first 1 to 4 hours after delivery of the newborn and placenta.
2. Intrapartum care refers to the medical and nursing care given to a pregnant woman and her family during labor and delivery.

B. Goals of intrapartum care

1. To promote physical and emotional well-being in the mother and fetus
2. To incorporate family-centered care concepts into the labor and delivery experience

C. National health goals.

Labor and birth are both high-risk periods for the mother and the fetus. Several national health goals speak to this risk. They are:

1. To reduce the number of maternal deaths to 3.3/100,000 live births from a baseline of 7.1/100,000
2. To reduce the number of fetal deaths at 20 or more weeks' gestation to 4.1/1,000 live births from a baseline of 6.8/1,000
3. To reduce fetal and infant deaths during the perinatal period (28 weeks' gestation to 7 days after birth) to 4.5/1,000 live births from a baseline of 7.5/1,000 live births (Department of Health and Human Services, 2000)

D. Factors affecting the intrapartum experience (See *Box* 9-1)

1. Previous experience with pregnancy
2. Cultural and personal expectations
3. Prepregnant health and biophysical preparedness for childbearing
4. Motivation for childbearing

BOX 9-1

Cultural competence in intrapartum care

Parameter	Cultural variation	Selected nursing intervention
Touch	Touch may or may not be acceptable in the laboring woman's culture	Determine early in the labor process whether therapeutic touch (back rub, effleurage) is an acceptable comfort measure.
Pain response	May be stoic and nonverbal; may scream or actively verbalize her discomfort, may moan softly; may thrash about	Assess facial expression, body posture and tension, activity level, and verbalization of pain to determine the level of discomfort.
Support person	May be husband, mother, sister, friend, other female family member, or doula	Respect the woman's choice of support person.
Language	May not speak or understand English	Provide an interpreter.
Placenta	May ask to have the placenta to take home; some cultures may bury it to ensure the child's health; some may cook and eat it to ensure the mother's health	Respect the client's request; observe standard precautions when supplying the mother with the placenta.

(Adapted from Pillitteri, A. [2003]. *Maternal & Child Health Nursing Care of the Childbearing & Childrearing Family,* 4th ed. Philadelphia: Lippincott Williams & Wilkins, Chapters 18 and 19.)

5. Socioeconomic readiness
6. Age of mother
7. Partnered versus unpartnered status
8. Extent of prenatal care
9. Extent of childbirth education

II. PHENOMENA AND PROCESSES OF LABOR AND DELIVERY

A. Onset of labor

1. Labor is the process by which the fetus and products of conception are expelled as the result of regular, progressive, frequent, and strong uterine contractions.
2. Theoretically, labor is thought to result from:
   a. Progesterone deprivation (*Table* 9-1)
   b. Oxytocin stimulation
   c. Fetal endocrine control
   d. Uterine decidua activation (release of a complex cascade of bioactive chemical agents into the amniotic fluid)

B. Factors affecting labor

1. **Passageway.** This refers to the adequacy of the pelvis and birth canal in allowing fetal descent; factors include:
   a. Type of pelvis (for example, gynecoid, android, anthropoid, or platypelloid)
   b. Structure of pelvis (for example, true versus false pelvis)
   c. Pelvic inlet diameters
   d. Pelvic outlet diameters
   e. Ability of the uterine segment to distend, the cervix to dilate, and the vaginal canal and introitus to distend
2. **Passenger.** This refers to the fetus and its ability to move through the passageway, which is based on the following:
   a. Size of the fetal head and capability of the head to mold to the passageway

TABLE 9-1
Possible causes of the onset of labor

Maternal factor theories	Fetal factor theories
▪ Uterine muscles stretch, causing release of prostaglandin. ▪ Pressure on the cervix stimulates nerve plexus, causing release of oxytocin by maternal posterior pituitary gland. This is known as the Ferguson reflex. ▪ Oxytocin stimulation in circulating blood increases slowly during pregnancy, rises dramatically during labor, and peaks during second stage. Oxytocin and prostaglandin work together to inhibit calcium binding in muscle cells, raising intracellular calcium and thus activating contractions. ▪ Estrogen/progesterone ratio shift—estrogen excites the uterine response, and progesterone quiets the uterine response. A decrease of progesterone allows estrogen to stimulate the contractile response of the uterus.	▪ Placental aging and deterioration triggers initiation of contractions. ▪ Fetal cortisol, produced by the fetal adrenal glands, rises and acts on the placenta to reduce progesterone formation and increase prostaglandin. ▪ Prostaglandin produced by fetal membranes (amnion and chorion) and the decidua stimulates contractions. When arachidonic acid stored in fetal membranes is released at term, it is converted to prostaglandin.

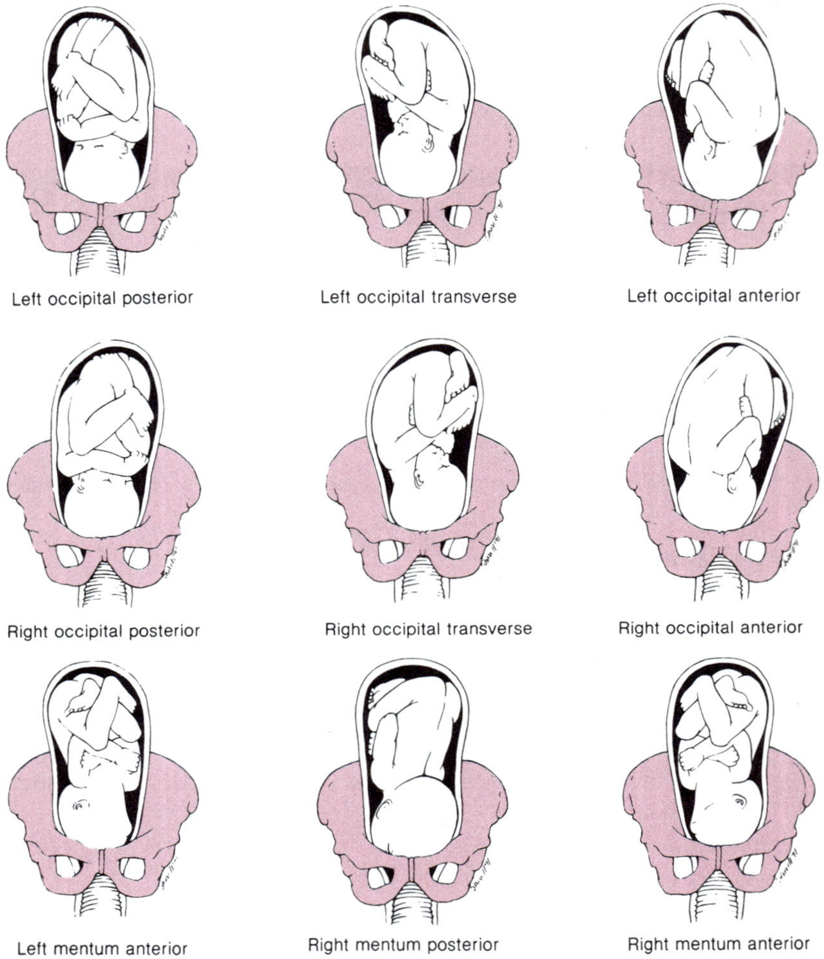

FIGURE 9-1
Fetal positions

b. Fetal presentation — the part of the fetus that enters the maternal pelvis first (for example, cephalic [vertex, face, brow]; breech [frank, single or double footling, complete]; or shoulder [transverse lie])

c. Fetal attitude — the relationship of fetal parts to one another

d. Fetal position — the relationship of a particular reference point of the presenting part and the maternal pelvis, described with a series of three letters (side of maternal pelvis [L, left; R, right; T, transverse], presenting part [O, occiput; S, sacrum; Sc, scapula; M, mentum], and part of the maternal pelvis [A, anterior; P, posterior]; *Figure* 9-1).

3. **Power.** This refers to the frequency, duration, and strength of uterine contractions to cause complete cervical effacement and dilation.
4. **Placental factors** refer to the site of placental insertion.
5. **Psyche** refers to the client's psychological state, available support systems, preparation for childbirth, experiences, and coping strategies.

C. Signs and symptoms of impending labor (premonitory signs)

1. **Lightening** is the descent of the fetus and uterus into the pelvic cavity 2 to 3 weeks before the onset of labor.
2. **Braxton Hicks contractions** are irregular, intermittent contractions that have occurred throughout the pregnancy, become uncomfortable, and produce a drawing pain in the abdomen and groin.
3. **Cervical changes** include softening, "ripening," and effacement of the cervix that will cause expulsion of the mucus plug (bloody show) and increased vaginal discharge
4. Rupture of amniotic membranes may occur before the onset of labor. If the woman suspects that her membranes have ruptured, she should contact her health care provider and go to the labor suite immediately so that she may be examined for prolapsed cord — a life-threatening condition for the fetus.
5. **Burst of energy or increased tension and fatigue** may occur right before the onset of labor.
6. **Weight loss** of about 1 to 3 pounds may occur 2 to 3 days before the onset of labor.
7. **Urinary frequency** returns.
8. **Backache**

D. Characteristics of true labor

1. Contractions occur at regular intervals (*Client and Family Teaching* 9-1).
2. Contractions start in the back and sweep around to the abdomen, increase in intensity and duration, and gradually have shortened intervals.
3. Walking intensifies contractions.
4. "Bloody show" (pink-tinged mucus released from the cervical canal as labor starts) is usually present.
5. Cervix becomes effaced and dilated.
6. Sedation does not stop contractions.

E. Characteristics of false labor

1. Contractions occur at irregular intervals.
2. Contractions are located chiefly in the abdomen, the intensity remains the same or is variable, and the intervals remain long.
3. Walking does not intensify contractions and often gives relief.
4. Bloody show usually is not present. If present, it is usually brownish rather than bright red and may be due to a recent pelvic examination or intercourse.

CLIENT AND FAMILY TEACHING 9–1

Comparison of false and true labor

False labor
- Contractions may be regular
- Decrease in frequency and intensity
- Longer intervals between contractions
- Discomfort in lower abdomen and groin
- Activity such as walking either has no effect or decreases contractions
- Contractions disappear while the woman is sleeping
- Sedation decreases or stops contractions
- Bloody show usually not present
- No appreciable change in the cervix

True labor
- Regular contractions
- Progressive frequency and intensity
- Shorter intervals between contractions
- Discomfort begins in back and radiates to the abdomen
- Activity such as walking increases contractions
- Contractions continue while the woman is sleeping
- Sedation does not stop contractions
- Bloody show usually present
- Progressive thinning and opening of the cervix

5. There are no cervical changes.
6. Sedation tends to decrease the number of contractions.

F. Stages of labor

1. The **first stage of labor** begins with the onset of regular contractions, which cause progressive cervical dilation and effacement. It ends when the cervix is completely effaced and dilated. It is composed of a latent, an active, and a transition phase.
   a. **Latent phase.** This phase begins with the onset of regular contractions, and effacement and dilation of the cervix to 3 to 4 cm. It lasts an average of 6.4 hours for nulliparas and 4.8 hours for multiparas. Contractions become increasingly stronger and more frequent.
   b. **Active phase.** Dilation continues from 3 to 4 cm to 7 cm. Contractions become stronger, more frequent, longer, and more painful.
   c. **Transition phase.** The culmination of the first stage is the transition phase during which the cervix dilates from 8 to 10 cm. The intensity, frequency, and duration of contractions peak, and there is an irresistible urge to push.
2. **Second stage (expulsive stage)**
   a. The second stage begins with complete dilation of the cervix and ends with delivery of the newborn. Duration may differ among primiparas (longer) and multiparas (shorter), but this stage should be completed within 1 hour after complete dilation.
   b. Contractions are severe at 2- to 3-minute intervals, with a duration of 50 to 90 seconds.
   c. The newborn exits the birth canal with help from the following cardinal movements, or mechanisms, of labor (*Figure* 9-2).
      - Descent
      - Flexion
      - Internal rotation
      - Extension
      - External rotation (restitution)
      - Expulsion
   d. "Crowning" occurs when the newborn's head or presenting part appears at the vaginal opening.
   e. Episiotomy (surgical incision in perineum) may be done to facilitate delivery and avoid laceration of the perineum.
3. **Third stage (placental stage)**
   a. This stage begins with delivery of the newborn and ends with delivery of the placenta. It occurs in two phases — placental separation and placental expulsion.
   b. Signs of placental separation include the uterus becoming globular, the fundus rising in the abdomen, lengthening of the cord, and increased bleeding (trickle or gush).
   c. Contraction of the uterus controls uterine bleeding and aids with placental separation and expulsion.
   d. Generally, oxytocic drugs are administered to help the uterus contract.
4. **Fourth stage (recovery and bonding)**
   a. This stage lasts from 1 to 4 hours after birth.
   b. The mother and newborn recover from the physical process of birth.

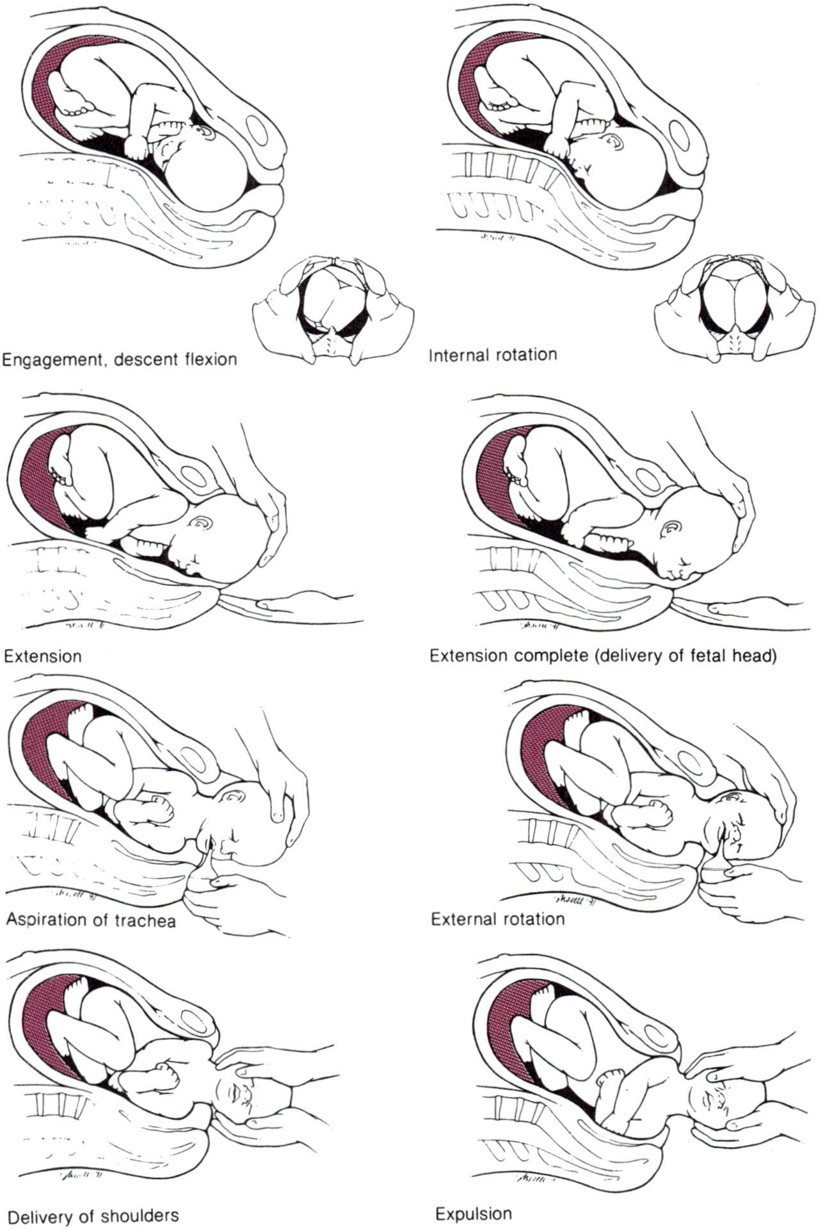

FIGURE 9-2
Cardinal movements of labor

c. The maternal organs undergo initial readjustment to the nonpregnant state.

d. The newborn body systems begin to adjust to extrauterine life and stabilize.

e. The uterus contracts in the midline of the abdomen with the fundus midway between the umbilicus and symphysis pubis.

III. INTRAPARTUM PAIN EXPERIENCE

A. Overview of pain

1. Intrapartum pain is a subjective experience of physical sensations associated with uterine contractions, cervical dilation and effacement, and fetal descent during labor and birth.
2. Physiologic responses to pain may include increased blood pressure, pulse, respirations, perspiration, pupil diameter, muscle tension (such as facial tension or fisted hands) or muscle activity (such as pacing, turning, or twisting).
3. Nonverbal expressions of pain may include withdrawal, hostility, fear, or depression.
4. Verbal expressions of pain may include statements of pain, moaning, and groaning.

B. Factors affecting perception of intrapartum pain

1. Previous experience with painful stimuli and personal expectations of the birth experience
2. Cultural concept of pain, specifically during childbirth, and how one should respond
3. Rapidly progressive uterine contractions
4. Fear, anxiety, and fatigue

C. Physiologic causes of intrapartum pain

1. Uterine anoxia due to compressed muscle cells during the contraction.
2. Compression of the nerve ganglia in the cervix and lower uterine segment during the contraction
3. Stretching of the cervix during dilation and effacement
4. Traction on, and stretching and displacement of the perineum
5. Pressure on the urethra, bladder, and rectum during fetal descent
6. Distention of the lower uterine segment
7. Stretching of the uterine ligaments

IV. INTRAPARTUM PAIN MANAGEMENT

A. Overview

1. The two goals of intrapartum pain management are:
   a. To provide maximal relief of pain with maximal safety for the mother and fetus
   b. To facilitate labor and delivery as a positive family experience
2. Pain relief may be achieved by using prepared childbirth methods (such as Lamaze), analgesics, or regional anesthetics.
3. Intervention for pain relief during labor depends on the following factors:
   a. Gestational age of the fetus
   b. Frequency, duration, and intensity of the contractions
   c. Labor progress
   d. Maternal response to pain and labor
   e. Allergies and sensitivities to analgesics and anesthetics

B. Nonpharmacologic pain management

1. Prepared childbirth methods can help the client feel more in control and relaxed, helping her "work with" the contractions; it may shorten labor.
2. Hypnosis may be useful in some clients.

3. Interventions aimed at supporting the client during labor may be helpful. These include:
   a. Providing information about the progress of labor
   b. Reinforcing techniques learned in prepared childbirth classes
   c. Directing breathing methods, abdominal lifting, pushing, relieving external pressure, distraction, cutaneous stimulation, and relaxation

C. Pharmacologic pain management

1. **Narcotic analgesics** provide effective pain relief and slight sedation (*Drug Chart* 9-1, page 134).
   a. Narcotic analgesics are systemic drugs that readily cross the placental barrier, with depressive effects on the neonate occurring 2 to 3 hours after intramuscular injection.
   b. Maternal side effects include nausea, vomiting, mild respiratory depression, and transient mental impairment.
   c. Fetal effects are reduced fetal heart rate (FHR) and decreased variability; neonatal effects are lowered Apgar score and respiratory depression.
   d. Opioid antagonists (such as naloxone [Narcan]) must be readily available in case of respiratory depression in the mother or newborn.
   e. The decision to administer a narcotic analgesic is based on the results of a vaginal examination; if birth is anticipated within 2 to 3 hours, the risk of neonatal narcosis may preclude the use of analgesics.
   f. The dosage is kept to the smallest effective dose.
2. **Barbiturates**
   a. These drugs cause maternal sedation and relaxation (see *Drug Chart* 9-1).
   b. Maternal side effects of barbiturates include nausea, vomiting, hypotension, restlessness, and vertigo.
   c. Neonatal side effects of barbiturates include central nervous system depression, prolonged drowsiness, and delayed establishment of feeding (for example, due to a poor sucking reflex or a poor sucking pressure).
   d. The rapid transfer of barbiturates across the placental barrier and the lack of an antagonist to counteract their effects make them generally inappropriate during active labor.
3. **Tranquilizers**
   a. These drugs decrease the anxiety and apprehension associated with pain and sometimes relieve the nausea associated with narcotic analgesics (see *Drug Chart* 9-1).
   b. Tranquilizers potentiate active sedative and analgesic effects, decreasing the dosage of analgesic and sedative drugs needed to produce the desired effect.
   c. Maternal side effects associated with tranquilizers include hypotension (which, in turn, decreases fetoplacental circulation), drowsiness, and dizziness.
   d. Fetal effects associated with tranquilizers include tachycardia and the loss of normal beat-to-beat variability on electronic fetal heart monitoring.
   e. Newborn effects associated with tranquilizers include hypotonia, hypothermia, generalized drowsiness, and a reluctance to feed for the first few days.
4. **Regional anesthesia (conduction anesthesia)**
   a. Types of regional anesthesia include spinal, epidural, paracervical, and pudendal blocks, and local infiltration (*Drug Chart* 9-2, page 135).
   b. These blocks provide pain relief with injected anesthetic agents at sensory nerve pathways.
   c. Adverse reactions may include maternal hypotension, allergic or toxic reaction, respiratory paralysis, and partial or total anesthetic failure.

DRUG CHART 9-1

Medications used for pain management during labor

Classifications	Uses	Selected interventions
Barbiturates secobarbital sodium (Seconal) pentobarbital (Nembutal)	▪ These drugs do not relieve pain. ▪ They are used to induce sleep, decrease anxiety, allow for rest, and inhibit uterine contractions.	▪ Sedatives should be given in early labor, when the birth is unlikely to occur within 12 to 24 hours. ▪ Sedatives may be given orally or by I.M. injection. ▪ These drugs may have an effect on neonatal CNS, causing decreased responsiveness and ability to suck.
Tranquilizers promethazine HCL (Phenergan) hydroxyzine HCL (Vistaril) propiomazine (Largon)	▪ These drugs decrease nausea and vomiting, relieve anxiety, and increase sedation.	▪ Tranquilizers are usually given in combination with a narcotic. ▪ Hydroxyzine is limited to I.M. injection. ▪ Promethazine may cause respiratory depression. ▪ These drugs are thought to potentiate the effects of narcotics, have a sedative effect on mother, do not appear to increase neonatal depression, and may cause respiratory depression in the mother.
Opioid analgesics meperidine (Demerol) morphine fentanyl	▪ These drugs do not eliminate pain. ▪ They decrease the perception of pain and allow for rest and relaxation between contractions.	▪ Opioids are the category of drugs most commonly administered parenterally during labor. ▪ Opioids should be given only after a labor pattern is established. ▪ Coaching is important to help the woman recognize the start of the contraction. ▪ Opioids may be administered every 3 to 4 hours by the I.V. or I.M. routes. ▪ Give I.V. slowly during a contraction to decrease transfer of the medication to the fetus. ▪ These drugs may decrease the frequency and duration of uterine contractions and may result in decreased fetal heart rate variability. In the newborn, respiratory depression, ineffective suck, abnormal reflexes, and decreased muscle tone may occur and last for several days.
Agonist/Antagonist nalbuphine (Nubain) butorphanol (Stadol) pentazocine (Talwin)	▪ These drugs block receptors responsible for respiratory depression, stimulate receptors that block painful sensations, and decrease maternal nausea and vomiting. ▪ They may be administered with local infiltration anesthesia.	▪ Monitor for the following side effects: CNS depression in the mother (drowsiness, dizziness, headache, orthostatic hypotension); respiratory depression in the mother; respiratory depression in the newborn; and other effects in the newborn (which are related to timing, amount, and route of dose before birth).
Opioid antagonist naloxone HCL (Narcan)	▪ These drugs reverse CNS depression and respiratory depression as a result of opioid administration.	▪ Administer dilute solution of Narcan (0.4 mg/10 ml) at a rate of 0.5 ml by direct I.V. push every 2 minutes. ▪ Give slowly to avoid seizures and severe pain. ▪ This drug crosses the placenta and antagonizes postoperative analgesia.

d. Nursing responsibilities during administration of regional anesthesia include:
- Assisting the anesthesiologist as requested
- Establishing a reliable intravenous line

DRUG CHART 9-2

Anesthetics used in labor and birth

Type	Drug	Usual dosage and route	Effect on mother	Effect on labor progress	Effect on fetus or newborn
Lumbar epidural block	**Local anesthestic** Bupivacaine (Marcaine) Ropivacaine (Naropin)	Administered for first stage of labor; with continuous block, anesthesia will last through delivery; injected at L3-4; fentanyl or morphine possibly added	Rapid onset (in minutes); lasting 60 to 90 minutes; loss of pain perception for labor contractions and delivery; possible maternal hypotension	Slowing of labor if given early; pushing feeling obliterated, resulting in possible prolonged second stage	May be some differences in response in first few days of life
Pudendal block	**Local anesthestic** Lidocaine (Xylocaine)	Administered just before delivery for perineal anesthesia; injected through vagina	Rapid anesthesia of perineum	None apparent	None apparent
Local infiltration of perineum	**Local anesthestic** Lidocaine (Xylocaine)	Injected just before the episiotomy incision	Anesthesia of perineum almost immediate	None apparent	None apparent
General intravenous anesthetic	**Thiopental**	Administered I.V. by anesthesiologist or nurse-anesthetist	Rapid anesthesia; also rapid recovery	Forceps required because abdominal pushing is no longer possible	Results in infant being born with CNS depression

(Adapted from Karch, AM [2004], *Lippincott's Nursing Drug Guide.* Philadelphia: Lippincott Williams & Wilkins.)

- Being prepared with medications and equipment for emergency situations if they arise

5. **General anesthesia** (inhalant [such as nitrous oxide and halothane] and intravenous [such as Pentothal]) usually is used during childbirth only if an emergency cesarean birth becomes necessary.

NURSING PROCESS OVERVIEW

V. FIRST AND SECOND STAGES OF LABOR

A. Maternal assessment

1. A complete **health history** should include:
   a. Name
   b. Age
   c. Physician
   d. Weight
   e. Allergies
   f. Blood type and Rh factor
   g. Previous medical conditions

h. Prenatal problems
i. Gravida and para status
j. Estimated date of delivery
k. Prenatal education
l. Method of newborn feeding

2. Screening for **risk factors** is essential and should include:
   a. Bleeding
   b. Premature rupture of membranes (if ruptured, determine time of rupture and note color and odor, if any)
   c. Hydramnios
   d. Abnormal presentation
   e. Multiple gestation
   f. Prolapsed cord
   g. Precipitous labor
   h. Meconium-stained amniotic fluid
   i. Fetal heart irregularities
   j. Postmaturity
3. **Physical assessment**
   a. Maternal vital signs, weight, and cardiac and respiratory status are monitored. The frequency of maternal vital signs and respiratory status assessment is as follows:
   - First stage latent. Blood pressure (BP), pulse, and respirations are assessed every hour (if the BP is greater than 140/90 or if the pulse is greater than 100, contact the primary care provider). Temperature is assessed every 4 hours (every 2 hours if the membranes are ruptured).
   - First stage active. BP, pulse and respirations are assessed every hour.
   - First stage transition. BP, pulse, and respirations are assessed every 30 minutes.
   - Second stage. BP and pulse are assessed every 5 to 15 minutes.

   b. Fundal height is measured.
   c. Status of labor (that is, contractions [onset, frequency, duration, and intensity], membranes, bleeding, cervical dilation, and fetal descent) is determined.
   ***d.* The client's need for comfort, analgesia, or anesthesia is assessed continuously (see sections III and IV).**
4. **Psychosocial assessment** should include anxiety, childbirth education, support systems, and the client's response to labor.
5. **Labor progress** assessment should include:
   a. Palpation or electronic monitoring (external with tocodynamometer and internal with intrauterine pressure catheter) is performed to assess the duration, frequency, and intensity of contractions. The frequency of contraction assessment is as follows.
   - First stage latent — every 30 minutes
   - First stage active — every 15 to 30 minutes
   - First stage transition — every 15 minutes
   - Second stage — each contraction

   b. Sterile vaginal examination is performed to assess cervical dilation (opening of external os from closed to 10 cm) and cervical effacement (thinning and shortening of the cervix, as measured from 0% [thick] to 100% [paper thin] effaced).
   c. Station is determined (that is, the relationship of the presenting part to the pelvic ischial spines).

B. Fetal assessment

1. Inspect the maternal abdomen to determine **fetal lie** — the relationship of the long axis (spine) of the fetus to the long axis of the mother. Fetal lie can be longitudinal or transverse.
   a. Longitudinal lie is when the long axis of the fetus is parallel to the long axis of the mother.
   b. Transverse lie is when the long axis of the fetus is perpendicular to the long axis of the mother.
2. Palpate the abdomen using the four Leopold maneuvers to determine **fetal position** and **possible size.**
3. Monitor **fetal status**
   a. Auscultate the FHR every 30 minutes during first stage latent; every 15 minutes during first stage active and first stage transition; and every 5 to 15 minutes during the second stage.
   - The normal range is between 120 and 160 beats per minute.
   - FHR decreases during contractions but returns to normal after 10 to 15 seconds.

   b. Assess changes in FHR to identify the following.
   - Early deceleration — slowing of the FHR early in the contraction. It is considered benign, mirrors the contraction, and is indicative of head compression.
   - Late deceleration — an indication of fetal hypoxia due to uteroplacental insufficiency. It usually begins at the peak of the contraction and ends after the contraction ends.
   - Variable deceleration — a transient decrease in FHR before, during, or after the contraction. It indicates cord compression and has a characteristic V or U pattern.
   - Bradycardia — an FHR less than 100 beats per minute or a drop of 20 beats per minute below baseline. It indicates cord compression or placental separation.
   - Tachycardia — an FHR greater than 160 beats per minute. It indicates fetal distress if it persists for more than 1 hour or is accompanied by late deceleration.
   - Loss of beat-to-beat variability — indicates fetal reaction to maternal drugs, fetal sleep, or fetal demise.

   c. Assess fetal acid-base status with fetal blood sampling or fetal scalp stimulation.
4. Continually assess the fetal response to the pain-relief methods used.

C. Nursing diagnoses

1. Health-Seeking Behaviors
2. Anxiety
3. Ineffective Individual Coping
4. Pain
5. Risk for Injury
6. Risk for Ineffective Airway Clearance (Newborn)
7. Risk for Hypoxia (Newborn)
8. Risk for Altered Parenting

D. Planning and outcome identification

1. The woman will be properly admitted to the labor and delivery unit.
2. The woman and her partner will understand normal labor process and progress.
3. The woman and her partner will implement good coaching, breathing, and other relaxation measures.
4. The mother will receive physical, emotional, and pharmacologic support as needed.
5. The woman will experience maximum safety.

6. The woman will be prepared for the birth of her child.
7. The newborn will receive essential immediate care.
8. The newborn and parents will experience early contact.

E. Implementation

1. **Perform admission procedures.**
   a. Collect urine specimen and other samples for laboratory testing as prescribed (such as hemoglobin, hematocrit, serologic test for syphilis, and type and crossmatch, if indicated).
   b. Perform perineal preparation and enema, if indicated.
   c. Notify attending physician or midwife, and report status.
   d. Obtain informed consent from the client.
2. **Provide client and family teaching throughout the first and second stages.**
   a. Explain how activity, toileting, and hydration needs will be met during labor.
   b. Explain equipment that will be used to monitor vital signs, labor, and fetal status.
   c. Explain the normal process and progress of labor and delivery to the woman and her support person.
   d. Explain to the woman that as the fetus descends in the birth canal, she will feel increased rectal pressure or the urge to push.
   e. Coach the woman regarding effective pushing effort. Explain the importance of assuming a position that facilitates expulsive efforts, maintains placental perfusion, and prevents or alleviates cord compression.
3. **Reinforce coaching, breathing, and other relaxation measures.**
4. **Provide physical, emotional, and pharmacologic support as needed throughout the first and second stages.**
   a. Provide pleasant, comfortable surroundings.
   b. Collaborate with the client and birth attendant to determine the most effective method of pain relief during each stage of the intrapartum period.
   c. Provide pharmacologic support as prescribed (see *Drug Chart* 9-1, page 134).
   d. Provide support during contractions by coaching breathing, giving back rubs, and offering cool cloths.
   e. Assist the client with pushing as indicated.
5. **Promote safety during the first and second stages of labor.**
   a. If the client's membranes are ruptured and the fetal head is not engaged, position the mother to prevent cord prolapse.
   b. Assess hydration status to avoid dehydration.
   c. Offer the client an opportunity to void every 1 to 2 hours to prevent trauma to the bladder during pushing and birth of the newborn.
   d. Interpret changes in the electronic fetal and maternal monitor strip, and take appropriate action.
6. **Prepare for the birth of the newborn.**
   a. Prepare for delivery when the perineal area is bulging in a primipara and when the cervix is dilated 7 to 8 cm in a multipara.
   b. Prepare the delivery area with equipment and supplies.
   c. Place the client in the birthing position.
   d. Assist the attending physician or nurse midwife with the birth; help the support person to be supportive, and check all vital signs and FHR.
7. **Implement immediate newborn care.**
   a. Establish and maintain a patent airway; suction with a bulb syringe or a DeLee mucus trap, and place the newborn on his side.

b. Compensate for poor newborn thermoregulation.
- Dry the newborn immediately with a warm blanket.
- Place the newborn under a radiant warmer.
- Wrap the newborn in a warmed, dry blanket or place the newborn on the mother's skin.

c. Determine the Apgar score at 1 and 5 minutes after delivery (*Table* 9-2).
d. Inspect the umbilical cord for two arteries and one vein.
e. Weigh and measure the newborn as his condition stabilizes.
f. Footprint the newborn, and fingerprint the mother.
g. Record the newborn's first voiding and stool passage.
h. Assess the newborn's gestational age.
i. Administer prophylactic eye medication to protect the conjunctivae from infection.
j. Administer vitamin K (phytonadione [AquaMEPHYTON]), if prescribed.

8. **Encourage initial parent-newborn bonding** by placing the newborn in the mother's arms with skin-to-skin contact.

F. Outcome evaluation

1. The woman is properly admitted to the labor and delivery unit.
2. The woman and her partner use their knowledge of normal labor process and progress.
3. The woman and her partner implement good coaching, breathing, and other relaxation measures.
4. The mother receives physical, emotional, and pharmacologic support as needed and verbalizes increased comfort.
5. The woman experiences maximum safety, and there are no complications.
6. The woman is prepared for the birth of her child.

TABLE 9-2
Apgar scoring chart*

	Score		
Sign	**0**	**1**	**2**
Heart rate	Absent	Slow (<100)	Normal (>100)
Respiratory effort	Absent	Slow, iregular weak cry	Good, strong cry
Muscle tone	Flaccid	Some flexion of extremitites	Well flexed
Reflex irritability			
Response to catheter in nostril	No response	Grimace	Cough or sneeze
Slap to sole of foot; withdrawal of foot	No response	Grimace	Cry and withdrawal of foot
Color	Blue, pale	Body pink, extremities blue	Completely pink

*The nurse and other members of the health care team use the Apgar score to measure the newborn's immediate adjustment to extrauterine life. Scores are assigned at 1 minute and again at 5 minutes after birth. Each sign is assigned a value. A score from 7–10 indicates that the newborn is doing well. A score of 4 or less indicates that the newborn may need assistance.

(From Apgar V. et al. (1958). *Evaluation of the newborn infant: Second report.* Journal of the American Medical Association, 168, 1985. Copyright 1958. American Medical Association; with permission.)

7. The newborn receives essential immediate care.
8. Parents hold and explore their infant.

NURSING PROCESS OVERVIEW

VI. THIRD AND FOURTH STAGES OF LABOR

A. Assessment **during the third and fourth stages focuses on the following:**

1. Maternal physiologic adjustment, including vital signs, bladder, uterine firmness, uterine fundus, perineum, and amount and color of lochia
2. Maternal emotional adjustment
3. Newborn physiologic adjustment, including respiratory effort and maintenance of body temperature
4. Signs of parent-newborn attachment
5. Mother's and newborn's breast-feeding attempts, if the mother is breast-feeding

B. Nursing diagnoses

1. Risk for Injury (Mother)
2. Ineffective Thermoregulation (Newborn)
3. Risk for Infection
4. Pain
5. Ineffective Breast-Feeding
6. Altered Family Coping

C. Planning and outcome identification

1. Physiologic adaptation will be achieved by the new mother.
2. Physiologic adaptation will be achieved by the newborn.
3. Potential complications will be detected.
4. Comfort measures will be provided as needed.
5. An opportunity to breast-feed will be provided.
6. A parent-newborn relationship and family integration will be established.
7. Accurate documentation of intrapartum care will be maintained.

D. Implementation

1. **Promote maternal physiologic adaptation.**
   - *a.* Initiate fundal massage gently, with adequate support to the lower uterine segment.
   - *b.* Evaluate vaginal bleeding and vital signs.
2. **Promote newborn physiologic adaptation.**
   - *a.* Suction secretions from the newborn's nose and mouth as necessary to maintain respirations.
   - *b.* Maintain the newborn's temperature by placing him in skin-to-skin contact with mother, covering him with warm blankets, or using a radiant warmer.
3. **Monitor the mother and newborn for potential complications.**
   - *a.* Observe mother for signs of hemorrhage and infection.
   - *b.* Observe infant for signs of respiratory distress, difficulty maintaining body temperature, and infection.

4. **Provide comfort measures.**
   a. Provide comfort measures for afterpains or perineal discomfort (such as analgesics, ice packs, and an opportunity to void).
   b. Place a warm blanket over the mother and newborn.
   c. Offer the mother warm liquids of her choice.
5. **Assist mother to breast-feed her newborn if she is breast-feeding.**
6. **Encourage parent-newborn attachment and family integration.**
   a. Place the newborn on the mother's abdomen, and encourage parents to touch the newborn.
   b. Promote family integration, when the parents are ready, by inviting siblings and other family members into the room.
   c. Help younger siblings to see and hold the newborn, when possible. (Toddlers are usually more interested in their mother than in the newborn.)
7. **Document intrapartum care; for example:**
   a. Time of delivery of newborn and placenta
   b. 1- and 5-minute Apgar scores
   c. Any immediate neonatal care provided
   d. Extent and repair of perineal lacerations or episiotomy
   e. Estimated maternal blood loss
   f. Medications administered before, during, and after delivery (to mother and neonate)
   g. Placement of identification bands, footprinting, and fingerprinting
   h. Maternal and newborn vital signs
   i. Neonatal care given
   j. Maternal or newborn voiding or bowel elimination
   k. Maternal and newborn breast-feeding attempts and responses
   l. Newborn's condition when transferred to the nursery
   m. Maternal condition when transferred to the postpartum unit

E. Outcome evaluation

1. Maternal physiologic adaptation is achieved.
   a. Maternal bleeding is within normal limits with firm uterine tone and normal maternal vital signs.
   b. The new mother verbalizes comfort with fundal massage.
2. Newborn physiologic adaptation is achieved. The newborn maintains normal respirations and body temperature.
3. Complications in the mother and newborn, if any, are promptly identified, and appropriate actions are taken.
4. The mother states that she is comfortable.
5. Mother states she was ready to breast-feed and that it was a positive experience.
6. Parent-newborn attachment, and family integration, is initiated.
   a. Parents and newborn begin interaction by face-to-face gazing and parental exploration of the newborn.
   b. Other family members visit the newborn.
7. Documentation of intrapartum care is accurate and complete.

Study questions

1. Which of the following best defines the intrapartum period?
1. Time from complete cervical dilation through delivery of the newborn
2. Period from the onset of contractions through complete cervical dilation
3. Period from the onset of contractions to the first 1 to 4 hours after delivery
4. Time from the 28th week of gestation through 28 days after birth of the newborn

2. Which of the following factors affecting labor is associated with the passageway?
1. Size of the fetal head and its ability to mold to the maternal pelvis
2. The presentation of the fetus in relation to the maternal pelvis
3. The structure of the maternal pelvis (for example, gynecoid versus android)
4. The frequency, duration, and strength of uterine contractions

3. Which of the following is an essential intrapartum fetal assessment?
1. Determination of the duration, frequency, and intensity of the contractions
2. Inspection of the maternal abdomen to determine fetal lie
3. Examination of the vagina to assess cervical dilation and effacement
4. Evaluation of the mother to determine knowledge about childbirth education

4. When describing fetal position, the first letter in the series denotes which of the following?
1. Presenting part of the fetus
2. Side of the maternal pelvis
3. Size of the maternal pelvis
4. Type of fetal delivery

5. Which of the following characteristics of contractions would the nurse expect to find in a client experiencing true labor?
1. Occurring at irregular intervals
2. Starting mainly in the abdomen
3. Gradually increasing intervals
4. Increasing intensity with walking

6. During which of the following stages of labor would the nurse assess "crowning"?
1. First stage
2. Second stage
3. Third stage
4. Fourth stage

7. Barbiturates are usually not given for pain relief during active labor for which of the following reasons?
1. The neonatal effects include hypotonia, hypothermia, generalized drowsiness, and reluctance to feed for the first few days.
2. These drugs readily cross the placental barrier, causing depressive effects in the newborn 2 to 3 hours after intramuscular injection.
3. They rapidly transfer across the placenta, and lack of an antagonist make them generally inappropriate during labor.
4. Adverse reactions may include maternal hypotension, allergic or toxic reaction, or partial or total respiratory failure.

8. Which of the following nursing interventions would the nurse perform during the third stage of labor?
1. Obtain a urine specimen and other laboratory tests.
2. Assess uterine contractions every 30 minutes.
3. Coach for effective client pushing.
4. Promote parent-newborn interaction.

9. Which of the following actions demonstrates the nurse's understanding about the newborn's thermoregulatory ability?
1. Placing the newborn under a radiant warmer
2. Suctioning with a bulb syringe

3. Obtaining an Apgar score
4. Inspecting the newborn's umbilical cord

10. Immediately before expulsion, which of the following cardinal movements occur?
1. Descent
2. Flexion
3. Extension
4. External rotation

11. The nurse is evaluating a client who is 34 weeks pregnant for spontaneous rupture of the membranes (SROM). Which findings indicate that SROM has occurred? Select all that apply:
1. Fernlike pattern when vaginal fluid is placed on a glass slide and allowed to dry
2. Acidic pH of fluid when tested with nitrazine paper
3. Presence of amniotic fluid in the vagina
4. Cervical dilation of 6 cm
5. Alkaline pH of fluid when tested with nitrazine paper
6. Contractions occurring every 5 minutes

Answer key

1. The answer is **3.**
The intrapartum period is defined as the time frame from the beginning of contractions to the first 1 to 4 hours after delivery of the newborn and placenta. The second stage of labor begins with complete cervical dilation and ends with the delivery of the newborn. The first stage of labor begins with the onset of contractions and ends when the cervix is completely dilated and effaced. The perinatal period refers to the time from the 28th week of gestation through the first 28 days after the birth of the newborn.

2. The answer is **3.**
The passageway refers to the pelvis and birth canal. Factors associated with the passageway include the structure and type of pelvis, pelvic diameters, and ability of the uterine segment, vaginal canal, and introitus to distend and the cervix to dilate. Size of the fetal head, ability to mold, and fetal presentation are factors associated with the passenger. The frequency, duration, and strength of uterine contractions are associated with the power.

3. The answer is **2.**
An essential fetal assessment is inspection of the maternal abdomen to determine fetal lie — the relationship of the long axis (spine) of the fetus to the long axis of the mother. Other fetal assessments include abdominal palpation to determine fetal position and possible size and auscultation of fetal heart rate. Determining the characteristics of contractions, vaginal examination to assess cervical dilation and effacement, and assessment of the mother's knowledge about childbirth education are assessments of maternal status.

4. The answer is **2.**
Fetal position, the relationship of a particular reference point of the presenting part and the maternal pelvis, is described by a series of three letters. The first letter denotes the side of the maternal pelvis, such as right, left, or transverse. The second letter denotes the presenting part, such as occiput, sacrum, or mentum. The third letter denotes the part of the maternal pelvis, such as anterior or posterior. Neither the size of the maternal pelvis or the type of fetal delivery is denoted by these three letters.

5. The answer is **4.**
With true labor, contractions increase in intensity with walking. In addition, true labor contractions occur at regular intervals, usually starting in the back and sweeping around to the abdomen. The interval of true labor contractions gradually shortens.

6. The answer is **2.**
Crowning, which occurs when the newborn's head or presenting part appears at the vaginal opening, occurs during the second stage of labor. During the first stage of labor, cervical dilation and effacement occur. During the third stage of labor, the newborn and placenta are delivered. The fourth stage of labor lasts from 1 to 4 hours after birth, during which time the mother and newborn recover from the physical process of birth and the mother's organs undergo the initial readjustment to the nonpregnant state.

7. The answer is **3.**
Barbiturates are rapidly transferred across the placental barrier, and lack of an antagonist makes them generally inappropriate during active labor. Neonatal side effects of barbiturates include central nervous system depression, prolonged drowsiness, delayed establishment of feeding (possibly due to poor sucking reflex or poor sucking pressure). Tranquilizers are associated with neonatal effects such as hypotonia, hypothermia, generalized drowsiness, and reluctance to feed for the first few days. Narcotic analgesics readily cross the placental barrier, causing depressive effects in the newborn 2 to 3 hours after intramuscular injection. Regional anesthesia is associated with such adverse reactions as maternal hypotension, allergic or toxic reaction, or partial or total respiratory failure.

8. The answer is **4.**
During the third stage of labor, which begins with the delivery of the newborn, the nurse would promote parent-newborn interaction by placing the newborn on the mother's abdomen and encouraging the parents to touch the newborn. Collecting a urine specimen and other laboratory tests are done on admission during the first stage of labor. Assessing uterine contractions every 30 minutes is performed during the latent phase of the first stage of labor. Coaching the client to push effectively is appropriate during the second stage of labor.

9. The answer is **1.**
The newborn's ability to regulate body temperature is poor. Therefore, placing the newborn under a radiant warmer aids in maintaining his body temperature. Suctioning with a bulb syringe helps maintain a patent airway. Obtaining an Apgar score measures the newborn's immediate adjustment to extrauterine life. Inspecting the umbilical cord aids in detecting cord anomalies.

10. The answer is **4.**
Immediately before expulsion or birth of the rest of the body, the cardinal movement of external rotation occurs. Descent, flexion, internal rotation, extension, and restitution (in this order) occur before external rotation.

11. The answers are **1, 3, 5.**
The fernlike pattern that occurs when vaginal fluid is placed on a glass slide and allowed to dry, the presence of amniotic fluid in the vagina, and an alkaline pH of fluid are all signs of ruptured membranes. The fernlike pattern seen when fluid is allowed to dry on a glass slide is the result of the high sodium and protein content of amniotic fluid. The presence of amniotic fluid in the vagina results from the expulsion of fluid from the amniotic sac. Cervical dilation and regular contractions are signs of progressing labor but do not indicate SROM.

10 Postpartum Care

I. OVERVIEW

A. Essential concepts

1. Postpartum care refers to the medical and nursing care given to a woman during the puerperium, which is the 6-week period after delivery, beginning with termination of labor and ending with the return of the reproductive organs to the nonpregnant state.
2. This period constitutes a physical and psychological adjustment to the process of childbearing and is sometimes referred to as the fourth trimester of pregnancy.
3. During this period, the uterus undergoes involution — the progressive changes in the uterus after delivery, leading to its return to near-prepregnant size and condition.
4. One aspect of postpartum care that commonly suffers with the trend toward earlier discharge is support in breast-feeding.

B. Goals of postpartum care

1. Promote normal uterine involution and return to the nonpregnant state.
2. Prevent or minimize postpartum complications.
3. Promote comfort and healing of pelvic, perianal, and perineal tissues.
4. Assist in restoration of normal body functions.
5. Increase understanding of physiologic and psychological changes.
6. Facilitate newborn care and self-care by the new mother.
7. Promote the newborn's successful integration into the family unit.
8. Support parenting skills and parent-newborn attachment.
9. Provide effective discharge planning, including appropriate referral for home care follow-up. (*Client and Family Teaching* 10-1 lists postpartum warning signs and symptoms to report to the physician.)

C. National health goals.

The first hour postpartum is an extremely dangerous one because of the possibility of hemorrhage. It is also the optimum time for breast-feeding. National health goals for this time period include:

1. Reduce the maternal mortality rate to 3.3/100,000 live births from a baseline of 7.1/100,000.
2. Reduce the proportion of births occurring within 24 months of a previous birth to 6% from a baseline of 11%
3. Increase the proportion of mothers who breast-feed their babies in the early postpartum period to 75% from a baseline of 64% (Department of Health and Human Services, 2000).

D. Factors affecting the postpartum experience (*Box* 10-1)

1. The nature of labor and delivery, and the birth outcome

CLIENT AND FAMILY TEACHING 10-1

Postpartum warning signs and symptoms to report to the physician

- Increased bleeding, clots, or passage of tissue
- Bright red vaginal bleeding anytime after birth
- Pain greater than expected
- Temperature elevation to 100.4° F
- Feeling of full bladder accompanied by inability to void
- Enlarging hematoma
- Feeling restless accompanied by pallor; cool, clammy skin; rapid heart rate; dizziness; and visual disturbance
- Pain, redness, and warmth accompanied by a firm area in the calf
- Difficulty breathing; rapid heart rate; chest pain; cough; feeling of apprehension; pale, cold, or blue skin color

BOX 10-1
Cultural competence in postpartum care

Country of origin	Cultural considerations
Chinese, Mexican, Korea, Southeast Asian women	May wish to eat only warm foods and drink hot drinks to restore the balance of hot and cold in their body and replace blood loss; may wish to avoid bathing, exercise, and hair washing for 7 to 30 days; may prefer to be cared for by family members; may prefer not to give baby colostrum
Arabic women	Eat special meals designed to restore energy; stay home for 40 days after delivery to avoid illness from exposure to outside air
Haitian women	May request the placenta to take home to bury or burn
Muslim women	Follow strict religious rules on modesty; must keep hair, arms to wrist, and legs to ankles covered at all times; cannot be alone with a man other than her husband or male relative; may require specially prepared meals (using halal meat)
Vietnamese women	May remain in bed for 10 days and wear a woolen cap to keep from getting cold; usually grandmother or nurse provides total care of mother and baby

2. Preparation for labor, delivery, and parenting
3. Abruptness of the transition to parenthood
4. The family's individual and collective experiences with childbearing and childrearing
5. Family members' role expectations
6. Sensitivity and effectiveness of nursing and other professional care
7. Risk factors for postpartum complications; risk factors may include:
   a. Preeclampsia or eclampsia
   b. Diabetes
   c. Cardiac problems
   d. Uterine overdistention (as a result of multiple births or hydramnios)
   e. Abruptio placentae or placenta previa
   f. Precipitous or prolonged labor, difficult delivery, or extended time spent in stirrups

II. POSTPARTUM BIOPHYSICAL CHANGES

A. Reproductive system changes

1. The **uterus** contracts firmly after delivery of the newborn, reducing its size by more than half. It remains this size for about 2 days, then decreases in size (involution) and descends about one fingerbreadth per day (*Figure* 10-1, page 148).
   a. At 10 to 14 postpartum days, the uterus cannot be palpated abdominally. It returns to near its nonpregnant size by 4 to 6 postpartum weeks. The site of placental attachment requires 6 to 7 weeks to heal; endometrial regeneration requires 6 weeks.
   b. Lochia, discharge from the uterus during the first 3 weeks after delivery, occurs in three types.
      – Lochia rubra is dark red discharge occurring in the first 2 to 3 days. It contains epithelial cells, erythrocytes, leukocytes, and decidua, and has a characteristic human odor.

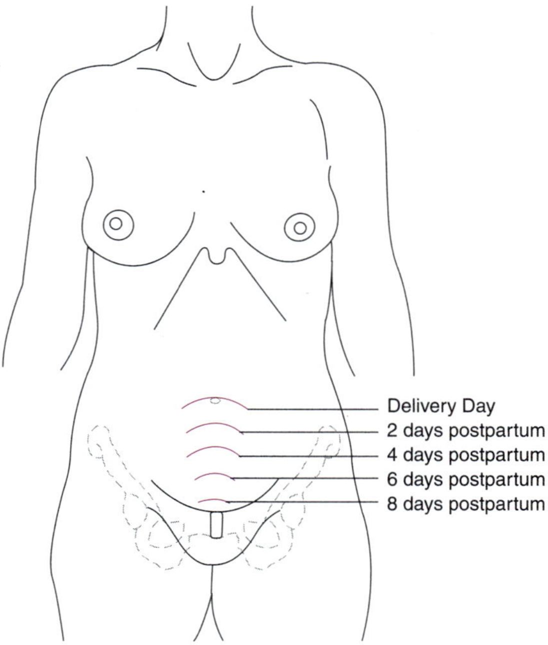

FIGURE 10-1
Uterine involution. The uterus decreases in size at a predictable rate after the birth. After 10 days it is no longer palpable because it is under the pubic bone.

- Lochia serosa is pink to brownish discharge, occurring from 3 to 10 days after delivery. It is a serosanguineous discharge containing decidua, erythrocytes, leukocytes, cervical mucus, and microorganisms. Lochia serosa has a strong odor.
- Lochia alba is an almost colorless to creamy yellowish discharge, occurring from 10 days to 3 weeks after delivery. It contains leukocytes, decidua, epithelial cells, fat, cervical mucus, cholesterol crystals, and bacteria. Lochia alba should have no odor.

2. The **cervix** becomes thicker and firmer; by the end of the first postpartum week, it is still dilated about 1 cm. Complete cervical involution may take 3 to 4 months. Childbirth results in a permanent change in the cervical os from round to elongated.
3. The **vagina** is smooth and swollen, with poor tone after delivery. Rugae reappear by 3 to 4 postpartum weeks. The estrogen index returns in 6 to 10 weeks.
4. The **perineum** appears edematous and bruised after delivery; episiotomy or lacerations may be present.
5. The **abdomen** remains soft and flabby for some time after delivery. Striae remain but are silvery white. Diastasis recti (separation of abdominal recti muscles) may occur in women with poor muscle tone.
6. **Breast** changes include the following:
   a. Rapid drop in estrogen and progesterone levels occurs, with an increase in secretion of prolactin after delivery.
   b. Colostrum is present at the time of delivery; breast milk is produced by the third or fourth postpartum day.

c. Larger and firmer breasts occur with lactation (primary engorgement). Congestion subsides in 1 or 2 days.

d. In the breast, prolactin stimulates alveolar cells to produce milk. Sucking of the newborn triggers a release of oxytocin and contractility of the myoepithelial cells, which stimulate milk flow; this is known as the letdown reflex. The average amount of milk produced in 24 hours increases with time.
- First week — 6 to 10 oz
- 1 to 4 weeks — 20 oz
- After 4 weeks — 30 oz

B. Endocrine system changes

1. Estrogen and progesterone levels decrease rapidly after delivery. This rapid drop in estrogen and progesterone after delivery of the placenta is responsible for many of the anatomic and physiologic changes during the puerperium.
2. Ovulation and resumption of menstruation are influenced by whether or not the client breast-feeds.
   a. Forty-five percent of lactating women resume menstruation by 12 weeks; 80% have one or more anovulatory cycles before the first ovulation.
   b. Forty percent of nonlactating women resume menstruation by 6 weeks after delivery; 65% by 12 weeks; and 90% by 24 weeks. Fifty percent ovulate during the first cycle.
3. Requirements for rest and sleep increase significantly.

C. Cardiovascular system changes

1. Transient bradycardia (50 to 70 beats per minute) occurs for 24 to 48 hours after delivery and may persist for 6 to 8 days.
2. Blood volume decreases to nonpregnant levels by 4 weeks after delivery.
3. Hematocrit rises by the third to seventh postpartum day.
4. Leukocytosis (20,000 to 30,000 white blood cells per mm^3) continues for several days after delivery.
5. Blood pressure remains stable and the pulse returns to nonpregnant rate by 3 months postpartum.

D. Immune system changes

1. Slight increases in maternal body temperature may occur without apparent cause following birth. However, the mother's temperature should remain within normal limits.
2. Any mother whose temperature reaches 38° C (100.4° F) in any two consecutive 24-hour periods during the first 10 postpartum days, excluding the first 24 postpartum hours, is considered to be febrile.

E. Respiratory system changes.

Pulmonary functions return to nonpregnant status by 6 months after delivery.

F. Renal and urinary system changes

1. Overdistention of the bladder is common owing to increased bladder capacity, swelling, bruising of tissues around the urethra, and diminished sensation to increased pressure.
   a. A full bladder displaces the uterus and can cause postpartum hemorrhage; bladder distention can lead to urine retention.
   b. Adequate bladder emptying generally resumes in 5 to 7 days after tissue swelling and bruising resolve.
2. The glomerular filtration rate remains elevated for about 7 days after delivery.

3. Dilated ureters and renal pelvis return to their nonpregnant states within 6 to 10 weeks after delivery.
4. Puerperal diaphoresis and diuresis occur within the first 24 hours after delivery.

G. GI system changes

1. Hunger and thirst are common after delivery.
2. GI motility and tone return to the nonpregnant state within 2 weeks after delivery.
3. Constipation commonly occurs during the early postpartum period owing to decreased intestinal muscle tone, perineal discomfort, and anxiety.
4. The client may return to her prepregnant weight in 6 to 8 weeks if weight gain during pregnancy was within the normal range.
5. Hemorrhoids are a common problem in the early postpartum period owing to pressure on the pelvic floor and straining during labor.

H. Musculoskeletal system changes

1. Most women ambulate 4 to 8 hours after delivery; early ambulation is encouraged to avoid complications, promote involution, and improve emotional outlook.
2. Relaxation and increased mobility of pelvic articulations occur 6 to 8 weeks after delivery.

I. Integumentary system changes

1. Melanin decreases gradually after delivery, causing a decrease in hyperpigmentation (coloration may not return to prepregnant status, however).
2. Visible vascular changes of pregnancy disappear as estrogen levels decrease.

III. POSTPARTUM PSYCHOSOCIAL ADAPTATION

A. Essential concepts

1. The postpartum period represents a time of emotional stress for the new mother, made even more difficult by the tremendous physiologic changes that occur.
2. Factors influencing successful transition to parenthood during the postpartum period include:
   a. Response and support of family and friends
   b. Relationship of the birthing experience to expectations and aspirations
   c. Previous childbearing and childrearing experiences
   d. Cultural influences
3. Rubin (1997) describes this period as occurring in three stages — taking-in, taking-hold, and letting-go.

B. Taking-in period

1. During this period, occurring 1 to 2 days after delivery, the new mother typically is passive and dependent; energies are focused on bodily concerns.
2. She may review her labor and delivery experience frequently.
3. Uninterrupted sleep is important if the mother is to avoid the effects of sleep deprivation, which include fatigue, irritability, and interference with normal restorative processes.
4. Additional nourishment may be needed because the mother's appetite is usually increased; poor appetite may be a clue that the restorative process is not progressing normally.

C. Taking-hold period

1. During this period, extending from 2 to 4 days after delivery, the mother becomes concerned with her ability to parent successfully and accepts increasing responsibility for her newborn.
2. The mother focuses on regaining control over her bodily functions — bowel and bladder function, strength, and endurance.
3. The mother strives to master newborn care skills (for example, holding, breast feeding or bottle feeding, bathing, and diapering). She may be sensitive to feelings of inadequacy and may tend to perceive nurses' suggestions as overt or covert criticism. The nurse should take this into account when providing instruction and emotional support.

D. Letting-go period

1. This period generally occurs after the new mother returns home; it involves a time of family reorganization.
2. The mother assumes responsibility for newborn care; she must adapt to demands of the newborn's dependency and to her decreased autonomy, independence, and (typically) social interaction.
3. Postpartum depression most commonly occurs during this period.

E. Postpartum depression

1. Many mothers experience a "let down" feeling after giving birth related to the magnitude of the birth experience and doubts about the ability to cope effectively with the demands of childrearing.
2. Typically, this depression is mild and transient, beginning 2 to 3 days after delivery and resolving within 1 to 2 weeks.
3. Rarely, relatively mild depression leads to postpartum psychosis, a pathologic condition.

NURSING PROCESS OVERVIEW

IV. THE POSTPARTUM PERIOD

A. Assessment

1. Associated findings
   a. Assess psychosocial adaptation, including:
   - Signs and symptoms of postpartum "blues," such as crying, despondency, loss of appetite, poor concentration, difficulty sleeping, and anxiety.
   - Evaluate integration of the newborn into the family.
   - Observe interactions of the new mother and other family members with the newborn.

   b. Evaluate nutritional status, including an ability to ingest food and fluids and adequacy of the diet to support involution and lactation.

   c. Evaluate the client's level of knowledge about newborn feeding (breast-feeding or bottle-feeding).
2. The **health history** should focus on family medical history, genetic history, and reproductive history.

3. **Physical examination.** Focus ongoing assessment on early identification of, and prompt intervention for, complications.
   a. During the critical first hour after delivery, carefully assess for hemorrhage by palpating the fundus frequently (at 15-minute intervals), inspecting the perineum for visible bleeding, and evaluating vital signs.
   b. Assess temperature, blood pressure, pulse, and respirations every 4 to 8 hours during the first few days postpartum. Note especially:
   - Mild temperature elevation, which may be due to dehydration, onset of lactation, or leukocytosis
   - Hypotension with a rapid, thready pulse (exceeding 100 beats/minute), which may signify hemorrhage and shock
   - Orthostatic hypotension due to cardiovascular readjustment to the nonpregnant state
   - Elevated blood pressure, possibly an early sign of pregnancy-induced hypertension

   c. Assess the fundus daily for firmness and location; make sure the client empties her bladder before palpating. Look for indications of subinvolution, which include:
   - Uterus not progressively decreasing in size or returning to the lower pelvis
   - Uterus remaining flabby and poorly contracted
   - Persistent backache or pelvic pain
   - Heavy vaginal bleeding

   d. Assess the amount and character of lochia daily to provide an essential index of endometrial healing. Report any abnormal findings, such as:
   - Fresh bleeding
   - Heavy, persistent, and malodorous lochia rubra

   e. Inspect the perineum, noting status of sutures (if any), tenderness, swelling, bruising, and hematoma; assess anal area for hemorrhoids and fissures.
   f. Handle the breasts gently and assess for firmness, tenderness, and warmth. Assess the nipples for cracks, fissures, and bleeding.
   g. Assess the degree of bladder distention frequently in the first 8 hours after delivery. Measure urine output; voiding small amounts on frequent, consecutive voidings indicates residual urine and a possible need for catheterization.
   h. Assess the status of bowel elimination and the return to predelivery patterns.
   i. Assess ambulation, rest and exercise patterns, and ability to perform activities of daily living.
   j. Assess peripheral circulation, noting varicosities, edema, and symmetry of size and shape, temperature, color, and range of motion. Note, particularly, signs of thrombophlebitis and the presence of Homans' sign.

B. Nursing diagnoses

1. Knowledge Deficit
2. Self-Care Deficit
3. Risk for Infection
4. Risk for Injury
5. Constipation
6. Altered Patterns of Urinary Elimination
7. Pain
8. Sleep Pattern Disturbance
9. Fatigue

10. Altered Parenting
11. Altered Role Performance
12. Anxiety

C. Planning and outcome identification

1. The woman and her partner will receive self-care and newborn care teaching.
2. The mother will receive adequate physical support and will progress toward recovery.
3. The mother will have adequate time for rest.
4. The mother will receive emotional and psychological support.

D. Implementation

1. **Provide self-care and newborn care teaching.**
   a. Instruct the client on sitting properly to relieve pain (that is, squeeze the buttocks together and contract pelvic floor muscles before sitting). Also instruct her to wear perineal pads loosely and to lie in the Sims position.
   b. Instruct the client to clean her breasts daily, with clean water if breast-feeding and with soap and water if bottle-feeding, and to wear a well-fitted bra.
   c. Assist with breast-feeding as needed; explain mechanisms involved in lactation, breast care, positioning of the mother and the newborn, and nursing techniques.
   d. Demonstrate how to clean the perineum after each voiding and defecation (that is, wiping from front to back, washing the hands, and applying a perineal pad from front to back).
   e. Teach the importance of adequate fluid intake, exercise, proper diet, and a regular defecation time.
   f. Support the client's attempts at ambulation and exercise; explain the advantages of early ambulation and regular exercise in preventing complications and strengthening muscles of the back, pelvic floor, and abdomen.
   g. Instruct the client to avoid constricting clothing that can impair circulation.
   h. Encourage the client to shower as soon as she can ambulate and to take tub baths, if desired, after 2 weeks. Recommend a daily shower to promote comfort and a sense of well-being.
   i. Demonstrate newborn care and safety measures.
   j. Advise the client to schedule a 4- to 6-week checkup to assess her general physical condition, progress of involution, and family adaptation to the newborn.
2. **Provide physical support to promote recovery from childbirth.**
   a. Monitor the cllient for complications and report and record increased pulse rate, decreased blood pressure, and elevated temperature.
   b. Gently massage the fundus, if boggy; express clots from the fundus as indicated.
   c. Apply ice or cold therapy to the episiotomy or lacerations immediately after delivery to decrease edema and provide anesthesia; thereafter, apply moist or dry heat therapy to promote comfort and healing.
   d. Apply anesthetic sprays, ointments, or witch hazel pads to the perineum to promote comfort; administer analgesia as ordered and indicated (*Drug Chart* 10-1, page 154); and offer sitz baths as needed.
   e. Treat breast pain of bottle-feeding client with analgesics and ice packs.
   f. Offer the opportunity to void within the first 4 to 8 hours after delivery and every 2 to 3 hours thereafter. If necessary, help stimulate urination by running water, placing the mother's hands in warm water, giving a warm beverage, providing privacy and support, or pouring warm water over the vulva.

DRUG CHART 10-1
Postpartum medications

Classifications	Uses	Selected interventions
Laxatives docusate (Colace, Surfak)	■ Used as a stool softener in the postpartal period to prevent constipation ■ It lowers the surface tension of feces, allowing water and lipids to penetrate the stool and soften it	■ Instruct the woman to swallow the medication with a full glass of water. ■ Instruct the woman regarding how to increase dietary fiber. ■ Promote activity as tolerated to improve intestinal motility. ■ Monitor for side effects, which may include occasional abdominal pain or diarrhea.
Biologicals rubella vaccine (Meruvax M-R-Vax II)	■ Used to prompt antibody formation in an individual who is not immune	■ Explain the medication to mother and obtain signature on appropriate form. ■ Instruct her to take acetaminophen for elevated temperature and achy feeling. ■ Caution her not to become pregnant for the next 3 months. ■ Tell her she may develop a rash. ■ Monitor for side effects, which may include measles-like rash, fever, headache, pain at the injection site, and malaise.
Rho (D) immune globulin (HypRho-D, Gamulin RH, Rhesonativ)	■ Prevents the production of anti-Rho(D) antibodies in the Rh-negative mother whose infant is Rh positive ■ Prevents hemolytic disease of the newborn	■ RhoGAM must be administered to the mother within 72 hours of delivery. ■ Type and cross match of the mother's blood and newborn's cord blood must be done before administration to determine the need for the drug. ■ Do not give RhoGAM to the newborn. ■ The dose may be given within 3-72 hours after a miscarriage or abortion. ■ Do not administer I.V. Administer into the deltoid muscle. ■ Monitor for side effects, which may include anemia, pain at the injection site, and fever. May decrease antibody response to some live virus vaccines, such as measles, mumps, and rubella.
Opioid analgesics oxycodone with acetaminophen (Percocet, Tylox)	■ Alters the perception of and response to painful stimuli; produces generalized CNS depression; decreases pain.	■ Assess the level of pain experienced by the patient. ■ Assess vital signs. ■ Assess bowel function. ■ Assess level of awareness before rooming-in begins. ■ Monitor for side effects, which may include dizziness, blurred vision, dry mouth, nausea, vomiting, constipation, and respiratory depression. ■ Explain to the mother that these drugs enter the breast milk.
Topical agents Dermoplast spray Americaine spray	■ Provides local anesthesia	■ Apply small amount of spray as needed to perineum.
Witch hazel pads Tucks	■ Relieves inflammation and itching	■ Apply one pad to perineum or hemorrhoids up to six times per day.

g. Provide adequate dietary fiber and fluids to promote bowel movements; if necessary, administer stool softeners, laxatives, suppositories, or enemas (see *Drug Chart* 10-1).

3. **Encourage the mother to rest.**

a. During hospitalization, limit visitors and adjust the routine to enable adequate rest.

b. Provide analgesia and position changes for comfort and promoting adequate rest; stressing the need for adequate rest to enhance coping ability.

CLIENT AND FAMILY TEACHING 10-2

Postpartum sexual activity

- Intercourse and your body do return to normal.
- Sexual intercourse may be resumed at about 2 to 4 weeks after birth.
- Sexual intercourse should not resume until vaginal bleeding has stopped and the episiotomy has healed.
- Sexual arousal may cause milk to leak from the breasts.
- Longer periods of foreplay will encourage lubrication. A natural vegetable oil may be used if additional lubrication is necessary.
- Alternative forms of sexual expression may be used.
- The couple should communicate openly with each other.
- Nap or lie down when the baby is napping.
- When the infant is weaned from the breast, your sex drive will usually return to normal.
- The contraceptive method of choice should be used, as directed, at the initiation of sexual activity.

4. **Provide emotional and psychological support** to promote maternal-infant and family-infant attachment.
   a. Encourage the mother to hold and explore her newborn.
   b. Facilitate visitation by partner and others.
   c. Provide time for parent-newborn contact, as indicated by the mother's and newborn's condition.
   d. Explain postpartum hormonal changes and how they can affect emotions and mood.
   e. Discuss expected newborn developmental milestones and expected maternal physical and psychological changes in the postpartum period.
   f. Discuss resumption of sexual activity and planning birth control, if desired. Typically, intercourse can be safely resumed after 3 weeks; other forms of sexual expression need not be affected (*Client and Family Teaching* 10-2).
   g. Explain the newborn's need to be touched, held, and spoken to often; discuss the newborn's responses to various stimuli.
   h. Allow the new parents to express feelings and concerns.

E. Outcome evaluation

1. The mother understands the importance of, and begins to implement, optimal self-care and newborn care.
2. The mother makes progress toward physical recovery from childbirth.
3. The mother gets adequate rest.
4. The mother and her partner adjust positively to childrearing and exhibit positive attachment to the infant.

Study questions

1. Which of the following would the nurse expect to find when assessing a client who delivered a newborn 12 hours ago?
1. Lochia alba
2. Soft, boggy fundus
3. Transient tachycardia
4. Complaints of hunger

2. When teaching a postpartum client about breast-related changes in the immediate postpartum period, on which of the following would the nurse base the teaching plan?
1. Estrogen and progesterone levels and secretion of prolactin rapidly increase.
2. Colostrum, present by 2 to 3 postpartum days, eventually changes to breast milk.
3. Estrogen and progesterone levels drop rapidly as prolactin secretion increases.

4. Rapid breast enlargement occurs to provide the newborn with sufficient breast milk.

3. Which of the following describes the rationale for preventing overdistention of the bladder?
1. A full bladder will displace the uterus and may cause postpartum hemorrhage.
2. A full bladder will prolapse, causing a great deal of discomfort for the new mother.
3. A full bladder will cause diaphoresis and lead to complaints of discomfort and pain.
4. A full bladder will rupture during palpation of the uterine fundus after delivery.

4. Which of the following factors most influences the new mother's successful transition to parenthood?
1. Early discharge, which offers the mother and newborn an opportunity to attain needed rest and sleep at home
2. The need of both parents to know that everything is okay and that no problems will occur
3. The new mother having full emotional support of family and friends and being emotionally ready for parenthood
4. The new mother understanding the signs and symptoms of "postpartum blues" and being able to deal with them

5. According to Rubin, during which of the following periods would the new mother frequently review her labor and delivery experience?
1. Letting-down
2. Letting-go
3. Taking-hold
4. Taking-in

6. Which of the following additional assessment findings would be most suspicious and lead the nurse to suspect postpartum "blues" in a client who is anxious and crying?
1. Loss of appetite, constipation, abdominal pain
2. Despondency, loss of appetite, difficulty sleeping
3. Increased appetite, urine retention, diarrhea
4. Poor concentration, constipation, diarrhea

7. While on a clinic visit, a client who is 2 weeks postpartum with her first child asks the nurse, "When can my husband and I have sex?" Which of the following responses would be most appropriate?
1. "It's okay now. I'm surprised your husband has been able to wait this long."
2. "Are you breast-feeding or bottle-feeding? That will make a difference."
3. "Typically, intercourse can be safely resumed 3 weeks after delivery."
4. "Why do you ask? Aren't you tired from taking care of the baby all day?"

8. When assessing lochia serosa, which of the following would the nurse expect?
1. Creamy yellow color
2. Characteristic odor
3. Serosanguineous appearance
4. White to colorless

9. After teaching a client about danger signs and symptoms to report to her doctor, which of the following client statements indicates the need for additional teaching?
1. "My vaginal discharge should be bright red for several days."
2. "My temperature should stay below 100.4° F."
3. "I'll call my doctor if I have trouble urinating."
4. "If I have any chest pain or trouble breathing, I'll call my doctor."

10. Which of the following would the nurse identify as the underlying cause for development of hemorrhoids in the early postpartum period?
1. Slowed return of GI motility to the prepregnant state.

2. Pressure on the pelvic floor and straining during labor
3. Elevation of glomerular filtration rate
4. Gradual decrease in melanin after delivery

11. The nurse observes several interactions between a mother and her neonate son. Which of the following behaviors of the mother would the nurse identify as evidence of mother-infant attachment? Select all that apply:
1. Talks and coos to her son
2. Cuddles her son close to her
3. Doesn't make eye contact with her son
4. Requests that the nurse take the baby to the nursery for feedings
5. Encourages the father to hold the baby
6. Takes a nap when the baby is sleeping

Answer key

1. The answer is 4.
Following delivery, the nurse would expect to find complaints of hunger and thirst. Additional assessment findings for this time period include lochia rubra; a fundus that is firm, located midline and at the level of the umbilicus or slightly lower; and transient bradycardia.

2. The answer is 3.
In the postpartum period, estrogen and progesterone levels drop rapidly, with an increase in the secretion of prolactin. Colostrum is present at the time of delivery, whereas breast milk is produced by the third or fourth postpartum day. At delivery, the breasts are typically soft and nontender. Primary engorgement, the development of larger and firmer breasts, usually occurs before the third postpartum day.

3. The answer is 1.
A full bladder will displace the uterus and can cause postpartum hemorrhage; bladder distention can lead to urine retention. In the early postpartum period, a full bladder also may prolapse or cause diaphoresis, leading to discomfort. However, these problems are not as life-threatening as hemorrhage. A full bladder will not rupture when the fundus is palpated.

4. The answer is 3.
The postpartum period represents a time of emotional stress for the new mother, made even more difficult by the tremendous physiologic changes that occur. One of the factors influencing successful transition to parenthood is response and support of family and friends. Early discharge and the parents' need to know that everything is okay are not associated with influencing the mother's transition to parenthood. Understanding is a difficult concept and therefore not measurable.

5. The answer is 4.
Rubin identifies three stages: taking-in, taking-hold, and letting-go. According to Rubin, during the taking-in period, the new mother may review her labor and delivery experience frequently. Many mothers do experience a "let-down" feeling after giving birth related to the magnitude of the birth experience and doubts about the ability to cope effectively with the demands of childrearing. However, Rubin does not describe a letting-down period. The letting-go stage, which generally occurs after the new mother returns home, is a time of family reorganization. During the taking-hold stage, the mother becomes concerned with her ability to parent successfully and accepts increasing responsibility for the newborn.

6. The answer is 2.
Assessment findings most characteristic of postpartum "blues" include crying, anxiety, despondency, loss of appetite, poor concentration, and difficulty sleeping. Constipation, abdominal pain, increased appetite, urine retention, diarrhea, and constipation may occur during the postpartum period, but these

conditions are not suspicious for postpartum "blues."

7. The answer is 3.
When questions related to the resumption of sexual activity arise, the best response would be that, typically, intercourse can be safely resumed after 3 weeks; other forms of sexual expression need not be affected. Although the newborn feeding method may affect sexual desire, it has no effect on the time when sexual relations can safely resume. Resuming sexual activity at 2 weeks is too early. The statement about being surprised about the husband's ability to wait is unprofessional. Asking the client why and then questioning that the client is too tired also is unprofessional.

8. The answer is 3.
Lochia serosa appears as pink to brownish, serosanguineous discharge with a strong odor occurring from 3 to 10 days after delivery. Lochia alba is typically almost colorless to creamy yellowish discharge occurring from 10 days to 3 weeks after delivery. Lochia rubra appears as dark red vaginal discharge with a characteristic odor, occurring in the first 2 to 3 days after delivery.

9. The answer is 1.
Bright red vaginal bleeding is a danger sign and needs to be reported immediately. Therefore, the client needs additional teaching to emphasize this point. Other danger signs and symptoms include a temperature above 100.4° F; feeling of a full bladder and difficulty urinating; increased bleeding, clots, or passage of tissue; pain greater than expected; enlarging hematoma; feeling restless accompanied by pallor, cool clammy skin, rapid heart rate, dizziness, and visual disturbances; pain, redness, and warmth accompanied by a firm area in the calf of the leg; difficulty breathing, rapid heart rate, chest pain, cough, feeling of apprehension, pale, cold, or blue skin color.

10. The answer is 1.
Hemorrhoids are common in the early postpartum period owing to the pressure on the pelvic floor and straining that occurs during labor. This condition may be exacerbated by constipation secondary to the decreased intestinal muscle tone, perineal discomfort, and anxiety after delivery. GI motility and tone return to the nonpregnant state in about 2 weeks. Elevation of the glomerular filtration rate affects urine output. A gradual decrease in melanin would lead to a decrease in hyperpigmentation.

11. The answer is 1, 2.
Talking, cooing, and cuddling with her son are positive signs that the mother is adapting to her new role as mother. Avoiding eye contact is a nonbonding behavior. Eye contact, touching, and speaking help establish attachment with the neonate. Feeding a neonate is an important role of a new mother and facilitates attachment. Encouraging the father to hold the neonate will facilitate attachment between the neonate and his father. Resting while the neonate sleeps will conserve energy and allow the mother to be awake and alert when her infant is awake; however, it is not evidence of bonding.

11 Newborn Care

I. OVERVIEW

A. Essential concepts

1. In the postpartum period, the newborn experiences complex biophysiologic and behavioral changes resulting from the transition to extrauterine life.
2. Nursing care of the newborn is based on knowledge of these changes and of the newborn's impact on the family unit.
3. The first few hours after birth represent a critical adjustment period for the newborn. In most settings, the nurse provides direct care to the newborn immediately after birth.
4. After the transition period, the nurse continues to evaluate the newborn at periodic intervals and to adjust nursing care plans according to ongoing findings.
5. The nurse must skillfully balance the family's need for privacy with the need to monitor the newborn's transition to extrauterine life.

B. Goals of newborn care

1. **Initial postpartum period**
   a. To establish and maintain an airway and support respirations
   b. To maintain warmth and prevent hypothermia
   c. To ensure safety and prevent injury or infection
   d. To identify actual or potential problems that may require immediate attention
2. **Continuing care**
   a. To continue protecting from injury or infection and identifying actual or potential problems that could require attention
   b. To facilitate development of a close parent-newborn relationship
   c. To provide parents with information about newborn care
   d. To assist parents in developing healthy attitudes about childrearing practices
3. **Safety and prevention of abduction of the newborn**
   a. To review the newborn identification procedures with the mother so she is informed of the safeguards being taken
   b. To observe that identification bands are in place when caring for the infant; to replace them immediately if they slide off during care, as they sometimes do
   c. To ask the mother to designate one person other than herself who may pick up the infant from the nursery and take him to the mother's room; to place an identification band on that person
   d. To refuse permission for anyone to remove the baby from the nursery or the mother's room without proper hospital identification
   e. To explain to the mother that she should never leave the baby unattended in her room but should bring the baby back to the nursery when she takes her shower or goes to the bathroom
   f. To instruct mothers, visitors, and staff to report any suspicious person who appears on the unit
   g. To place alarms or observation cameras in hallways or on doors that provide access to the unit but are difficult to monitor otherwise
   h. To use identification bands for the infant that have an embedded microchip, which will sound an alarm if the newborn is removed from the unit without permission; to deactivate the microchip upon discharge

C. Factors affecting newborn adaptation

1. Antepartum experiences of the mother and newborn (such as exposure to toxic substances and parental attitudes toward childbearing and childrearing)

2. Intrapartum experiences of the mother and newborn (such as length of labor, type of intrapartum analgesia or anesthesia)
3. Newborn's physiologic capacity to make the transition to extrauterine life
4. Ability of health care providers to assess and respond appropriately in the event of problems

II. TRANSITION TO EXTRAUTERINE LIFE

A. Essential concepts

1. Immediate initiation of respiration and changes in the circulatory patterns are essential for extrauterine life.
2. Within 24 hours after birth, the newborn's renal, GI, hematologic, metabolic, and neurologic systems must function sufficiently for progression to, and maintenance of, extrauterine life.

B. Transition period

1. This is a phase of instability during the first 6 to 8 hours of life through which all newborns pass, regardless of gestational age or nature of labor and delivery.
2. In the first period of reactivity (immediately after birth), respiration is rapid (may reach 80 breaths per minute), and transient nostril flaring, retractions, and grunting may occur. The heart rate may reach 180 beats per minute during the first few minutes of life.
3. Following this initial response, the newborn becomes quiet, relaxes, and falls asleep; this first sleep (known as the sleep phase) occurs within 2 hours of birth and lasts from a few minutes to several hours.
4. The second period of reactivity, starting when the newborn awakes, is marked by hyperresponsiveness to stimuli, skin color changes from pink to slightly cyanotic, and a rapid heart rate.
5. Oral mucus may cause major choking, gagging, and coughing problems.

C. Respiratory adaptation

1. Initial respirations are triggered by physical, sensory, and chemical factors.
   a. Physical factors include the effort required to expand the lungs and fill the collapsed alveoli (such as change in pressure gradients).
   b. Sensory factors include temperature, noise, light, sound, and a drop in temperature.
   c. Chemical factors include changes in the blood (such as decreased O_2 level, increased CO_2 level, and decreased pH) as a result of the transitory asphyxia during delivery.
2. The newborn respiratory rate ranges between 30 and 60 breaths per minute.
3. Oral mucous secretions may cause the newborn to cough and gag, especially during the first 12 to 18 hours.
4. Newborns are obligatory nose breathers. The reflex response to nasal obstruction, opening the mouth to maintain an airway, is not present in most newborns until 3 weeks after birth.

D. Cardiovascular adaptation

1. Various anatomic changes take place after birth; some are immediate, and others occur with time (*Table* 11-1, page 162).
2. Peripheral circulation is sluggish, causing acrocyanosis (cyanosis of the hands and feet and around the mouth). The feet may be cold to touch.
3. Pulse rate is 120 to 160 beats per minute while awake and 100 beats per minute while asleep.

TABLE 11-1
Changes in fetal circulation at birth

Structure	Before birth	After birth
Umbilical vein	Brings arterial blood to the heart	Obliterated; becomes round ligament of liver
Umbilical arteries	Bring arteriovenous blood to placenta	Obliterated; become vesical ligaments on anterior abdominal wall
Ductus venosus	Shunts arterial blood into inferior vena cava	Obliterated; becomes ligamentum venosum
Ductus arteriosus	Shunts arterial and some venous blood from pulmonary artery to aorta	Obliterated; becomes ligamentum arteriosum
Foramen ovale	Connects right and left auricles (atria)	Obliterated usually; at times open
Lungs	Contain no air and very little blood; filled with fluid	Filled with air and well supplied with blood
Pulmonary arteries	Bring little blood to lungs	Bring much blood to lungs
Aorta	Receive blood from both ventricles	Receives blood only from left ventricle
Inferior vena cava	Brings venous blood from body and arterial blood from placenta	Brings blood only to right auricle

4. Blood pressure averages 80/46 mm Hg and varies with the size of the newborn and the newborn's activity level.
5. *Table* 11-2 lists normal newborn hematologic values.

E. Thermoregulation and metabolic changes

1. The newborn's temperature may drop several degrees after delivery because the external environment is cooler than the intrauterine environment.
2. A limited supply of subcutaneous fat and a large skin surface area in relation to body weight predispose the newborn to heat transfer with the environment.
3. Rapid heat loss in a cool environment occurs by conduction, convection, radiation, and evaporation.
4. Cold stress (hypothermia) in the newborn, with its associated metabolic acidosis, can be lethal even for a vigorous, full-term newborn.

F. Neurologic adaptation

1. The newborn's neurologic system is not fully developed anatomically or physiologically.
2. The newborn exhibits uncoordinated movements, labile temperature regulation, poor control over musculature, easy startling, and tremors of the extremities.
3. Neonatal development is rapid; as the newborn grows, more complex patterns of behavior (such as head control, smiling, and purposeful reaching) will develop.
4. Newborn reflexes are important indicators of normal development (*Table* 11-3, pages 164 and 165).

G. GI adaptation

1. Digestive enzymes are active at birth and can support extrauterine life by 36 to 38 weeks' gestation.

TABLE 11-2
Neonatal blood values

Parameter	Normal range
Hemoglobin	▪ 14–20 g/dl
Red blood cells	▪ 5.0–7.5 million/mm^3
Hematocrit	▪ 43%–63%
White blood cells (WBCs)	▪ 10,000–30,000/mm^3
Neutrophils	▪ 40%–80%
Eosinophils	▪ 2%–3%
Lymphocytes	▪ 20%–40%
Monocytes	▪ 3%–10%
Immature WBCs	▪ 3%–10%
Platelets	▪ 150,000–350,000/mm^3
Reticulocytes	▪ 3%–7%
Blood volume	▪ Total blood volume at term 80–85 ml/kg of body weight ▪ Third day after early cord clamping: 82.3 ml/kg ▪ Third day after late cord clamping: 92.6 ml/kg

2. The necessary muscular and reflex developments for transporting food are present at birth.
3. Digestion of protein and carbohydrates is readily accomplished; fat digestion and absorption are poor owing to the inadequacy of pancreatic enzymes and lipase.
4. Salivary glands are immature at birth; little saliva is manufactured until the newborn is 3 months old.
5. A meconium bowel movement, which is greenish black, viscous, and contains occult blood, is excreted within 24 hours in 90% of normal newborns.
6. Wide variations occur among newborns regarding interest in food, symptoms of hunger, and amount of food ingested at any one sitting. The newborn stomach holds 60 to 90 ml.
7. Some newborns nurse immediately when put to the breast; others take up to 48 hours for effective feeding.
8. Random hand-to-mouth movement and finger sucking have been observed in utero; these actions are well developed at birth and are intensified with hunger.

H. Kidney adaptation

1. The glomerular filtration rate is relatively low at birth owing to inadequate surface area of the glomerular capillaries.
2. Although these limitations do not compromise the healthy newborn, they do restrict the capacity of the newborn to respond to stressors.
3. Decreased ability to excrete drugs and excessive fluid loss can rapidly lead to acidosis and fluid imbalances.

TABLE 11-3
Newborn reflexes

Reflex	Normal response	Abnormal response
Rooting and sucking	■ Newborn turns head in direction of stimulus, opens mouth, and begins to suck when cheek, lip, or corner of mouth is touched with finger or nipple.	■ Weak or no response occurs with prematurity, neurologic deficit or injury, or central nervous system (CNS) depressions secondary to maternal drug ingestion (such as narcotics).
Swallowing	■ Newborn swallows in coordination with sucking when fluid is placed on back of tongue.	■ Gagging, coughing, or regurgitation of fluid may occur; possibly associated with cyanosis secondary to prematurity, neurologic deficit, or injury; typically seen after laryngoscopy.
Extrusion	■ Newborn pushes tongue outward when tip of tongue is touched with finger or nipple.	■ Continuous extrusion of tongue or repetitive tongue thrusting occurs with CNS anomalies and seizures.
Moro	■ Bilateral symmetrical extension and abduction of all extremities, with thumb and forefinger injury (brachial plexus) or forming characteristic "c," are followed by adduction of extremities and return to relaxed flexion when newborn's position changes suddenly or when newborn is placed on back on flat surface.	■ Asymmetrical response is seen with peripheral nerve injury (brachial plexus) or fracture of clavicle or long bone of arm or leg. ■ No response occurs in cases of severe CNS injury.
Stepping	■ Newborn will step with one foot and then the other in walking motion when one foot is touched to flat surface.	■ Asymmetrical response is seen with CNS or peripheral nerve injury or fracture of long bone of leg.
Prone crawl	■ Newborn will attempt to crawl forward with both arms and legs when placed on abdomen on flat surface.	■ Asymmetrical response is seen with CNS or peripheral nerve injury or fracture of long bone of leg.
Tonic neck or "fencing"	■ Extremities on side to which head is turned will extend, and opposite extremities will flex when newborn's head is turned to one side while resting. ■ Response may be absent or incompleted immediately after birth.	■ Persistent response after 4th month may indicate neurologic injury. Persistent absence seen in CNS injury and neurologic disorders.
Startle	■ Newborn abducts and flexes all extremities and may begin to cry when exposed to sudden movement or loud noise.	■ Absence of response may indicate neurologic deficit or injury. Complete and consistent absence of response to loud noises may indicate deafness. ■ Response may be absent or diminished during deep sleep.
Crossed extension	■ Newborn's opposite leg will flex and then extend rapidly as if trying to deflect stimulus to other foot when placed in supine position; newborn will extend one leg in response to stimulus on bottom of foot.	■ Weak or absent response is seen with peripheral nerve injury or fracture of long bone.
"Blink"	■ Newborn will blink in response to bright light or sudden movement toward the eye.	■ Persistent blinking and failure to habituate suggest neurologic deficit.

TABLE 11-3
Newborn reflexes *(continued)*

Reflex	Normal response	Abnormal response
Palmar grasp	▪ Newborn's finger will curl around object and hold on momentarily when finger is placed in palm of newborn's hand.	▪ Response is diminished in prematurity. ▪ Asymmetry occurs with peripheral nerve damage (brachial plexus) or fracture of humerus. ▪ No response occurs with severe neurologic deficit.
Plantar grasp	▪ Newborn's toes will curl downward when a finger is placed against the base of the toes.	▪ Diminished response occurs with severe neurologic deficit.
Babinski sign	▪ Newborn's toes will hyperextend and fan apart from dorsiflexion of big toe when one side of foot is stroked upward from heel and across ball of foot.	▪ No response occurs with CNS deficit.

Adapted from Pillitteri, A. (2003). *Maternal and Child Health Nursing,* 4th ed. Philadelphia: Lippincott Williams & Wilkins. pp. 636-638.

4. Most newborns void in the first 24 hours after birth and two to six times per day for the first 1 to 2 days; thereafter, they void 5 to 20 times in 24 hours.
5. Urine may be cloudy from mucus and urate; a reddish stain (brick dust) may be noticed on the diaper owing to uric acid crystals.

I. Hepatic adaptation

1. During fetal life and to some degree after birth, the liver continues to aid in blood formation.
2. During the neonatal period, the liver produces substances that are essential for blood coagulation.
3. Iron stores from the mother are sufficient to carry the newborn through the fifth month of extrauterine life; at this time, the newborn becomes susceptible to iron deficiency.
4. The liver also controls the amount of circulating unconjugated bilirubin, a pigment derived from the hemoglobin and released with the breakdown of red blood cells.
5. Unconjugated bilirubin can leave the vascular system and permeate other extravascular tissues (such as the skin, sclera, and oral mucous membranes), resulting in a yellow coloring termed *jaundice* or *icterus.*
6. In protracted cold stress, anaerobic glycolysis occurs, resulting in increased acid production. Metabolic acidosis develops, and if there is a defect in respiratory function, respiratory acidosis also develops. Excessive fatty acids displace the bilirubin from the albumin-binding sites. The increased level of circulating unbound bilirubin that results increases the risk of kernicterus, even at serum bilirubin levels of 10 mg/dl or less.

J. Immune system adaptation

1. The newborn cannot limit an invading organism at the portal of entry.
2. The immaturity of a number of protective systems significantly increases the risk of infection in the newborn period.
   a. The inflammatory response is reduced qualitatively and quantitatively.
   b. Phagocytosis is sluggish.

c. The acidity of the stomach and the production of pepsin and trypsin are not fully developed until 3 to 4 weeks of age.

d. Immunoglobulin A (IgA) is missing from the respiratory and urinary tracts; unless the newborn is breast-fed, IgA is absent from the GI tract as well.

3. Infection represents a leading cause of morbidity and mortality during the neonatal period.

NURSING PROCESS OVERVIEW

III. THE NORMAL NEWBORN

A. Assessment – neonatal health history

1. Comprehensive knowledge of the pregnancy, labor, and delivery is essential to understanding the significance of physical findings in the newborn.
2. A systematic approach helps ensure that pertinent data are not overlooked.
3. Major categories of data include:
   a. Maternal prenatal history and care
   b. Maternal blood type and Rh factor, history of isoimmunization, and antibody titers
   c. Maternal screening test results (such rubella titer, hepatitis antigen screen, venereal disease research laboratory, chlamydia screen, gonorrhea cultures, herpes cultures, and human immunodeficiency virus screen)
   d. Labor history, including onset, length, and complications
   e. Rupture of membranes, including color and amount of fluid, presence of meconium, and relationship to time of delivery
   f. Fetal monitoring record (such as evidence of fetal distress, fetal scalp sampling, and blood gas analysis results)
   g. Delivery history, including length of second stage of labor and medications and anesthetic (amount and when administered)
   h. Newborn history (such as need for resuscitation and Apgar scores at 1 and 5 minutes)
   i. Newborn laboratory results (such as hematocrit, blood type, and blood glucose level)

B. Assessment – physical examination

1. **General appearance**
   a. Posture
   b. Skin condition, including color, turgor, wrinkling, vernix caseosa, milia, lanugo, erythema toxicum, and birthmarks
   c. Respiratory effort, including rate, use of accessory muscles, nasal flaring, and grunting
2. **Vital signs and anthropometric assessment**
   a. Respiratory rate. While the newborn is quiet, count breaths for 60 seconds before determining apical rate. The normal rate is 30 to 60 breaths per minute.
   b. Heart rate. Count the apical rate for 60 seconds over the cardiac apex; the normal rate is 120 to 160 beats per minute.
   c. Temperature. Take the temperature every 30 minutes until the newborn is stable, and every 4 hours thereafter.
      - Take an axillary temperature with the thermometer held in the axillary fold for at least 3 minutes. The normal newborn temperature range is 36.4° to 37.2° C (97.5°

to 99° F). Axillary temperatures are the preferred method and are considered to be a close estimation of rectal temperature

- Take a tympanic temperature with an electronic sensor inserted in the ear canal to measure the temperature of blood circulating in the internal carotid artery; accurate findings are available in seconds.
- Take a rectal temperature (not preferred owing to risk of trauma to rectal mucosa), if necessary, with the thermometer inserted 0.25 to 0.5 inch and with the newborn's legs stabilized with the nurse's hand.

d. Size. Compare the newborn's size (weight, length, and head circumference) with standards, such as those established by Lubchenko and colleagues. These models can be used to identify newborns with an excellent chance for normal growth or newborns at risk for various reasons. For example, they may be small at term or small for gestational age or out of proportion with other measurements (suggesting special problems, such as dwarfism or fused suture lines).

- Weight. Weigh the newborn at the same time each day before feeding; 95% of full-term newborns weigh 2,500 to 4,250 g. Newborns initially lose between 5% and 10% of birth weight in the first few days of life. They require 120 calories/kg/day and 140 to 160 ml/kg/day of fluid in order to regain their birth weight and continue to grow.
- Length. Place the newborn on a flat surface and extend the legs fully before measuring; average full-term length is 50 cm (20 inch).
- Head circumference. Measure around the fullest part of the occiput; average head circumference is 35.5 cm.

e. Chest circumference. Place the measure over the nipples and across the lower border of the scapulae; average circumference is 33 cm, usually 2 to 3 cm smaller than the head.

f. Blood pressure. Although it is not routinely measured at birth, blood pressure assessed by Doppler ultrasound is the most accurate method in the newborn. It measures systolic, diastolic, and mean arterial pressures; average blood pressure at birth is 80/46 mm Hg.

3. Detailed physical examination

a. Head and face

- Head size is in proportion to the body (normally about 25% of total body size).
- Molding may be present.
- Symmetry of features is assessed.
- Ocular hypertelorism, wide-spaced eyes — a distance of more than 3 cm between the inner canthi of the eyes may be detected.

b. Fontanels

- The anterior fontanel is normally diamond-shaped, 3 to 4 cm long and 2 to 3 cm wide; it closes at 18 months.
- The posterior fontanel is normally triangle-shaped and smaller than the anterior fontanel; it closes by 8 to 12 weeks.
- A tense, bulging fontanel may indicate increased intracranial pressure.
- A sunken fontanel is characteristic of dehydration.

c. Eyes

- Color usually appears blue or gray owing to scleral thinness.
- Transient strabismus and nystagmus are common findings.
- Doll's eye phenomenon may be seen when the head is turned and eye movements lag behind.

d. Nose and mouth
- Nasal patency is determined by closing the newborn's mouth and compressing one nostril at a time or by advancing a nasogastric tube.
- Mucus secretions, if excessive, may indicate a tracheoesophageal fistula.
- Precocious teeth, sucking calluses, and inclusion cysts (Epstein pearls) may be apparent.

e. Ears and neck
- Ear pliability and flexibility. In a full-term newborn, the ears are normally soft and pliable, and recoil readily when bent forward.
- Low-set ears (the top of the ear below the level of the eyes' canthi) may indicate a chromosomal or organ abnormality.
- Hearing is normally well developed once the eustachian tube is cleared.
- The neck size is normally short, with many thick folds.
- Neck webbing is associated with chromosomal abnormalities.

f. Chest
- Contour is normally round and symmetrical.
- Breast engorgement may be evident 2 to 3 days after birth owing to maternal hormones.
- Respirations are normally shallow, symmetrical, and synchronous with abdominal movement.
- Breath sounds may reveal crackles and rhonchi.
  - Crackles may be present during the transitional period, representing fetal lung fluid and areas of atelectasis. These areas should clear within several hours.
  - Rhonchi indicate fluid, mucus, or meconium in the larger bronchi and are possibly associated with life-threatening conditions such as meconium aspiration.
- Heart sounds. About 90% of all murmurs are transient and are related to incomplete closure of the foramen ovale or ductus arteriosus.

g. Abdomen
- The contour is normally rounded and protuberant owing to weak abdominal musculature.
- The umbilical cord normally appears white and gelatinous in the first few hours, with two arteries and one vein apparent; it begins to dry within a few hours.
- A shrunken, scaphoid appearance indicates diaphragmatic hernia.
- Bowel sounds are normally present within one hour after birth and are audible when the newborn is quiet.

h. Genitalia (female)
- Labia minora may have vernix and smegma in the creases.
- Labia majora normally cover the labia minora and clitoris.
- The clitoris is normally prominent.
- Vaginal discharge may be present because of maternal hormones; this is called pseudomenstruation.
- The hymenal tag is normally present.

i. Genitalia (male)
- Rugae are normally present on the scrotum, and both testes are descended into the scrotum.
- The urinary meatus is normally located at the tip of the glans penis. *Epispadias* is the term used to describe the condition in which the meatus is located on the dorsal surface. *Hypospadias* is the term used to describe the condition in which the meatus is located on the ventral surface.

j. Back and buttocks
- The spine is normally flat and round. Tufts of hair or small indentations at the sacrum or base of the spine are associated with spina bifida occulta.
- There is a patent anal opening.

k. Upper extremities
- The upper extremities are normally well flexed, with symmetrical movement.
- The grasp reflex is normally present.
- Partial or complete muscle flaccidity of the arm may indicate trauma to the brachial plexus.
- Brachial pulses are normally present.

l. Lower extremities
- The lower extremities are normally short, bowed, and well flexed.
- Femoral and pedal pulses are normally present.

C. Assessment – neurologic assessment (newborn reflexes)

1. Blink, cough, sneeze, and gag reflexes are present at birth and remain unchanged through adulthood.
2. Several other reflexes are normally present at birth, reflecting neurologic immaturity; they disappear in the first year (see *Table* 11-3, pages 164 and 165). Absence of these reflexes may indicate a serious neurologic problem.
3. Sensory behaviors

a. Vision
- The infant can see objects about 6 to 8 inches away.
- The infant prefers black and white patterns.
- The infant is sensitive to light.
- The infant can track parents with his eyes.
- The infant has immature muscle coordination.

b. Hearing. The infant can detect sounds once the eustachian tubes are clear.

c. Taste
- Taste buds develop before birth.
- The infant prefers sweet to bitter or sour tastes.

d. Touch
- The infant can feel pressure, pain, and touch immediately, or shortly after, birth.
- The infant is sensitive to being cuddled.

e. Smell
- After mucus and amniotic fluids are cleared from nasal passages, the infant can differentiate pleasant from unpleasant odors.
- The infant can distinguish his mother's wet breast pad from another mother's at 1 week.

D. Gestational age assessment

1. Systematic assessment of physical signs and neurologic traits helps estimate the newborn's gestational age.

a. Physical and neuromuscular maturity may be estimated by using a standard, such as the Ballard assessment criteria. The Ballard scale assigns scores to 13 parameters, including neonatal postures and postural angles, and developmental hallmarks, such as plantar creases and genital characteristics. The total score reflects an assigned gestational age. For example, a score of 10 correlates with 28 gestational weeks; 15, with 30 weeks; 20, with 32 weeks; and so forth.

b. The Dubowitz scale is a more extensive gestational rating scale.

2. To a large extent, the degree of maturity at birth determines the ability of the newborn to survive.
3. Determining gestational age provides information about system maturity and guides assessment of potential complications.

E. Assessment – behavioral capabilities

1. Individual personalities, behavioral characteristics, and temperament play an important role in the ultimate relationship the newborn will form with parents and others.
2. By their actions, newborns encourage or discourage attachment and caretaking activities.
3. Awareness of the newborn's unique behavioral responses is important if parents are to learn to react to their newborn in ways that promote health.
4. Brazelton and others have devised scales to evaluate newborn behavior.

F. Nursing diagnoses

1. Transition period
   a. Ineffective Airway Clearance
   b. Ineffective Thermoregulation
   c. Risk for Infection
   d. Risk for Injury
   e. Potential for Altered Growth and Development
2. Continuing care
   a. Altered Nutrition: Less Than Body Requirements
   b. Risk for Ineffective Breast-Feeding
   c. Fluid Volume Deficit
   d. Risk for Altered Parent-Infant Attachment
   e. Knowledge Deficit
   f. Health-Seeking Behaviors Related to Newborn Needs
   g. Ineffective Coping
   h. Noncompliance With the Treatment Regimen

G. Planning and outcome identification

1. **Transition period**
   a. A patent airway will be maintained in the newborn.
   b. A neutral thermal environment will be achieved in the newborn.
   c. The newborn will be protected from infection and injury.
   d. Actual or potential problems will be identified and managed.
2. **Continuing care**
   a. The newborn will begin to take nourishment.
   b. The newborn will void and have a bowel movement within 24 hours.
   c. Parent-newborn attachment will occur.
   d. The family will receive information about newborn care.
   e. The newborn will undergo routine procedures.
   f. The parents will keep appointments for follow-up assessments of their newborn.

H. Implementation – transition period

1. **Maintain airway patency.** Keep a bulb syringe in the crib to suction mucus, formula, or breast milk from the mouth quickly in order to maintain a clear airway.
2. **Maintain a neutral thermal environment.**
   a. Place the newborn under a radiant warmer using a skin sensor to monitor temperature as needed.

TABLE 11-4
LATCH breast-feeding charting system

	0	1	2
L Latch	▪ Too sleepy ▪ No latch achieved ▪ Stimulate to suck	▪ Repeated attempts ▪ Holds nipple in mouth ▪ Rhythmic sucking	▪ Grasps breast ▪ Tongue down
A Audible swallowing	▪ None	▪ A few with stimulation	▪ Spontaneous and intermittent if < 24 hr old ▪ Spontaneous and frequent if > 24 hr old
T Type of nipple	▪ Inverted	▪ Flat	▪ Everted
C Comfort	▪ Engorged ▪ Cracked or bleeding ▪ Large blisters or bruises ▪ Severe discomfort	▪ Filing ▪ Reddened ▪ Small blisters or bruises ▪ Mild to moderate discomfort	▪ Soft ▪ Nontender
H Hold (positioning)	▪ Full assist (staff holds infant) ▪ Place pillows for comfort	▪ Minimal assist ▪ Explain one side, then the other	▪ Mother holds and feeds infant without assistance

From Simpson, KR & Creehan, PA. (1996). *AWHONN's Perinatal Nursing.* Philadelphia: Lippincott Williams & Wilkins. p. 344.

b. Delay bathing until the newborn's temperature is stable.
c. Apply a stockinette cap to prevent heat loss from the newborn's head.

3. **Protect from infection.**
a. Prevent infection by using aseptic technique and by administering prophylactic ophthalmic antibiotics as indicated.
b. Protect from nosocomial infection by performing handwashing as appropriate, and by observing "clean" dress code (scrub suits and cover gown).

4. **Identify actual or potential problems.**
a. Protect from hypoglycemia.
- Observe for jitteriness, tremors, eye rolling, weakness, high-pitched cry, and poor muscle tone.
- Use a standard glucose test.
- Report result to the primary care provider if glucose values are less than 40 mg/dl.

b. Protect from cardiac or other congenital problems.
- Report episodes of central cyanosis, apnea, and respiratory difficulty immediately.
- Carry out screening tests for congenital conditions as appropriate.

I. Implementation – continuing care

1. **Promote adequate hydration and nutrition.**
a. Support establishment of a feeding pattern (*Tables* 11-4 and 11-5, page 172).
b. Feed the newborn according to established protocol (such as breast milk, glucose water, or formula).
c. Adjust the type of formula to prevent problems with bowel elimination.
d. Assist with breast- or bottle-feedings as needed.
e. Observe the mother's ease and comfort in feeding the newborn.

TABLE 11-5
Pattern of infant feedings with formula

Age of Infant	Number of feedings	Volume per feeding	Total
Birth to 2 wks	6–10	½–2 oz (60–90 ml)	3–20 oz (90–600 ml)
2 wks–1 mo	6–8	3–4 oz (90–120 ml)	18–32 oz (540–960 ml)
1–3 mo	5–6	5–6 oz (150–180 ml)	25–36 oz (750–1080 ml)
3–7 mo	4–5	6–7 oz (180–210 ml)	24–35 oz (750–1080 ml)
7–12 mo	3–4	7–8 oz (210–240 ml)	21–32 oz (750–1080 ml)

From Simpson, KR & Creehan, PA. (1996). *AWHONN's Perinatal Nursing*. Philadelphia: Lippincott Williams & Wilkins. p. 348.

2. **Promote normal elimination patterns.**
   a. Support a feeding pattern with no less than 2 hours and no more than 5 hours between feedings.
   b. If the newborn is formula-fed, select a type that the infant can tolerate without excessive regurgitation or constipation.
   c. Measure amount of formula ingested at each feeding.
   d. Measure amount of time the infant was fed from each breast at each feeding.
3. **Promote positive parent-newborn attachment.**
   a. Support parent-newborn attachment.
   b. Provide opportunities for parent-infant interaction and observe behaviors.
4. **Provide family teaching about newborn care.**
   a. Prepare short teaching sessions to allow the mother and baby to rest frequently.
   b. Recognize that discharge may occur as early as 6 hours after delivery, and plan teaching accordingly.
   c. Give parents printed information regarding self-care, infant care and safety, and the recommended immunization schedule.
   d. Cover the following topics in teaching sessions.
   - Bathing
   - Cord care
   - Care of the uncircumcised male
   - Circumcision care
   - Diapering and dressing
   - Dealing with crying
   - Formula preparation, sterilization, and bottle-feeding techniques
   - Breast-feeding techniques (and breast feeding and returning to work issues; *Client and Family Teaching* 11-1)
   - Burping
   - Elimination patterns
   - Prevention and care of diaper rash
   - Swaddling or wrapping
   - Handling and carrying
   - Temperature measurement
   - Safety considerations

CLIENT AND FAMILY TEACHING 11-1

Breast-feeding and the workplace

- Arrange for child care near your work place, if possible.
- Discuss with your supervisor the possibility of using your lunch period for breast-feeding.
- Many states have passed laws allowing breast-feeding in public places.
- Cover yourself and your infant with a small blanket so that you are not exposed.
- If you can't arrange to breast-feed during work hours, pump your breasts at least once a day to maintain milk supply. You can rent a small electric pump for this purpose.
- Breast milk can be safely stored in a refrigerator or iced container for 24 to 48 hours.
- Plastic containers are best for storing breast milk.
- Any reminder of a baby may cause your breasts to leak. Wear breast pads and store a change of clothes at work. Placing the heel of your hand on the breast with gentle pressure may stop leaking.
- Drink four to six 8-ounce glasses of fluid each day.
- Plan to breast-feed your infant before leaving the day-care facility.
- Relax and enjoy your baby.

  - Signs and symptoms of illness
  - Administration of common medications (such vitamins and antipyretics)
  - Clearing nasal passages with a bulb syringe.

e. Observe the mother's ease and comfort in performing newborn care, such as diapering and holding the baby.

5. **Prepare the newborn for (and perform if so ordered) routine procedures** (such as identifying the newborn, administering vitamin K [*Drug Chart* 11-1, page 174], and circumcision). Inform parents of procedures and witness informed consent signatures as needed.
6. **Make follow-up appointments and arrange for home visits for the family before discharge.** If indicated, write out and give parents a list of various follow-up appointments (such as ambulatory laboratory studies to assess for phenylketonuria and bilirubin).

J. Outcome evaluation

1. **Transition period**

a. The newborn breathes without assistance, as evidenced by normal respirations between 30 and 60 breaths per minute within 2 hours of birth.

b. The newborn maintains a stable temperature, as evidenced by axillary temperature of 36.4° to 37.2° C (97.5° to 99° F) within 1 to 2 hours of birth.

c. The newborn shows no evidence of infection or injury.

d. Actual or potential problems are identified and managed.

  - The newborn does not develop symptoms of hypoglycemia, or evident symptoms resolve without further complications within 12 to 24 hours.
  - The newborn demonstrates normal cardiac output, as evidenced by a regular heart rate of 120 to 160 beats per minute within 2 hours of birth.
  - The newborn continues to make physical and behavioral adaptations and is screened for congenital conditions, as appropriate, within the first week of life.

2. **Continuing care**

a. The newborn begins to take nourishment within 4 to 8 hours of birth.

  - The mother demonstrates an ability to feed the newborn by the time of discharge and states she is satisfied with her choice (*Table* 11-6, page 175).
  - The newborn feeds every 2 to 4 hours, is content, sleeps between feedings, and regains his birth weight by 7 to 14 days after birth.

DRUG CHART 11-1
Medications used in the newborn

Classifications	Used for	Selected Interventions
Vitamins phytonadione (K) (AquaMEPHYTON, Mephyton)	▪ Prophylaxis and treatment of hemorrhagic disease of the newborn. It is a necessary component for the production of coagulation factors II, VII, IX, and X, which are produced by microorganisms in the intestinal tract.	▪ Prepare the medication for injection immediately after birth. ▪ Administer the injection into large muscle (newborn thigh). ▪ Assess for signs of bleeding such as black tarry stool, hematuria, or bleeding from the cord. ▪ Monitor for side effects, including local irritation and pain, swelling, or both at the site of injection.
Anti-infectives erythromycin base (Akne-mycin, Ilotycin)	▪ Inhibits bacterial protein synthesis. Prophylaxis for ophthalmia neonatorium from *Neisseria gonorrhoeae* or *Chlamydia trachomatis.*	▪ Wash hands; cleanse eye of debris if necessary. ▪ Store at room temperature in a sealed container. ▪ Apply a ¼-inch long, narrow strip along the lower conjunctival surface of each eye from inner canthus outward. ▪ Do not touch applicator tip to the eye. ▪ Report redness or swelling to physician. ▪ Monitor for side effects, including edema, inflammation, and drainage. ▪ This drug is contraindicated in herpes and fungal infections.
Biologicals hepatitis B immune globulin (HBIG) (H-BIG, H-BIG IV, HyperHep) hepatitis B vaccine (Engerix-B, Recombivax-HB)	▪ Provides immunization against hepatitis B. Used for neonates born to mothers who are HB_3 Ag+. (Also used for adult as postexposure prophylaxis.) ▪ Provides active immunity to hepatitis B. Used for all neonates. (Also used for adults at risk of becoming infected with hepatitis B.)	▪ Rotate the vial; do not shake it. ▪ Give the first dose within 12 hours after birth. ▪ The second dose is administered at 1 month of age. ▪ The third dose is given at 6 months of age. ▪ Administer the vaccine with epinephrine 1:1000 on hand to treat laryngospasm (allergic reactions). ▪ Provide a written record of immunization. ▪ Provide comfort measures as needed. ▪ Monitor for side effects, including local irritation (redness, warmth, tenderness, and swollen area) and low grade fever (99.8° F; 37.7° C).

b. The newborn voids and has a bowel movement within 24 hours.
- The newborn voids six to eight times daily and has two to three bowel movements.
- The newborn demonstrates urinary and bowel elimination patterns within normal limits for mode of feeding.

c. Parent-newborn attachment is evident.
- The newborn and parents demonstrate positive interaction, as evidenced by touching, eye contact, and responsiveness to each other.
- Parents demonstrate growing comfort and ease in handling their newborn by the time of discharge.

d. Mother and partner correctly demonstrate infant care.

e. Appointments for follow-up care are made and kept. The mother and infant progress as expected.

TABLE 11-6
Developing cultural competence

Here are some examples of cultural beliefs and practices regarding baby care.*

Umbilical cord

People of Latin American or Filipino cultural background may use an abdominal binder or bellyband to protect against dirt, injury, and umbilical hernia. They may also apply oils to the stump of the cord or tape metal to the umbilicus to ward off evil spirits.

People of northern European ancestry may expect a sterile cutting of the cord at birth. They may allow the stump to air-dry and discard the cord once it falls off.

Some Latin American cultures cauterize the stump with a hot flame, hot coal, or the like.

In Kenya, women may express colostrum to the cord stump.

In Ecuador, the cord is left long in girls to prevent a small uterus and problems with childbirth.

Parent-infant contact

People of Asian ancestry may pick up the baby as soon as it cries, or they may carry the baby at all times.

Some Native Americans, notably the Navajos, may use cradle boards.

Korean mothers may be reluctant to pick up or touch their infant, deferring infant care to the paternal grandmother.

The Muslim father traditionally calls praise to Allah in the newborn's right ear and cleans the infant after birth.

Feeding

Some people of Asian heritage may breast-feed their babies for the first 1 to 2 years of life. Many Cambodian refugees practice breast-feeding on demand without restriction, or if formula-feeding, provide a "comfort bottle" in between feedings.

People of Iranian heritage may breast-feed female babies longer than male babies.

Some people of African ancestry may wean their babies after they begin to walk.

Most Korean mothers resist breast-feeding in the hospital, contending that they do not have "milk," and state that they will begin breast-feeding at home.

Some Asians, Hispanics, Eastern Europeans, and Native Americans may delay breast-feeding because they believe colostrum is "bad."

Circumcision

People of Muslim and Jewish ancestry practice circumcision as a religious ritual.

Many natives of Africa and Australia practice circumcision as a puberty rite.

Native Americans and people of Asian and Latin American cultures rarely perform circumcision.

Only 15% of the world's male population is circumcised.

Health and illness

Some people from Latin American cultural backgrounds may believe that touching the face or head of an infant when admiring it will ward off the "evil eye." They may also neglect to cut the baby's nails to avoid nearsightedness and instead put mittens on the baby's hands to prevent scratching. They also may believe that fat babies are healthy.

Some people of Asian heritage may not allow anyone to touch the baby's head without asking permission.

Some Orthodox Jews believe that saying the baby's name before the formal naming ceremony will harm the baby.

Some Asian and Haitians delay naming their infants.

Some people of Vietnamese ancestry believe that cutting a baby's hair or nails will cause illness.

*Note: The information is meant only to provide examples of some of the behaviors that may be found within certain cultures. Not all members of a culture practice the behaviors described.

From Olds, S., London, M., Ladewig, P., and Davidson, M. (2004). *Maternal-Newborn Nursing & Women's Health Care,* 7th ed. Upper Saddle River, New Jersey: Pearson Education, Inc., p. 276.

Study questions

1. Which of the following would the nurse identify as a goal of newborn care in the initial postpartum period?
1. To facilitate development of a close parent-newborn relationship
2. To assist parents in developing healthy attitudes about childrearing practices
3. To identify actual or potential problems requiring immediate or emergency attention
4. To provide the parents of the newborn with information about well-baby programs

2. Before birth, which of the following structures connects the right and left auricles of the heart?
1. Umbilical vein
2. Foramen ovale
3. Ductus arteriosus
4. Ductus venosus

3. After birth, which of the following structures receives blood only from the left ventricle?
1. Aorta
2. Inferior vena cava
3. Pulmonary arteries
4. Ductus arteriosus

4. The initial respirations in the newborn are a result of which of the following?
1. A rise in temperature
2. A change in pressure gradients
3. Increased blood pH
4. Decreased blood CO_2 level

5. Which of the following when present in the urine may cause a reddish stain on the diaper of a newborn?
1. Mucus
2. Uric acid crystals
3. Bilirubin
4. Excess iron

6. Which of the following would the nurse identify as correct about the newborn's immune system?
1. The risk of infection in the newborn is relatively low.
2. Phagocytosis occurs fairly rapidly in the newborn.
3. The newborn is unable to limit invading organisms at their point of entry.
4. Immunoglobulin A (IgA) is present in the GI and respiratory tracts.

7. When assessing the newborn's heart rate, which of the following ranges would be considered normal if the newborn were sleeping?
1. 80 beats per minute
2. 100 beats per minute
3. 120 beats per minute
4. 140 beats per minute

8. Which of the following is true regarding the fontanels of the newborn?
1. The anterior is triangle-shaped; the posterior is diamond-shaped.
2. The posterior closes at 18 months; the anterior closes at 8 to 12 weeks.
3. The anterior is larger in size when compared to the posterior fontanel.
4. The anterior is bulging; the posterior appears sunken.

9. Which of the following groups of newborn reflexes are present at birth and remain unchanged through adulthood?
1. Blink, cough, rooting, and gag
2. Blink, cough, sneeze, and gag
3. Rooting, sneeze, swallowing, and cough
4. Stepping, blink, cough, and sneeze

10. Which of the following describes the Babinski reflex?
1. The newborn's toes will hyperextend and fan apart from dorsiflexion of the big toe when one side of foot is stroked upward

from the heel and across the ball of the foot.
2. The newborn abducts and flexes all extremities and may begin to cry when exposed to sudden movement or loud noise.
3. The newborn turns his head in the direction of stimulus, opens his mouth, and begins to suck when cheek, lip, or corner of mouth is touched
4. The newborn will attempt to crawl forward with both arms and legs when he is placed on his abdomen on a flat surface.

11. Which of the following laboratory test results would the nurse consider as abnormal?
1. Hemoglobin, 16 g/dl
2. White blood cell count, 15,000/mm^3
3. Platelets, 75,000/mm^3
4. Red blood cell count, 5.6 million/mm^3

12. The first period of reactivity in the newborn begins at birth. Which of the following are characteristic of this period?
Select all that apply:
1. This period lasts about 30 minutes.
2. The infant is awake and alert.
3. A strong suck is present.
4. Respirations may be increased to 80/minute.
5. Flaring of nares and grunting are common.
6. Bowel sounds are present.

Answer key

1. The answer is 3.
In the initial postpartum period, one of the goals of newborn care is to identify actual and potential problems that might require immediate attention. Other goals include establishing and maintaining an airway and supporting respirations, maintaining warmth and preventing hypothermia, and ensuring safety and preventing injury or infection. Continuing-care goals include facilitating the development of a close parent-newborn relationship, assisting parents to develop healthy attitudes, and providing parents with information about well-baby programs. All of these tasks should be carried out only after the initial goals are met.

2. The answer is 2.
The foramen ovale is an opening between the right and left auricles (atria) that should close shortly after birth so the newborn will not have a murmur or mixed blood traveling through the vascular system. The umbilical vein, ductus arteriosus, and ductus venosus are obliterated at birth.

3. The answer is 1.
Before birth, the aorta carries blood from both of the ventricles. After birth, the aorta receives blood from the left ventricle. The inferior vena cava empties into the right auricle. The pulmonary arteries carry blood to the lungs. The ductus arteriosus is obliterated after birth.

4. The answer is 2.
Initial respirations are triggered by physical, sensory, and chemical factors. Physical factors include the change in pressure gradients. Sensory factors include a drop in temperature, noise, light, and sound. Chemical factors include the decreased oxygen level, increased carbon dioxide level, and decreased pH as a result of the transitory asphyxia that occurs during delivery.

5. The answer is 2.
Uric acid crystals in the urine may produce the reddish "brick dust" stain on the diaper. Mucus would not produce a stain. Bilirubin and iron are from hepatic adaptation.

6. The answer is 3.
The newborn cannot limit the invading organism at the port of entry. In addition, the newborn's risk of infection is increased significantly because of the immaturity of a number of the protective systems. Phago-

cytosis is sluggish and IgA is absent in the respiratory and urinary tracts (unless the newborn is breast-fed) and the GI tract.

7. The answer is 2.
The normal heart rate for a newborn that is sleeping is about 100 beats per minute. If the newborn were awake, the normal heart rate would range from 120 to 160 beats per minute.

8. The answer is 3.
The anterior fontanel is larger than the posterior fontanel. Additionally, the anterior fontanel, which is diamond-shaped, closes at 18 months, whereas the posterior fontanel, which is triangle-shaped, closes at 8 to 12 weeks. Neither fontanel should appear bulging, which may indicate increased intracranial pressure, or sunken, which may indicate dehydration.

9. The answer is 2.
Blink, cough, sneeze, swallowing, and gag reflexes are all present at birth and remain unchanged through adulthood. Reflexes such as rooting and stepping subside within the first year.

10. The answer is 1.
With the Babinski reflex, the newborn's toes hyperextend and fan apart from dorsiflexion of the big toe when one side of the foot is stroked upward from the heel and across the ball of the foot. With the startle reflex, the newborn abducts and flexes all extremities and may begin to cry when exposed to sudden movement or loud noise. With the rooting and sucking reflex, the newborn turns his head in the direction of stimulus, opens his mouth, and begins to suck when the cheek, lip, or corner of mouth is touched. With the crawl reflex, the newborn will attempt to crawl forward with both arms and legs when he is placed on his abdomen on a flat surface.

11. The answer is 3.
Normally, neonatal platelets should range from 150,000 to 350,000/mm^3. Thus, a platelet level of 75,000/mm^3 would be abnormal. A hemoglobin level of 16 g/dl, white blood cell count of 15,000/mm^3, and a red blood cell count of 5.6 million/mm^3 are within acceptable normal ranges.

12. The answer is 1, 2, 3, 4, 5.
Immediately after birth the infant is awake and alert and his eyes are open. A strong sucking reflex is present and the newborn may appear hungry. Bursts of random movement alternating with immobility are likely. The heart rate is rapid and irregular. Respirations may be as high as 80/minute accompanied by grunting and nasal flaring. This first period of reactivity lasts about 30 minutes after birth. It is an optimum opportunity for the mother to begin breast-feeding. Bowel sounds are usually absent at this time.

12 Antepartum Complications

I. ESSENTIAL CONCEPTS

A. Although most pregnancies progress to successful delivery without complications, various factors can alter the physiologic processes of pregnancy and compromise the well-being of the mother or the developing fetus.

B. These complications may occur at any time during pregnancy and can result from preexisting maternal medical problems or from the pregnancy itself.

C. Significant complications of pregnancy include:

1. Spontaneous abortion
2. Gestational trophoblastic disease (hydatidiform mole)
3. Ectopic pregnancy
4. Incompetent cervix
5. Hyperemesis gravidarum
6. Anemia
7. Placenta previa
8. Abruptio placentae
9. Preeclampsia and eclampsia
10. Gestational diabetes
11. Hemolytic disease of the fetus and newborn
12. Infections

D. Maternal conditions that can significantly affect the fetus or the progress of pregnancy include diabetes mellitus, cardiac disease, hypertensive disease, hematologic disorders (such as anemia or hemoglobinopathies), infections, sexually transmitted diseases, smoking, and substance abuse.

E. Major goals of prenatal nursing are screening for, and preventing, complications and developing therapeutic interventions.

F. Early and consistent prenatal care results in improved fetal and maternal outcome, regardless of complications that may occur. Evaluate each pregnancy to identify at-risk clients as early as possible. Remember that risk assessments must be updated throughout the pregnancy because a gestation categorized as low risk initially may become high risk later.

NURSING PROCESS OVERVIEW

II. ANTEPARTUM COMPLICATIONS

A. Assessment

1. Health history

a. Elicit a description of symptoms, including onset, duration, location, and precipitating factors, if known. Cardinal signs and symptoms of antepartum complications may include (*Client and Family Teaching* 12-1):

- Dizziness
- Nausea and vomiting
- Headache
- Fatigue
- Abdominal pain or cramping
- Uterine contractions before the end of week 37 of gestation

CLIENT AND FAMILY TEACHING 12-1

Antepartum danger signs and symptoms to report immediately

Instruct the client to report the following signs and symptoms to her health care provider immediately.

Sign or symptom	Possible indication
Sudden gush of fluid from the vagina	Rupture of membranes, impending labor, or route for infection
Spotting or bleeding from the vagina	Labor, placenta previa, abruptio placentae, ectopic pregnancy, or hydatidiform mole
Headache with visual disturbance, epigastric pain, swelling of hands and face, or sudden weight gain	Pregnancy-induced hypertension, preeclampsia, or eclampsia
Uterine pain	Labor, abruptio placentae, and urinary tract infection
Fever, rash, malaise, or other flulike symptoms	Infection by an organism
Unusual, foul-smelling, or purulent discharge from the vagina	Infection by an organism
Pain on urination, frequency of urination, and backache	Urinary tract infection
Family history of diabetes, dizziness, confusion, thirst, glycosuria, or polyuria	Diabetes mellitus
Exposure to a communicable disease	Possible infection by an organism
Sudden lower abdominal pain, minimal vaginal bleeding, confusion, pallor, rapid pulse, or severe shoulder pain	Possible ectopic pregnancy

b. Explore personal and family history for risk factors for antepartum complications.

2. **Physical examination**

a. **Vital signs**
- Measure weight for excessive loss or gain.
- Measure for increased blood pressure.
- Measure for rapid pulse.
- Measure for increased temperature.

b. **Inspection**
- Assess for vaginal bleeding.
- Inspect for premature rupture of the membranes (PROM).
- Assess the skin for rash; pale, dry skin; or edema.
- Inspect the oral cavity for overall dental health and signs of poor nutrition (such as rough, tender tongue; fissures at the corners of the mouth; pale mucous membrane; and swollen or inflamed gingiva).

c. **Palpation**
- Palpate the uterus to determine whether it is abnormally soft or hard, and whether it is larger or smaller than expected for gestational age.
- Palpate the cervix to detect preterm cervical dilation.

d. **Auscultate** the fetal heart rate (FHR) to detect abnormally fast or slow rates.

3. **Laboratory studies and diagnostic tests**
   a. A **complete blood count** is the most routinely performed test in the laboratory. It provides information about the number, type, and health of red blood cells (RBCs) and white blood cells, and the hematocrit and hemoglobin value.
   b. A **pregnancy test** (human chorionic gonadotropin [hCG]) may be performed on maternal urine or serum. A positive test indicates that a pregnancy probably exists. There are other factors that can yield a positive test result (medications, tumors, premature menopause, and blood in the urine).
   c. **Serum alpha-fetoprotein measurement.** Alpha-fetoprotein is the predominant protein in fetal plasma. A small amount crosses the placental barrier into the maternal serum, and some is excreted into the amniotic fluid. Therefore, it can be measured in maternal serum or in amniotic fluid. An abnormal concentration of alpha-fetoprotein in either amniotic fluid or maternal serum is associated with such fetal anomalies as open neural tube defects (anencephaly and spina bifida).
   d. **Ultrasound** refers to the use of high-frequency sound waves passed through the maternal abdomen. These sound waves are deflected by fetal structures and allow visualization of fetal movement, fetal heart movement, and respiratory effort. They can also be used throughout pregnancy to determine fetal age, visualize the placenta, and locate pockets of amniotic fluid for amniocentesis.
   e. **Blood glucose and glycosolated hemoglobin.** A blood glucose test indicates the concentration of glucose in the blood, represented in milligrams of glucose per deciliter of blood. Glycosolated hemoglobin measures the amount of glucose attached to hemoglobin. It reflects the average blood glucose level over the past 4 to 6 weeks and is usually reported as a single digit.
   f. The **indirect Coombs' test** is used in the search for agglutination of Rh-positive RBCs to determine whether antibodies are present in maternal blood. It is used to anticipate hemolytic disease of the newborn.
   g. **Amniocentesis** refers to aspiration of a sample of amniotic fluid for examination of fetal cells. This may be used to determine chromosomal abnormalities or fetal lung maturity, or to diagnose fetal hemolytic disease.
   h. **Serologic tests** are used to determine the presence and type of sexually transmitted diseases.
   i. **Cultures** are disease and site specific, and are used to determine the type of infectious agent present and to identify medications to which these agents are susceptible.

B. Nursing diagnoses. (Both general and complication-specific are listed. Planning and outcome identification, implementation, and outcome evaluation are focused on general diagnoses.)

1. **General diagnoses**
   a. Pain
   b. Anxiety
   c. Fear
   d. Ineffective Individual Coping
   e. Ineffective Family Coping: Compromised
   f. Altered Family Processes
   g. Powerlessness
   h. Knowledge Deficit
   i. Noncompliance

2. **Complication-specific diagnoses**
   a. Fluid Volume Deficit
   b. Anticipatory Grieving
   c. Dysfunctional Grieving
   d. Risk for Infection
   e. Situational Low Self-Esteem
   f. Altered Nutrition: Less Than Body Requirements
   g. Altered Nutrition: More Than Body Requirements
   h. Constipation
   i. Activity Intolerance
   j. Decreased Cardiac Output
   k. Altered Tissue Perfusion: Uteroplacental

C. Planning and outcome identification

1. The client and fetus (if applicable) will make a full recovery and will not develop additional complications.
2. The client and family will express their fears and anxieties, and will exhibit functional grieving.
3. The client and family will understand the complication and treatment regimen.
4. The client and family will comply with the treatment regimen.

D. Implementation

1. **Ensure that appropriate physical needs are addressed and monitor for additional complications.**
   a. Assist the woman in planning for adequate rest, activity, and nutrition.
   b. Assist the couple in setting realistic goals based on the mother's health and the restrictions required by the complication.
2. **Address emotional and psychosocial needs.**
   a. Assess the client's feeling about herself and the pregnancy and assist the woman in maintaining her self-esteem.
   b. Encourage verbalization of any grief, loss, and potential guilt feelings.
   c. Offer emotional support to the client and her family as they go through a normal grieving process due to a crisis to their pregnancy, or a loss of their pregnancy.
   d. Evaluate the client and her family's support system.
   e. Assess for an appropriate coping response.
3. **Provide client and family teaching.**
   a. Provide information about the actual complication and the expected outcome, if possible.
   b. Instruct the couple about specific signs and symptoms to report.
   c. Provide printed instructions on various self-care measures (such as use of medications, dietary and activity restrictions, and rest) to manage the existing problem and prevent additional complications.
   d. Explain the need, purpose, and procedure for various diagnostic tests.
4. **Promote compliance.**
   a. Allow for choice among alternative treatments when possible.
   b. Include the partner and other family members in decision-making when possible.

E. Outcome evaluation

1. The client and fetus (if applicable) recover fully and do not develop additional complications.
2. The client and family express their fears and anxieties, and exhibit functional grieving.

3. The client and family understand the complications and treatment regimen.
4. The client and family comply with the treatment regimen.

III. SPONTANEOUS ABORTION

A. Description

1. Spontaneous abortion is the expulsion of the fetus and other products of conception from the uterus before the fetus is capable of living outside of the uterus.
2. Types of spontaneous abortions
   a. A threatened abortion is characterized by cramping and vaginal bleeding in early pregnancy with no cervical dilation. It may subside or an incomplete abortion may follow.
   b. An imminent or inevitable abortion is characterized by bleeding, cramping, and cervical dilation. Termination cannot be prevented.
   c. An incomplete abortion is characterized by expulsion of only part of the products of conception (usually the fetus). Bleeding occurs with cervical dilation.
   d. A complete abortion is characterized by complete expulsion of all products of conception.
   e. A missed abortion is characterized by early fetal intrauterine death without expulsion of the products of conception. The cervix is closed, and the client may report dark brown vaginal discharge. Pregnancy test findings are negative.
   f. Recurrent (habitual) abortion is spontaneous abortion of three or more consecutive pregnancies.

B. Etiology.

Spontaneous abortion may result from unidentified natural causes or from fetal, placental, or maternal factors.

1. **Fetal factors**
   a. Defective embryologic development
   b. Faulty ovum implantation
   c. Rejection of the ovum by the endometrium
   d. Chromosomal abnormalities
2. **Placental factors**
   a. Premature separation of the normally implanted placenta
   b. Abnormal placental implantation
   c. Abnormal placental function
3. **Maternal factors**
   a. Infection
   b. Severe malnutrition
   c. Reproductive system abnormalities (such as incompetent cervix)
   d. Endocrine problems (such as thyroid dysfunction)
   e. Trauma
   f. Drug ingestion

C. Pathophysiology.

The fetal or placental defect or the maternal condition results in the disruption of blood flow, containing oxygen and nutrients, to the developing fetus. The fetus is compromised and subsequently expelled from the uterus.

D. Assessment findings

1. **Associated findings.** The client and family may exhibit a grief reaction at the loss of pregnancy, including:

   a. Crying
   b. Depression
   c. Sustained or prolonged social isolation
   d. Withdrawal
2. **Clinical manifestations** include common signs and symptoms of spontaneous abortion.
   a. Vaginal bleeding in the first 20 weeks of pregnancy
   b. Complaints of cramping in the lower abdomen
   c. Fever, malaise, or other symptoms of infection
3. **Laboratory and diagnostic study findings**
   a. Serum beta hCG levels are quantitatively low.
   b. Ultrasound reveals the absence of a viable fetus.

E. Implementation

1. Provide appropriate management and prevent complications.
   a. Assess and record vital signs, bleeding, and cramping or pain.
   b. Measure and record intravenous fluids, and laboratory test results. In instances of heavy vaginal bleeding, prepare for surgical intervention (D&C) if indicated.
   c. Prepare for RhoGAM administration to an Rh-negative mother, as prescribed. Whenever the placenta is dislodged (birth, D&C, abruption) some of the fetal blood may enter maternal circulation. If the woman is Rh-negative, enough fetal Rh-positive blood cells may enter her circulation to cause isoimmunization, the production of antibodies against Rh-positive blood, thus endangering the well-being of future pregnancies. Because the blood type of the conceptus is not known, all women with Rh-negative blood should receive RhoGAM after an abortion (see *Drug Chart* 10-1, page 154).
   d. Recommend iron supplements and increased dietary iron as indicated to help prevent anemia.
2. Provide client and family teaching.
   a. Offer anticipatory guidance relative to expected recovery, the need for rest, and delay of another pregnancy until the client fully recovers.
   b. Suggest avoiding intercourse until after the next menses or using condoms when engaging in intercourse.
   c. Explain that in many cases, no cause for the spontaneous abortion is ever identified.
3. Address emotional and psychosocial needs.

IV. GESTATIONAL TROPHOBLASTIC DISEASE (HYDATIDIFORM MOLE)

A. Description

1. Hydatidiform mole is an alteration of early embryonic growth causing placental disruption, rapid proliferation of abnormal cells, and destruction of the embryo.
2. There are two distinct types of hydatidiform moles — complete and partial.
   a. In a complete mole, the chromosomes are either 46XX or 46XY but are contributed by only one parent and the chromosome material is duplicated. This type usually leads to choriocarcinoma.
   b. A partial mole has 69 chromosomes. There are three chromosomes for every pair instead of two. This type of mole rarely leads to choriocarcinoma.

B. Etiology. The etiology of hydatidiform moles is unknown. Genetic, ovular, or nutritional abnormalities could be responsible for trophoblastic disease.

C. Pathophysiology

1. A hydatidiform mole is a placental tumor that develops after pregnancy has occurred; it may be benign or malignant. The risk of malignancy is greater with a complete mole.
2. The embryo dies and the trophoblastic cells continue to grow, forming an invasive tumor.
3. It is characterized by proliferation of placental villi that become edematous and form grapelike clusters. The fluid-filled vesicles grow rapidly, causing the uterus to be larger than expected for the duration of pregnancy.
4. Blood vessels are absent, as are a fetus and an amniotic sac.

D. Assessment findings

1. **Clinical manifestations**
   a. Vaginal bleeding (may contain some of the edematous villi)
   b. Uterus larger than expected for the duration of the pregnancy
   c. Abdominal cramping from uterine distention
   d. Signs and symptoms of preeclampsia before 20 weeks' gestation
   e. Severe nausea and vomiting
2. **Laboratory and diagnostic study findings**
   a. hCG serum levels are abnormally high.
   b. Ultrasound reveals characteristic appearance of molar growth.

E. Nursing management

1. **Ensure physical well-being of the client through accurate assessment and interventions.**
   a. Review pertinent history and history of this pregnancy.
   b. Prepare for suction curettage evacuation of the uterus (induction of labor with oxytocic agents or prostaglandins is not recommended because of the increased risk of hemorrhage).
   c. Administer intravenous fluids as prescribed.
2. Provide client and family teaching.
   a. Ensure appropriate follow-up and self-care by explaining that frequent follow-up physical and pelvic examinations are necessary to assess the possibility of recurrence of the problem or progression to choriocarcinoma. Also explain that hCG levels should be monitored for 1 year.
   b. Discuss the need to prevent pregnancy for at least 1 year after diagnosis and treatment.
   c. Inform the client that hormonal birth control agents are not recommended because they suppress pituitary luteinizing hormone, which may interfere with serum hCG measurement.
   d. Describe and emphasize signs and symptoms that must be reported (irregular vaginal bleeding, persistent secretion from the breast, hemoptysis, and severe persistent headaches). These symptoms may indicate spread of the disease to other organs.
3. Address emotional and psychosocial needs.

V. ECTOPIC PREGNANCY

A. Description. Implantation of products of conception in a site other than the uterine cavity (such as fallopian tube, ovary, cervix, or peritoneal cavity)

B. Etiology. Ectopic pregnancy can result from conditions that hinder ovum passage through the fallopian tube and into the uterine cavity, such as:

1. Salpingitis
2. Diverticula
3. Tumors
4. Adhesions from previous surgery
5. Transmigration of the ovum from one ovary to the opposite fallopian tube

C. Pathophysiology. The uterus is the only organ capable of containing and sustaining a pregnancy. When the fertilized ovum implants in other locations, the body is unable to maintain the pregnancy.

D. Assessment findings

1. **Associated findings**
   a. Suspect ectopic pregnancy in a client whose history includes a missed menstrual period, spotting or bleeding, pelvic or shoulder pain, use of intrauterine device, pelvic infections, tubal surgery, or previous ectopic pregnancy.
   b. Be aware of grief and loss behaviors in the client and family.
2. Common **clinical manifestations.** (The client with ectopic pregnancy may report signs and symptoms of a normal pregnancy or may have no symptoms at all.)
   a. Dizziness and syncope (faintness)
   b. Sharp abdominal pain and referred shoulder pain
   c. Vaginal bleeding
   d. Adnexal mass and tenderness
   e. A ruptured fallopian tube can produce life-threatening complications, such as hemorrhage, shock, and peritonitis.
3. **Laboratory and diagnostic study findings**
   a. Blood samples for hemoglobin value, blood type and group, and crossmatching.
   b. A pregnancy test reveals elevated serum quantitative beta hCG.
   c. Ultrasound will confirm extrauterine pregnancy.

E. Nursing management

1. **Ensure that appropriate physical needs are addressed and monitor** for complications. Assess vital signs, bleeding, and pain.
2. **Provide client and family teaching to relieve anxiety.**
   a. Explain the condition and expected outcome.
      - Maternal prognosis is good with early diagnosis and prompt treatment such as laparotomy to ligate bleeding vessels and repair or remove the damaged fallopian tube.
      - Pharmacologic agents, such as methotrexate followed by leucovorin, may be given orally when ectopic pregnancy is diagnosed by routine sonogram before the tube has ruptured. A hysterosalpingogram usually follows this therapy to confirm tubal patency.
      - Rh-negative women must receive RhoGAM to provide protection from isoimmunization for future pregnancies (see *Drug Chart* 10-1, page 154).

b. Describe self-care measures, which depend on the treatment.

3. **Address emotional and psychosocial needs.**

VI. INCOMPETENT CERVIX

A. Description

1. Incompetent cervix is characterized by a painless dilation of the cervical os without contractions of the uterus.
2. Incompetent cervix commonly occurs at about the 20th week of pregnancy.

B. Etiology

1. History of traumatic birth
2. Repeated dilatation and curettage
3. Client's mother treated with diethylstilbestrol when pregnant with the client
4. Congenitally short cervix
5. Uterine anomalies
6. Unknown etiology

C. Pathophysiology. The connective tissue structure of the cervix is not strong enough to maintain closure of the cervical os during pregnancy.

D. Assessment findings

1. **Associated findings**
   a. History of cervical trauma
   b. History of repeated, spontaneous, second trimester terminations
   c. Possibly spontaneous rupture of the membranes
2. A common **clinical manifestation** is appreciable cervical dilation with prolapse of the membranes through the cervix without contractions.

E. Nursing management

1. **Provide client and family teaching.** Describe problems that must be reported immediately (pink-tinged vaginal discharge, increased pelvic pressure, and rupture of the membranes).
2. **Maintain an environment to preserve the integrity of the pregnancy.**
   a. Prepare for cervical cerclage, if appropriate.
   b. Maintain activity restrictions as prescribed.
   c. Discuss the need for vaginal rest (no intercourse or orgasm)
3. **Prepare for the birth if membranes are ruptured.**
4. Address emotional and psychosocial needs.

VII. HYPEREMESIS GRAVIDARUM

A. Description. Hyperemesis gravidarum is severe and excessive nausea and vomiting during pregnancy, which leads to electrolyte, metabolic, and nutritional imbalances in the absence of other medical problems.

B. Etiology. The etiology of hyperemesis gravidarum is obscure. Suggested causative factors include:

1. High levels of hCG in early pregnancy
2. Metabolic or nutritional deficiencies
3. More common in unmarried white women and first pregnancies

4. Ambivalence toward the pregnancy or family-related stress
5. Thyroid dysfunction

C. Pathophysiology

1. Continued vomiting results in dehydration and ultimately decreases the amount of blood and nutrients circulated to the developing fetus.
2. Hospitalization may be required for severe symptoms when the client needs intravenous hydration and correction of metabolic imbalances.

D. Assessment findings. Signs and symptoms occur during the first 16 weeks of pregnancy and are intractable.

1. **Clinical manifestations** include:
   a. Unremitting nausea and vomiting
   b. Vomitus initially containing undigested food, bile, and mucus; later containing blood and material that resembles coffee grounds
   c. Weight loss
2. Other common signs and symptoms include:
   a. Pale, dry skin
   b. Rapid pulse
   c. Fetid, fruity breath odor from acidosis
   d. Central nervous system effects, such as confusion, delirium, headache, and lethargy, stupor, or coma

E. Nursing management

1. **Promote resolution of the complication.**
   a. Make sure the client receives nothing by mouth until cessation of vomiting
   b. Administer intravenous fluids as prescribed; they may be given on an ambulatory basis when dehydration is mild.
   c. Measure and record fluid intake and output.
   d. Encourage small frequent meals and snacks once vomiting has subsided.
   e. Administer antiemetics as prescribed.
2. **Address emotional and psychosocial needs.** Maintain a nonjudgmental atmosphere in which the client and family can express concerns and resolve some of their fears.

VIII. ANEMIA

A. Description

1. Hemoglobin value of less than 11 mg/dl or hematocrit value less than 33% during the second and third trimesters
2. Mild anemia (hemoglobin value of 11 mg/dl) poses no threat but is an indication of a less than optimal nutritional state.
3. Iron deficiency anemia is the most common anemia of pregnancy, affecting 15% to 50% of pregnant women. It is identified as physiologic anemia of pregnancy.

B. Etiology. Causes of anemia include:

1. Nutritional deficiency (such as iron deficiency or megaloblastic anemia, which includes folic acid deficiency and B_{12} deficiency)
2. Acute and chronic blood loss
3. Hemolysis (such as sickle cell anemia, thalassemia, or glucose-6-phosphate dehydrogenase [G6PD])

C. Pathophysiology

1. The hemoglobin level for nonpregnant women is usually 13.5 g/dl. However, the hemoglobin level during the second trimester of pregnancy averages 11.6 g/dl as a result of the dilution of the mother's blood from increased plasma volume. This is called *physiologic anemia* and is normal during pregnancy.
2. Iron cannot be adequately supplied in the daily diet during pregnancy. Substances in the diet, such as milk, tea, and coffee, decrease absorption of iron. During pregnancy, additional iron is required for the increase in maternal RBCs and for transfer to the fetus for storage and production of RBCs. The fetus must store enough iron to last 4 to 6 months after birth.
3. During the third trimester, if the woman's intake of iron is not sufficient, her hemoglobin level will not rise to a value of 12.5 g/dl and nutritional anemia may occur. This will result in decreased transfer of iron to the fetus.
4. Hemoglobinopathies, such as thalassemia, sickle cell disease, and G6PD, lead to anemia by causing hemolysis or increased destruction of RBCs.

D. Assessment findings

1. **Associated findings.** In clients with a hemoglobin level of 10.5 g/dl, expect complaints of excessive fatigue, headache, and tachycardia.
2. **Clinical manifestations**
   a. Signs of iron deficiency anemia (hemoglobin level below 10.5 g/dl) include brittle fingernails, cheilosis (severely chapped lips), or a smooth, red, shiny tongue.
   b. Women with sickle cell anemia experience painful crisis episodes.

E. Nursing management

1. **Provide client and family teaching. Discuss using iron supplements and increasing dietary sources of iron as indicated.**
2. Prepare for blood typing and crossmatching, and for administering packed RBCs during labor if the client has severe anemia.
3. Provide support and management for clients with hemoglobinopathies.
   a. In a client who has thalassemia or who carries the trait, provide support, especially if the woman has just learned that she is a carrier. Also assess for signs of infection throughout the pregnancy.
   b. In a pregnant client with sickle cell disease, assess iron and folate stores and reticulocyte counts; complete screening for hemolysis; provide dietary counseling and folic acid supplements; and observe for signs of infection.
   c. In a pregnant client with G6PD, provide iron and folic acid supplementation and nutrition counseling, and explain the need to avoid oxidizing drugs.

IX. PLACENTA PREVIA

A. Description

1. The placenta implants in the lower uterine segment, near the cervical os. The degree to which it covers the os leads to three different classifications.
   a. Total placenta previa occurs when the placenta completely covers the internal os.
   b. Partial placenta previa occurs when the placenta partially covers the internal os.
   c. Low-lying or low-implantation placenta previa occurs when the placental border reaches the border of the internal os.
2. The incidence of placenta previa is three to six per 1,000 deliveries.

B. Etiology. Predisposing factors include:

1. Multiparity (80% of affected clients are multiparous)
2. Advanced maternal age (older than age 35 in 33% of cases)
3. Multiple gestation
4. Previous cesarean birth
5. Uterine incisions
6. Prior placenta previa (incidence is 12 times greater in women with previous placenta previa)

C. Pathophysiology

1. Pathologic process seems to be related to the conditions that alter the normal function of the uterine decidua and its vascularization.
2. Bleeding, which results from tearing of the placental villi from the uterine wall as the lower uterine segment contracts and dilates, can be slight or profuse.

D. Assessment findings

1. Associated findings. In cases of suspected placenta previa, a vaginal examination is delayed until ultrasound results are available and the client is moved to the operating room for what is termed a double-set-up procedure. The operating room is needed because the examination can cause further tearing of the villi and hemorrhage, which can be fatal to the client and fetus.
2. Common **clinical manifestations** include:
   a. Bright red, painless vaginal bleeding
   b. Soft, nontender abdomen; relaxes between contractions, if present.
   c. FHR stable and within normal limits
3. **Laboratory and diagnostic study findings.** Transabdominal ultrasonography confirms suspicion of placenta previa.

E. Nursing management

1. **Ensure the physiologic well-being of the client and fetus.**
   a. Take and record vital signs, assess bleeding, and maintain a perineal pad count. Weigh perineal pads before and after use to estimate blood loss.
   b. Observe for shock, which is characterized by a rapid pulse, pallor, cold moist skin, and a drop in blood pressure.
   c. Monitor the FHR.
   d. Enforce strict bed rest to minimize risk to the fetus.
   e. Observe for additional bleeding episodes.
2. Provide client and family teaching
   a. Explain the condition and management options. To ensure an adequate blood supply to the mother and fetus, place the woman at bed rest in a side-lying position. Anticipate the order for a sonogram to localize the placenta. If the condition of mother or fetus deteriorates, a cesarean birth will be required.
   b. Prepare the client for ambulation and discharge (may be within 48 hours of last bleeding episode).
   c. Discuss the need to have transportation to the hospital available at all times.
   d. Instruct the client to return to the hospital if bleeding recurs and to avoid intercourse until after the birth.
   e. Instruct the client on proper handwashing and toileting to prevent infection.
3. Address emotional and psychosocial needs.
   a. Offer emotional support to facilitate the grieving process, if needed.

b. After birth of the newborn, provide frequent visits with the newborn so that mother can be certain of the infant's condition.

X. ABRUPTIO PLACENTAE

A. Description. Abruptio placentae is premature separation of a normally implanted placenta after the 20th week of pregnancy, typically with severe hemorrhage.

B. Etiology

1. The cause of abruptio placentae is unknown.
2. Risk factors include:
   a. Uterine anomalies
   b. Multiparity
   c. Preeclampsia
   d. Previous cesarean birth
   e. Renal or vascular disease
   f. Trauma to the abdomen
   g. Previous third trimester bleeding
   h. Abnormally large placenta
   i. Short umbilical cord

C. Pathophysiology. The placenta detaches in whole or in part from the implantation site. This occurs in the area of the decidua basalis.

D. Assessment findings

1. **Associated findings.** Severe abruptio placentae may produce such complications as:
   a. Renal failure
   b. Disseminated intravascular coagulation
   c. Maternal and fetal death
2. Common **clinical manifestations** include:
   a. Intense, localized uterine pain, with or without vaginal bleeding.
   b. Concealed or external dark red bleeding
   c. Uterus firm to boardlike, with severe continuous pain
   d. Uterine contractions
   e. Uterine outline possibly enlarged or changing shape
   f. FHR present or absent
   g. Fetal presenting part may be engaged.
3. **Laboratory and diagnostic study findings.** Ultrasound may be able to identify the extent of abruption. However, the absence of an ultrasound finding does not rule out the presence of abruption.

E. Nursing management

1. **Continuously evaluate maternal and fetal physiologic status, particularly:**
   a. Vital signs
   b. Bleeding
   c. Electronic fetal and maternal monitoring tracings
   d. Signs of shock — rapid pulse, pallor, cold and moist skin, decrease in blood pressure
   e. Decreasing urine output
   f. Never perform a vaginal or rectal examination or take any action that would stimulate uterine activity.

2. **Assess the need for immediate delivery.** If the client is in active labor and bleeding cannot be stopped with bed rest, emergency cesarean birth may be indicated.
3. **Provide appropriate management**
   a. On admission, place the woman on bed rest in a lateral position to prevent pressure on the vena cava.
   b. Insert a large-gauge intravenous catheter into a large vein for fluid replacement. Obtain a blood sample for fibrinogen level.
   c. Monitor the FHR externally and measure maternal vital signs every 5 to 15 minutes. Administer oxygen to the mother by mask.
   d. Prepare for cesarean birth, which is the method of choice.
4. Provide client and family teaching.
5. Address emotional and psychosocial needs. Outcome for the mother and fetus depends on the extent of the separation, amount of fetal hypoxia, and amount of bleeding.

XI. PREGNANCY-INDUCED HYPERTENSION (PIH; PREECLAMPSIA AND ECLAMPSIA)

A. Description

1. **Preeclampsia** is a hypertensive disorder of pregnancy developing after 20 weeks' gestation and characterized by edema, hypertension, and proteinuria.
2. **Eclampsia** is an extension of preeclampsia and is characterized by the onset of seizure activity.

B. Etiology

1. The cause of preeclampsia is unknown.
2. Possible contributing factors include:
   a. Genetic or immunologic
   b. Primigravid status
   c. Conditions that create excess trophoblastic tissue, such as multiple gestation, diabetes, or hydatidiform mole.
   d. Age younger than 18 or older than 35

C. Pathophysiology.

Preeclampsia is a multisystem, vasospastic disease process characterized by hemoconcentration, hypertension, and proteinuria.

D. Assessment findings

1. **Clinical manifestations of mild preeclampsia**
   a. Blood pressure exceeding 140/90 mm Hg; or increase above baseline of 30 mm Hg in systolic pressure or 15 mm Hg in diastolic pressure on two readings taken 6 hours apart
   b. Generalized edema in the face, hands, and ankles (a classic sign)
   c. Weight gain of about 1.5 kg (3.3 lb) per month in the second trimester or more than 1.3 to 2.3 kg (3 to 5 lb) per week in the third trimester
   d. Proteinuria 1+ to 2+, or 300 mg/dl, in a 24 hour sample
2. Warning signs of worsening preeclampsia
   a. Rapid rise in blood pressure
   b. Rapid weight gain
   c. Generalized edema
   d. Increased proteinuria

TABLE 12-1
Significant laboratory findings in PIH

Test	Findings
Blood	
Hematocrit	37%–47%
Renal function	
Serum uric acid	4.5–6 mg/dl > 10 mg/dl (severe pregnancy-induced hypertension [PIH])
Creatinine	< 1 mg/dl 2–3 mg/dl (severe PIH)
Creatinine clearance	>130–180 ml/min
BUN	< 10 mg/dl 10–16 mg/dl (severe PIH)
Coagulation	
Platelets	< 150,000 ml (severe PIH)
Fibrin degradation products	Absent

From Lowdermilk, D. & Perry S. (2004). *Maternity and Women's Healthcare.* 8th ed. St. Louis: Mosby, p. 844.

e. Epigastric pain, marked hyperreflexia, and severe headache, which usually precede convulsions in eclampsia
f. Visual disturbances
g. Oliguria (less than120 ml in 4 hours)
h. Irritability
i. Severe nausea and vomiting

3. **Clinical manifestations of severe preeclampsia**
   a. Blood pressure exceeding 160/110 mm Hg noted on two readings taken 6 hours apart with the client on bed rest
   b. Proteinuria exceeding 5 g/24 hours
   c. Oliguria (less than 400 ml/24 hours)
   d. Headache
   e. Blurred vision, spots before eyes, and retinal edema
   f. Pitting edema of the sacrum, face, and upper extremities
   g. Dyspnea
   h. Epigastric pain
   i. Nausea and vomiting
   j. Hyperreflexia
4. **Eclampsia** exists once the patient has experienced a grand mal seizure. The patient may progress to more serious complications, such as cerebral hemorrhage, liver rupture, and coma.
5. **Laboratory and diagnostic study findings.** Abnormal test results are provided in *Table* 12-1.

E. Nursing management

1. **Monitor for, and promote the resolution of, complications.**
   a. Monitor vital signs and FHR.
   b. Minimize external stimuli; promote rest and relaxation.
   c. Measure and record urine output, protein level, and specific gravity.
   d. Assess for edema of face, arms, hands, legs, ankles, and feet. Also assess for pulmonary edema.
   e. Weigh the client daily.
   f. Assess deep tendon reflexes every 4 hours.
   g. Assess for placental separation, headache and visual disturbance, epigastric pain, and altered level of consciousness.
2. **Provide treatment as prescribed.**
   a. Mild preeclampsia treatment consists of bed rest in left lateral recumbent position, balanced diet with moderate to high protein and low to moderate sodium, and administration of magnesium sulfate (*Drug Chart* 12-1, page 196).
   b. Severe preeclampsia treatment consists of complete bed rest, balanced diet with high protein and low to moderate sodium, fluid and electrolyte replacements, administration of magnesiuum sulfate and the antihypertensive hydralazine.
   c. Treatment of eclampsia consists of administration of magnesium sulfate and hydralazine as well as sedative anticonvulsants, such as diazepam, phenobarbital, or phenytoin.
3. **Institute seizure precautions.** Seizures may occur up to 72 hours after delivery.
4. The only absolute treatment of preeclampsia and eclampsia is delivery of the infant.
5. Address emotional and psychosocial needs.

XII. GESTATIONAL DIABETES

A. Description

1. Gestational diabetes is abnormal carbohydrate, fat, and protein metabolism that is first diagnosed during pregnancy, regardless of the severity.
2. Gestational diabetes is further classified as:
   a. Gestational diabetes characterized by an abnormal glucose tolerance test (GTT) without other symptoms. Fasting glucose is normal and the diabetes is controlled by diet.
   b. Gestational diabetes characterized by abnormal GTT and elevated fasting glucose. This type of gestational diabetes must be controlled by insulin.
3. About 15,000 infants are born to mothers with diabetes each year. Since 1980, the International Workshop-Conference on Gestational Diabetes and the American Diabetic Association have recommended universal screening for gestational diabetes between 24 and 28 weeks of gestation.

B. Etiology.

Gestational diabetes is a disorder of late pregnancy (typically), caused by the increased pancreatic stimulation associated with pregnancy.

C. Pathophysiology

1. In gestational diabetes mellitus, insulin antagonism by placental hormones, human placental lactogen, progesterone, cortisol, and prolactin leads to increased blood glucose levels. The effect of these hormones peaks at about 26 weeks' gestation. This is called the diabetogenic effect of pregnancy.

DRUG CHART 12-1

Medications used for antepartum complications

Classifications	Used for	Selected interventions
Anticonvulsants sedatives, hypnotics, skeletal muscle relaxants, CNS depressants	Promotes relaxation and rest; prevents seizures; relieves anxiety	▪ Infuse drugs slowly over time. ▪ Always administer as a "piggy back" infusion. ▪ Assess vital signs every 5–15 min. ▪ Assess deep-tendon reflexes every 30–60 min. ▪ Strict intake and output (urine = 30 ml/hr). ▪ Count respirations every 5–15 min (rate at least 12/min). ▪ Strict bed rest ▪ Have Valium and calcium gluconate prepared at bedside for immediate use.
Magnesium sulfate	Prevents seizures and blocks neuromuscular transmission.	▪ Monitor for side effects, including flushing, thirst, absence of deep tendon reflexes, respiratory depression, cardiac arrhythmias, decreased urinary output, or cardiac arrest.
Diazepam (Valium, Vazepam)	Stops seizure activity	▪ Monitor for side effects, including lethargy, blurred vision, respiratory depression, nausea, vomiting, and hypotension.
Electrolytes calcium gluconate 10% (Kalcinate)	Antidote for magnesium intoxication	▪ Monitor for side effects, including syncope, bradycardia, and cardiac arrest.
Antihypertensives hydralazine hydrochloride (Apresoline)	Relaxes arterial smooth muscle to reduce blood pressure	▪ Monitor for side effects, including headache, dizziness, drowsiness, epigastric pain, and hypotension.
diazoxide (Hyperstat)	Peripheral vasodilator; used for severe hypertension	▪ Monitor for side effects, including precipitous drop in blood pressure, tachycardia, angina, hyperglycemia, and sodium and water retention.
Antidiabetics/hormones Insulin injection (Humulin R, Velosulin Human, and Regular—[intermediate and short-acting insulin])	Lowers blood glucose by increasing transport into cells and promoting the conversion of glucose to glycogen; inhibits the release of free fatty acids and promotes the conversion of amino acids to protein in muscle	▪ Take a daily fasting blood glucose level. ▪ Sliding scale coverage based on serum and urinary glucose ▪ Assess for signs and symptoms of hypo- and hyperglycemia. ▪ Educate the client and family about blood testing, self-injection, and dietary restrictions. ▪ Demonstrate mixing two kinds of insulin in the same syringe. ▪ Monitor for side effects, including urticaria, hypoglycemia, allergic reaction, and a local reaction at the injection site.

2. The pancreatic beta cell functions are impaired in response to the increased pancreatic stimulation and induced insulin resistance.
3. Pregnancy complicated by diabetes puts the mother at increased risk for the development of complications, such as spontaneous abortion, hypertensive disorders, preterm labor, infection, and birth complications.

4. The effects of diabetes on the fetus include hypoglycemia, hyperglycemia, and ketoacidosis. Hyperglycemic effects can include:
   a. Congenital defects
   b. Macrosomia
   c. Intrauterine growth restriction
   d. Intrauterine fetal death
   e. Delayed lung maturity
   f. Neonatal hypoglycemia
   g. Neonatal hyperbilirubinemia

D. Assessment findings

1. **Associated findings** include a poor obstetric history, including spontaneous abortions, unexplained stillbirth, unexplained hydramnios, premature birth, low birth weight or birth weight exceeding 4,000 g (8 lb, 13 oz), and birth of a newborn with congenital anomalies.
2. Common clinical manifestations include:
   a. Glycosuria on two successive office visits
   b. Recurrent monilial vaginitis
   c. Macrosomia of the fetus on ultrasound
   d. Polyhydramnios
3. **Laboratory and diagnostic study findings.**
   a. Fasting blood sugar test will reveal elevated blood glucose levels.
   b. A 50-g glucose screen (blood glucose level is measured 1 hour after client ingests a 50-g glucose drink) reveals elevated blood glucose levels. The normal plasma threshold is 130 to 140 mg/dl.
   c. A 3-hour oral glucose tolerance test (performed if 50-g glucose screen results are abnormal) reveals elevated blood glucose levels (*Table* 12-2).
   d. The glycosylated hemoglobin (HbA1c) test (measures glycemic control in the 4 to 6 weeks before the test is performed; performed on women with preexisting diabetes) results reflect enzymatic bonding of glucose to hemoglobin A amino acids. This is a useful indicator of overall blood glucose control. The upper normal level of HbA1c is 6% of total hemoglobin. Women with HbA_1c levels greater than 10% are at the most significant risk for having a fetus with malformations.

TABLE 12-2
Normal glucose tolerance test values for pregnancy

Test timing	Venous plasma	Whole blood
Fasting	95 mg/dl	≤ 95 mg/dl
1 hr	180 mg/dl	≤ 140 mg/dl
2 hr	155 mg/dll	≤ 130 mg/dl
3 hr	140 mg/dl	—

e. Screens for fetal (and later, neonatal) complications, including:
- Maternal serum alpha-fetoprotein level to assess risk of neural tube defects in newborn.
- Ultrasonography to detect fetal structural anomalies, macrosomia, and hydramnios.
- Nonstress test (as early as 30 weeks), contraction stress test, and biophysical profile because of risk of unexplained intrauterine fetal demise in the antepartum period.
- Lung maturity studies (by amniocentesis) to determine lecithin-sphingomyelin (L/S) ratio and to detect phosphatidylglycerol (PG); the adequacy of L/S and PG, predictor of the newborn's ability to avoid respiratory distress (see "Newborn of a diabetic mother" in Chapter 15).

E. Nursing management

1. Establish an initial database, and maintain serial documentation of test results throughout the pregnancy.
2. Provide client and family teaching.
   a. Assess the client's understanding of gestational diabetes mellitus and its implications for daily life.
   b. As needed, explain the effects of gestational diabetes on the mother and fetus.
   c. Point out the need for frequent laboratory testing and follow-up for mother and fetus, for example, to prevent infection and assess other potential complications.
   d. Discuss and demonstrate insulin self-injection (see *Drug Chart* 12-1, page 196).
   e. Demonstrate how to self-monitor blood glucose level. Explain that blood is generally tested daily before meals and at bedtime.
   f. Explain the need to test urine for ketones, which are harmful to the fetus.
   g. Point out the importance of keeping daily records of blood glucose levels, insulin dose, dietary intake, periods of exercise, periods of hypoglycemia, kind and amount of treatment, and daily urine test results.
   h. Discuss potential complications and their management.
   - Diabetic ketoacidosis is a multisystem disorder resulting from hyperglycemia in which plasma glucose levels exceed 350 mg/dl in the nonpregnant state or are 200 mg/dl or more during pregnancy.
   - Hypoglycemia is a disorder caused by too much insulin, insufficient food, excess exercise, diarrhea, or vomiting. *Client and Family Teaching* 12-2 lists signs and symptoms of hypoglycemia and hyperglycemia.
     - Discuss the management of hypoglycemia (administering 12 fluid oz of orange juice [or 20 g of carbohydrates] and waiting 20 minutes before repeating the procedure).
     - Report any episode to the health care provider as soon as possible.

   i. Explain the need for continued evaluation during the postpartum period until blood glucose levels are within normal limits.
3. **Arrange for the client to consult a dietitian to discuss the prescribed diabetic diet and to ensure adequate caloric intake. Energy needs are usually calculated at a rate of 30 to 35 calories per kilogram of ideal body weight.**
4. Address emotional and psychosocial needs. Intervene appropriately to allay anxiety regarding diabetes and childbirth.

CLIENT AND FAMILY TEACHING 12-2

Signs and symptoms of hypoglycemia and hyperglycemia

Hypoglycemia

- Shakiness, dizziness
- Sweating
- Pallor; cold, clammy skin
- Disorientation, irritability
- Headache
- Hunger
- Blurred vision
- Nervousness
- Weakness, fatigue
- Shallow respirations, but normal pulse rate
- Urine negative for glucose and acetone
- Blood glucose level < 60 mg/dl

Hyperglycemia

- Fatigue
- Flushed, hot skin
- Dry mouth, excessive thirst
- Frequent urination
- Rapid, deep respirations; fruity odor
- Depressed reflexes
- Drowsiness, headache

5. **Prepare the client for intensive frequent intrapartum assessment, which may include:**
   a. Fetal monitoring
   b. Intravenous infusion of glucose, insulin, and oxytocin
   c. Evaluation for diabetic ketoacidosis (signs and symptoms include altered level of consciousness, labored breath sounds, fruity breath odor, and ketonuria)
   d. Intravenous fluid and electrolyte replacement therapy
   e. Invasive maternal cardiac monitoring
6. **Identify and make referral to support groups and resources available to the client and family.**

XIII. HEMOLYTIC DISEASE OF THE FETUS AND NEWBORN

A. Description

1. Hemolytic disease of the fetus and newborn is an immune reaction of the mother's blood against the blood group factor on the fetus's RBCs.
2. When RhoGAM (Rh immune globulin) became available in the 1960s to treat isoimmunization in Rh-negative women, the incidence of hemolytic disease in the fetus and newborn dropped significantly.

B. Etiology

1. Hemolytic disease occurs most frequently when the mother does not have the Rh factor present in her blood but the fetus has this factor. Another common cause of hemolytic disease is ABO incompatibility. In most cases of ABO incompatibility, the mother has blood type O and the fetus has blood type A. It may also occur when the fetus has blood type B or AB.
2. Hemolysis is occasionally caused by maternal anemias such as thalassemia or from other blood group antigens (anti-D).

C. Pathophysiology

1. This disorder occurs when the fetus has a blood group antigen that the mother does not possess. The mother's body forms an antibody against that particular blood group

antigen, and hemolysis begins. The process of antibody formation is called maternal sensitization.

2. The fetus has resulting anemia from the hemolysis of blood cells. The fetus compensates by producing large numbers of immature erythrocytes, a condition known as erythroblastosis fetalis, hemolytic disease of the newborn, or hydrops fetalis. *Hydrops* refers to the edema and *fetalis* refers to the lethal state of the infant.
3. In Rh incompatibility, the hemolysis usually begins in utero. It may not affect the first pregnancy but all pregnancies that follow will experience this problem. In ABO incompatibility, the hemolysis does not usually begin until the birth of the newborn.

D. Assessment findings

1. Clinical manifestations

a. The hemolytic response in ABO incompatibility usually begins at birth with a resulting newborn jaundice.

b. Rh incompatibility may lead to:
- Hydramnios in the mother
- Excess bilirubin levels in the amniotic fluid
- Varying degrees of hemolytic anemia (erythroblastosis) in the fetus. If the condition is left unmanaged, 25% of affected infants may die or suffer permanent brain damage.

2. Laboratory and diagnostic study findings

a. The indirect Coombs' test can aid in the search for agglutination of Rh-positive RBCs to determine if antibodies are present.

b. Amniocentesis is used to determine optical density and estimate fetal hemolysis. Spectrophotometer readings are made of the amniotic fluid collected. The readings are obtained to determine fluid density. They are plotted on a graph and correlated with gestational age. The amount of bilirubin resulting from the hemolysis of RBCs can then be estimated.

c. An antibody titer should be drawn at the first prenatal visit on all Rh-negative women. It should also be drawn at 28 and 36 weeks of pregnancy and again at delivery or abortion. The normal value is 0. The result is usually reported as a ratio; normal is 1:8. If the titer is absent or minimal (1:8), no therapy is needed. A rising titer indicates the need for RhoGAM and vigilant monitoring of fetal well-being.

E. Nursing management

1. Administer RhoGAM to the unsensitized Rh-negative client as appropriate (see *Drug Chart 10-1,* page 154).

a. Administer RhoGAM at 28 weeks' gestation, even when titers are negative, or after any invasive procedure such as amniocentesis. RhoGAM protects against the effects of early transplacental hemorrhage (as recommended by the American College of Gynecologists).

b. When the Rh-negative mother is in labor, crossmatch for RhoGAM, which must be given within 72 hours of delivery of the newborn.

2. **Provide management for the sensitized Rh-negative mother and Rh-positive fetus.**

a. Focus management of the sensitized Rh-negative mother on close monitoring of fetal well-being, as reflected by Rh titers, amniocentesis results, and sonography.

b. If there is evidence of erythroblastosis, notify the perinatal team of the possibility for delivery of a compromised newborn.

3. **Provide management for ABO incompatibility.**
   a. Phototherapy usually can resolve the newborn jaundice associated with ABO incompatibility.
   b. In addition, initiation of early feeding and exchange blood transfusions may be immediate measures required to reduce indirect bilirubin levels.
4. Provide client and family teaching.

XIV. INFECTIONS DURING PREGNANCY

A. Description

1. Maternal infections during pregnancy may significantly contribute to fetal morbidity and mortality.
2. Two of the most common groups of infections present during pregnancy are sexually transmitted infections and TORCH infections.
   a. Sexually transmitted infections include:
   - Chlamydia
   - Gonorrhea
   - Group B streptococcus
   - Hepatitis B
   - Human papillomavirus
   - Syphilis
   - Trichomonas
   - Candidiasis
   - Bacterial vaginosis
   - Human immunodeficiency virus

   b. TORCH infections include:
   - Toxoplasmosis
   - Other infections — hepatitis A, infectious hepatitis, hepatitis C, or syphilis
   - Rubella
   - Cytomegalovirus
   - Herpes simplex virus

B. Etiology

1. Infections in this category may be caused by various viruses. Other organisms, such as bacteria, spirochetes, protozoa, or yeast, also may cause maternal infections, which are harmful to the developing fetus. Even though the infection in the mother may be very mild, the effects on the fetus can be catastrophic.
2. The infectious organism may be acquired during sexual intercourse, through the use of contaminated articles such as needles, from human body fluids (semen, saliva, blood, urine, cervical mucus, breast milk, and stool), by eating undercooked meat, or by contact with infected cat feces in the litter box, sand box, or garden soil.
3. Most organisms cross the placental barrier and infect the fetus, causing birth anomalies. The fetus may also acquire the organism as it travels the birth canal during labor, causing illness after birth.

C. Pathophysiology

1. These infectious organisms are capable of crossing the placental barrier and adversely affecting the development of the fetus. Spontaneous abortion or fetal and newborn abnormalities may occur.
2. In some instances, the infection can also cause infertility or sterility in the mother.

D. Assessment findings for sexually transmitted diseases

1. **Associated findings**
   a. Previous history of sexually transmitted disease or pelvic inflammatory disease
   b. Numerous sexual partners
   c. Use of intravenous drugs or partners who use intravenous drugs
2. **Common clinical manifestations**
   a. PROM
   b. Preterm birth
   c. Systemic fetal infection
3. **Laboratory and diagnostic study findings.** Serologic and culture testing will reveal infection.

E. Assessment findings for TORCH infections

1. Common clinical manifestations
   a. Influenza-type symptoms
   b. Rash
   c. Lymphedema and lymphadenopathy
2. **Laboratory and diagnostic study findings.** Serologic and culture testing will reveal infection.

F. Implementation

1. **Carefully screen for infections during pregnancy and treat possible infections as ordered.**
   a. At the first prenatal visit, the pregnant woman should have a rubella titer drawn. A titer of 1:8 provides evidence of immunity. If the titer is below 1:8, rubella vaccine is offered to the woman before discharge postpartum (see *Drug Chart* 10-1, page 154). Those women who require the vaccine should be cautioned not to become pregnant for at least 3 months after receiving the vaccine.
   b. Cytomegalovirus currently has no effective therapy. This is important to remember because the highest rate of maternal infections occurs between the ages of 15 and 35. Usually, the infection is a symptomatic.
   c. Women who are presumed to be susceptible to varicella-zoster (chickenpox) should have immune testing. Varicella-zoster immune globulin should be administered to those who are susceptible or who have been exposed. Varicella-zoster immune globulin should be administered to the exposed newborn within 72 hours of birth.
   d. All pregnant women should be screened for HbsAg, the hepatitis B surface antigen. The hepatitis B immune globulin can prevent infection in both mother and newborn. An initial injection can be given to the newborn, followed by doses at 1 month and 6 months of age. Adults receive three injections given over a 6- to 12-month period (see *Drug Chart* 11-1, page 174).
2. **Provide client and family teaching** regarding the diagnosis of infection to promote compliance with the treatment plan.
   a. Explain how maternal infections are acquired and transmitted to the developing fetus during pregnancy.
   b. Demonstrate proper hand-washing technique, stressing that it is the single most successful means of preventing infection.
   c. Discuss hygienic and dietary measures that reduce the risk of infection.
   d. Explain the organism, test, treatment, and fetal effects of the specific infection to the client and family.

e. Include the client in planning solutions for possible fetal effects.
f. Discuss "safe sex" with the client and partner.
g. Seek the couple's input for development of a plan for follow-up care.

Study questions

1. Which of the following statements best describes hyperemesis gravidarum?
1. Severe anemia leading to electrolyte, metabolic, and nutritional imbalances in the absence of other medical problems
2. Severe nausea and vomiting leading to electrolyte, metabolic, and nutritional imbalances in the absence of other medical problems
3. Loss of appetite and continuous vomiting that commonly results in dehydration and ultimately decreasing maternal nutrients.
4. Severe nausea and diarrhea that can cause GI irritation and possibly internal bleeding

2. In which of the following clients would the nurse suspect anemia?
1. Client in her first trimester with a hemoglobin level of 12 g/dl
2. Client in her second trimester with a hemoglobin level of 11 g/dl
3. Client in her third trimester with a hemoglobin level of 8 g/dl
4. Client in her first trimester with a hemoglobin of 10.5 g/dl

3. Which of the following would the nurse identify as a classic sign of PIH?
1. Edema of the feet and ankles
2. Edema of the hands and face
3. Weight gain of 1 lb/week
4. Early morning headache

4. Which of the following medications would the nurse expect to administer for prevention of hemolytic disease of the fetus and newborn?
1. Magnesium sulfate
2. Diazepam
3. Rohm
4. Phenobarbital

5. In which of the following types of spontaneous abortions would the nurse assess dark brown vaginal discharge and a negative pregnancy test?
1. Threatened
2. Imminent
3. Missed
4. Incomplete

6. Which of the following factors would the nurse suspect as predisposing a client to placenta previa?
1. Multiple gestation
2. Uterine anomalies
3. Abdominal trauma
4. Renal or vascular disease

7. Which of the following would the nurse assess in a client experiencing abruptio placentae?
1. Bright red, painless vaginal bleeding
2. Concealed or external dark red bleeding
3. Palpable fetal outline
4. Soft and nontender abdomen

8. Which of the following is described as premature separation of a normally implanted placenta during the second half of pregnancy, usually with severe hemorrhage?
1. Placenta previa
2. Ectopic pregnancy
3. Incompetent cervix
4. Abruptio placentae

9. Which of the following best describes gestational trophoblastic disease?
1. A hypertensive disorder of pregnancy that develops after 20 weeks' gestation and is characterized by edema, hypertension, and proteinuria
2. The implantation of products of conception in the fallopian tubes, ovaries, cervix, or peritoneal cavity

3. Expulsion of the fetus and other products of conception from the uterus before the fetus is viable
4. An alteration of early embryonic growth, causing placental disruption, rapid proliferation of abnormal cells, and destruction of the embryo

10. When obtaining the history for a pregnant client, she tells the nurse that her mother took diethylstilbesterol (DES) when the client's mother was pregnant with the client. The nurse would know that the client is at risk for which of the following?

1. Placenta previa
2. Incompetent cervix
3. Preeclampsia
4. Severe eclampsia

11. When providing chest thrusts to alleviate choking in a pregnant woman, the rescurer would stand behind her and encircle her chest with his arms. Identify the area where the fist would be placed.

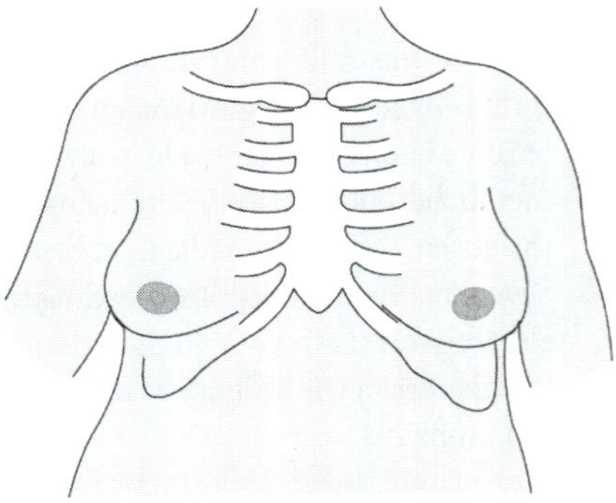

Answer key

1. The answer is 2.
The description of hyperemesis gravidarum includes severe nausea and vomiting, leading to electrolyte, metabolic, and nutritional imbalances in the absence of other medical problems. Hyperemesis is not a form of anemia. Loss of appetite may occur secondary to the nausea and vomiting of hyperemesis, which, if it continues, can deplete the nutrients transported to the fetus. Diarrhea does not occur with hyperemesis.

2. The answer is 3.
Anemia during pregnancy is described as a hemoglobin level of 10 g/dl or less during the second and third trimesters. Thus, the nurse would suspect anemia in the client in her third trimester with a hemoglobin of 8 g/dl. Hemoglobin levels of 12 g/dl, 11 g/dl, and 10.5 g/dl are above the cut-off range for the diagnosis of anemia during pregnancy.

3. The answer is 2.
Edema of the hands and face is a classic sign of PIH. Many healthy pregnant women experience foot and ankle edema. A weight gain of 2 lb or more per week indicates a problem. Early morning headache is not a classic sign of PIH.

4. The answer is 3.
Hemolytic disease of the fetus and newborn is an immune reaction by the mother's blood against the blood group factor on the fetus's RBCs. RhoGAM would be given at 28 weeks' gestation to protect the fetus. Magnesium sulfate, diazepam, and phenobarbital would be given to treat PIH.

5. The answer is 3.
In a missed abortion, there is early fetal intrauterine death, and products of conception are not expelled. The cervix remains closed; there may be a dark brown vaginal discharge, negative pregnancy test, and cessation of uterine growth and breast tenderness. A threatened abortion is evidenced with cramping and vaginal bleeding in early pregnancy, with no cervical dilation. An imminent abortion presents with bleeding, cramping, and cervical dilation. An incomplete abortion involves only expulsion of part of the products of conception and bleeding occurs with cervical dilation.

6. The answer is **1.**
Multiple gestation is one of the predisposing factors that may cause placenta previa. Uterine anomalies, abdominal trauma, and renal or vascular disease may predispose a client to abruptio placentae.

7. The answer is **2.**
A client with abruptio placentae may exhibit concealed or dark red bleeding, possibly reporting sudden intense localized uterine pain. The uterus is typically firm to boardlike, and the fetal presenting part may be engaged. Bright red, painless vaginal bleeding, a palpable fetal outline, and a soft nontender abdomen are manifestations of placenta previa.

8. The answer is **4.**
Abruptio placentae is described as premature separation of a normally implanted placenta during the second half of pregnancy, usually with severe hemorrhage. Placenta previa refers to implantation of the placenta in the lower uterine segment, causing painless bleeding in the third trimester of pregnancy. Ectopic pregnancy refers to the implantation of the products of conception in a site other than the endometrium. Incompetent cervix is a condition characterized by painful dilation of the cervical os without uterine contractions.

9. The answer is **4.**
Gestational trophoblastic disease refers to an alteration of early embryonic growth, causing placental disruption, rapid proliferation of abnormal cells, and destruction of the embryo. PIH refers to a hypertensive disorder of pregnancy that develops after 20 weeks' gestation and is characterized by edema, hypertension, and proteinuria. Ectopic pregnancy refers to the implantation of products of conception in the fallopian tubes, ovaries, cervix, or peritoneal cavity. Spontaneous abortion refers to the expulsion of the fetus and other products of conception from the uterus before the fetus is viable.

10. The answer is **2.**
One of the causes of incompetent cervix may be that the woman's mother took DES during pregnancy. Use of DES is not associated with placenta previa, preeclampsia, or severe eclampsia.

11. Place the thumb side of your fist on the middle of the woman's sternum. Placement of the fist against the sternum ensures a solid structure for compression. Grab the fist with the other hand and perform backward thrusts until the foreign body is expelled. Pressure on the chest compresses the ribs, increasing chest and lung pressure. The increased pressure is sufficient to force the object to move upward and dislodge it from the airway.

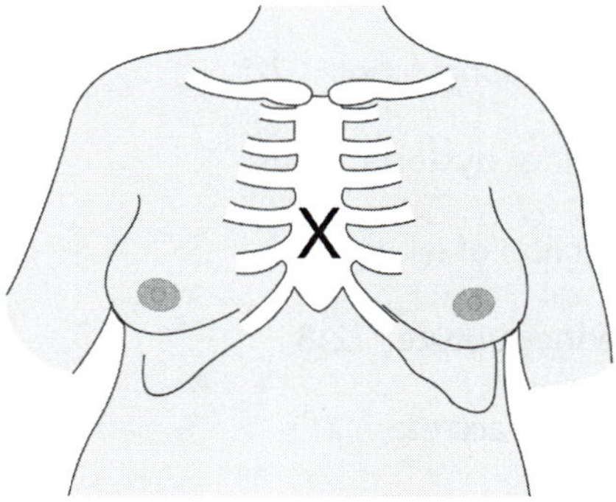

13 Intrapartum Complications

I. ESSENTIAL CONCEPTS

A. Problems that can be anticipated because of maternal or fetal conditions or that can be stabilized and corrected without emergency intervention are increasingly managed in facilities designed to accommodate high-risk maternal and fetal clients.

B. When the expectant mother is the best "incubator" for the high-risk newborn, she may be transported to a tertiary care facility before the onset of labor and the actual birth.

C. Because intrapartum emergencies commonly develop rapidly, on-the-spot nursing assessment and intervention are crucial.

D. Principles of nursing care during normal labor (see Chapter 9) apply to complicated labor as well.

NURSING PROCESS OVERVIEW

II. INTRAPARTUM COMPLICATIONS

A. Assessment

1. Health history

a. Elicit a description of symptoms, including onset, duration, location, and precipitating factors or events. Cardinal signs and symptoms may include:
- A sudden gush of fluid from the vagina
- Any copious vaginal bleeding
- Presence of uterine contractions with or without abdominal pain
- Decreased fetal movement

b. Explore maternal and family history for risk factors for intrapartum complications.
- Maternal risk factors include:
  - Age younger than 18
  - History of preterm labors
  - Poor obstetric history
  - Multiple pregnancy
  - Hydramnios
  - Smoking
  - Poor hygiene
  - Poor nutrition
  - Employment
- Family risk factors may include:
  - History of diabetes
  - History of complications of birth in other family members

c. Assess the family's responses to high-risk pregnancy, labor, and a potential crisis situation.

d. Assess maternal, paternal, and family bonding and the potential for perinatal loss and grief.

2. Physical examination

a. **Vital signs**
- Measure maternal blood pressure, pulse, and respirations in the presence of vaginal fluid leakage or bleeding to assess for infection.
- Measure maternal vital signs to identify presence of shock.

- Monitor fetal heart rate (FHR) to determine fetal status.

b. Inspection
- Inspect the perineum for characteristics of vaginal discharge. Observe for color, odor, consistency, and amount.
- Observe size and shape of the uterus.
- At delivery, visually inspect the placenta for abnormal characteristics.

c. Palpation
- Monitor uterine activity to determine progress of labor.
- Evaluate the cervix for readiness for, or progress in, labor. Do not perform a vaginal examination if bleeding is present.

3. Laboratory and diagnostic studies

a. Ultrasound is used to determine fetal status, localize the placenta, and determine amniotic fluid volume.

b. Kleihauer-Betke or fetal cell blood test is used to determine whether the blood cells are maternal or fetal. Maternal cells remain colorless when stained. Fetal cells become purple-pink when stained.

c. Nitrazine test tape and presence of ferning are used to determine if there is rupture of the amniotic sac. Nitrazine paper turns green-blue in the presence of amniotic fluid. On microscopic examination of a sample of fluid, a ferning pattern, similar to frost on a window, appears on the dried slide. This is characteristic of a high-estrogen fluid.

d. Electronic uterine monitoring will demonstrate the presence of uterine contractions.

e. Complete blood count will document the presence of anemia or infection.

B. Nursing diagnoses.

In addition to complication-specific diagnoses, the following nursing diagnoses are common to care of the at-risk intrapartum client.

1. Anxiety
2. Fear
3. Ineffective Compromised Family Coping
4. Anticipatory Grieving
5. Self-Esteem Disturbance
6. Spiritual Distress
7. Knowledge Deficit
8. Pain
9. Risk for Injury

C. Planning and outcome identification

1. Threats to optimal physical and emotional pregnancy outcome will be determined.
2. The client will be physically comfortable, and the client and family will have a healthy response to their high-risk pregnancy status and potential complications.
3. The client and family will understand their pregnancy complication and the necessary treatments.

D. Implementation

1. Assess maternal and fetal physiologic status to detect early maternal or fetal changes requiring early intervention.

   a. Perform ongoing assessment during the intrapartum period (see Chapter 9).

   b. Expect the unexpected, and be prepared to provide critical care nursing if needed.

   c. Accurately document the assessed problem and subsequent nursing interventions and their effectiveness.

2. **Provide physical and emotional support.**
   a. Observe the client and family for emotional response and ability to cope with discomfort and pain.
   b. Provide comfort measures.
   c. Coordinate physical care for client with emotional needs of the client and family. (Typically, clients with intrapartum complications require intravenous fluids and various procedures and treatments, such as electronic monitoring, central venous lines, medications, and urinary catheterization.)
   d. Assess and support the client's and family's psychosocial and emotional needs, particularly in relation to potential loss and grief.
   e. Encourage and support coping mechanisms, including aspects of loss and grief.
3. **Provide client and family education.**
   a. Provide information on status of mother and infant to help relieve anxiety.
   b. Provide anticipatory guidance for the client and her partner.

E. Outcome evaluation

1. The client and fetus maintain normal physiologic status; any deviations that arise are identified and corrected early.
2. The couple demonstrates greater comfort, decreased fear and anxiety, and increased use of coping techniques.
3. The client and partner express understanding of their pregnancy complication and the necessary procedures to be performed.

III. PREMATURE RUPTURE OF MEMBRANES (PROM)

A. Description. PROM is rupture of the chorion and amnion before the onset of labor. The gestational age of the fetus and estimates of viability affect management.

B. Etiology. The precise cause and specific predisposing factors are unknown.

C. Pathophysiology

1. PROM is associated with malpresentation, possible weak areas in the amnion and chorion, subclinical infection, and possibly incompetent cervix.
2. Basic and effective defense against the fetus contracting an infection is lost and the risk of ascending intrauterine infection, known as chorioamnionitis, is increased.
3. The leading cause of death associated with PROM is infection.
4. When the latent period (time between rupture of membranes and onset of labor) is less than 24 hours, the risk of infection is low.

D. Assessment findings

1. **Clinical manifestations**
   a. PROM is marked by amniotic fluid gushing from the vagina. The fluid may merely trickle or leak from the vagina in the absence of contractions.
   b. Pooling of amniotic fluid in the vagina will be visualized during a speculum examination.
   c. Maternal fever, fetal tachycardia, and malodorous discharge may indicate infection.
2. **Laboratory and diagnostic study findings.** Rupture of membranes is confirmed by the following.
   a. Ferning is evident.
   b. Nitrazine test tape turns blue-green.

E. Nursing management

1. **Prevent infection and other potential complications.**
   a. Make an early and accurate evaluation of membrane status, using sterile speculum examination and determination of ferning. Thereafter, keep vaginal examinations to a minimum to prevent infection.
   b. Obtain smear specimens from vagina and rectum as prescribed to test for beta-hemolytic streptococci, organisms that increases the risk to the fetus.
   c. Determine maternal and fetal status, including estimated gestational age. Continually assess for signs of infection.
   d. Maintain the client on bed rest if the fetal head is not engaged. This method may prevent cord prolapse if additional rupture and loss of fluid occur. Once the fetal head is engaged, ambulation can be encouraged.
2. Provide client and family education.
   a. Inform the client, if the fetus is at term, that the chances of spontaneous labor beginning are excellent; encourage the client and partner to prepare themselves for labor and birth.
   b. If labor does not begin or the fetus is judged to be preterm or at risk for infection, explain treatments that are likely to be needed.

IV. PRETERM LABOR

A. Description. Preterm labor is labor that begins after 20 weeks' gestation and before 37 weeks' gestation.

B. Etiology. Among the many causes of preterm labor are:

1. PROM
2. Preeclampsia
3. Hydramnios
4. Placenta previa
5. Abruptio plyacentae
6. Incompetent cervix
7. Trauma
8. Uterine structural anomalies
9. Multiple gestation
10. Intrauterine infection (chorioamnionitis)
11. Congenital adrenal hyperplasia
12. Fetal death
13. Maternal factors, such as stress (physical and emotional), urinary tract infections, and dehydration

C. Pathophysiology. The uterus begins the process of contraction prior to term gestational age.

D. Assessment findings. Clinical manifestations of preterm labor are basically the signs of true labor that occur when the gestational age of the fetus is greater than 20 and less than 37 weeks.

1. Low back pain
2. Suprapubic pressure
3. Vaginal pressure
4. Rhythmic uterine contractions

5. Cervical dilation and effacement
6. Possible rupture of membranes
7. Expulsion of the cervical mucus plug
8. Bloody show

E. Nursing management

1. Assess the mother's condition and evaluate signs of labor.
   a. Obtain a thorough obstetric history.
   b. Obtain specimens for complete blood count and urinalysis.
   c. Determine frequency, duration, and intensity of uterine contractions.
   d. Determine cervical dilation and effacement.
   e. Assess status of membranes and bloody show.
2. Evaluate fetus for distress, size, and maturity (sonography and lecithin-sphingomyelin ratio).
3. Perform measures to manage or stop preterm labor.
   a. Place the client on bed rest in the side-lying position.
   b. Prepare for possible ultrasonography, amniocentesis, tocolytic drug therapy, and steroid therapy (*Drug Chart* 13-1, pages 212 and 213).
   c. Administer tocolytic (contraction-inhibiting) medications as prescribed.
   d. Assess for side effects of tocolytic therapy (such as decreased maternal blood pressure, dyspnea, chest pain, and FHR exceeding 180 beats/minute).
4. Provide physical and emotional support. Provide adequate hydration.
5. Provide client and family education.

V. VASA PREVIA

A. Description. Vasa previa is a rare developmental disorder made up of two separate disorders.

1. Velamentous insertion of the umbilical cord, in which the umbilical blood vessels course through the amnion and chorion and meet to form the umbilical cord a distance from the placental surface. This places the fragile umbilical vessels at risk for tearing and hemorrhage.
2. The fragile unprotected umbilical vessels cross the internal os and are in front of the presenting fetal head, thus creating a vasa previa.

B. Etiology. Uncertain. However, it may be due to uneven growth of the placenta or abnormal implantation of the blastocyte.

C. Pathophysiology. The fetal vessels rupture or are compressed, leading to fetal hypoxia.

D. Assessment findings

1. Associated findings
   a. Vasa previa is of no danger to the mother.
   b. Once the umbilical vessels rupture, fetal demise is virtually certain.
2. Clinical manifestations
   a. Vessels are occasionally palpated during a vaginal examination.
   b. Minimal bright red vaginal bleeding is evident.
   c. Fetal bradycardia occurs.
3. Laboratory and diagnostic study findings
   a. Ultrasound may reveal vasa previa.
   b. Kleihauer-Betke or fetal cell blood test will confirm the presence of fetal blood cells.

DRUG CHART 13-1
Medications used for intrapartum complications

Classifications	Used for	Selected interventions
Tocolytics ritodrine HCL (Yutopar) terbutaline sulfate (Brethine)	▪ Terminates preterm labor ▪ Acts on beta-2 receptor sites	▪ Assess maternal and fetal heart rates continuously during infusion. ▪ Always use an infusion control mechanism to maintain a specified flow rate. ▪ Always administered as a "piggy back" I.V. ▪ Measure intake and output (I&O) every hour. Output should be 30 ml/hour or more. ▪ Assess maternal blood pressure (BP) continuously during infusion of these drugs. ▪ Monitor for the following side effects: hypotension, increased heart rate, hypokalemia, pulmonary edema, nausea, vomiting, headache, and increased serum glucose.
Calcium channel blocker nifedipine (Procardia)	▪ Inhibits contraction of smooth muscle	▪ Assess maternal and fetal heart rates continuously during administration. ▪ Measure I&O every hour. Output should be 30 ml/hour or more. ▪ Assess maternal BP continuously during administration of these drugs. ▪ Monitor for the following side effects: headache, jitteriness, shakiness, dyspnea, palpitations, chest pain, and tachycardia.
Nonsteroidal anti-inflammatory drug (NSAID) indomethacin (Indocin)	▪ Prostaglandin antagonist that can be used to inhibit uterine contractions	▪ Assess maternal and fetal heart rates continuously during administration. ▪ Measure I&O every hour. Output should be 30 ml/hour or more. ▪ Assess maternal BP continuously during administration of these drugs. ▪ Monitor for the following side effects: headache, nausea, vomiting, prolonged bleeding time, blurred vision, and syncope.
Anticonvulsant magnesium sulfate ($MgSO_4$)	▪ A CNS depressant that halts uterine contractions ▪ Muscle relaxant; prevents seizures	▪ Assess maternal and fetal heart rates continuously during infusion. ▪ Always use an infusion control mechanism to maintain a specified flow rate. ▪ Always administer as a "piggy back" I.V. ▪ Measure I&O every hour. Output should be 30 ml/hour or more. ▪ Assess maternal BP continuously during infusion of these drugs. ▪ Assess deep-tendon reflexes every 1 to 4 hours during continuous infusion of $MgSO_4$. ▪ Discontinue $MgSO_4$ if deep tendon reflexes are absent or if respirations fall below 14/minute. ▪ Monitor for the following side effects, including flushing, thirst, respiratory depression, decreased or absent deep-tendon reflexes, decreased urinary output, respiratory arrest, and cardiac arrest.

DRUG CHART 13-1

Medications used for intrapartum complications *(continued)*

Classifications	Used for	Selected interventions
Electrolyte calcium gluconate (10% solution)	▪ Used as an antidote for effects of magnesium sulfate electrolyte ▪ Maintains nervous and muscle cell permeability ▪ Acts as an activator in the transmission of nerve impulses and contraction of cardiac, skeletal, and smooth muscle	▪ Assess maternal and fetal heart rates continuously during infusion. ▪ Always use an infusion control mechanism to maintain a specified flow rate. ▪ Always administer as a "piggy back" I.V. ▪ Measure I&O every hour. Output should be 30 ml/hour or more. ▪ Assess maternal BP continuously during infusion of these drugs. ▪ Monitor for the following side effects: bradycardia, tingling, syncope, nausea, vomiting, phlebitis at I.V. site, and cardiac arrest.
Prostaglandin dinoprostone (Prepidil, Prostin E_2 [suppository or gel])	▪ Stimulates uterine smooth muscle to contract ▪ Initiates softening, effacement, and dilatation of the cervix	▪ Suppository (prostaglandin) is inserted every 2 hours times 3. ▪ Keep the suppository cold and bring it to room temperature before insertion. After insertion, have the client remain dorsal recumbent for 15–30 minutes. ▪ The gel is inserted into the cervical os by catheter two times; 6 hours apart. ▪ Monitor for the following side effects: headache, nausea, vomiting, hypotension, hypertension, dyspnea, and uterine hyperstimulation.
Oxytocic oxytocin (Pitocin, Syntocinon [I.V. drip])	▪ Used for induction of labor	▪ Oxytocin is infused at a rate of 1–2 mU/minute and increased by 1–2 mU/minute every 15–30 minutes until a contraction pattern is established. ▪ Monitor vital signs and fetal heart rate closely. ▪ Assess the contractile pattern. ▪ Limit I.V. fluids to 150 ml/hour. ▪ Mix 10 IU oxytocin in 1,000 ml Ringer's lactate and hang as a "piggy back" solution. ▪ Always use the infusion port closest to the client. ▪ Monitor for water intoxication.
Corticosteroid anti-inflammatory immunosuppressant (Betamethasone, Celestone)	▪ Hastening fetal lung maturity ▪ Preventing respiratory distress syndrome in the newborn	▪ Give to mother 12–24 hours before delivery. ▪ Administer initial dose I.M. ▪ May repeat in 24 hours and again in 2 weeks. ▪ Assist with measures to halt preterm labor. ▪ Observe for burning, itching, and irritation at the injection site. ▪ Adverse effects include swelling, tachycardia, sodium and fluid retention, increased risk of infection with long-term use. ▪ Initial dose is 12.5 mg I.M.

E. Nursing management

1. **Identify and assist with treatment of the disorder.**
   a. Monitor FHR and status during labor.
   b. Assist with diagnosis of the condition.
   c. Anticipate and assist with emergency cesarean birth.

2. Provide physical and emotional support.
3. Provide client and family education. Explain emergency procedures to the client and family.

VI. UMBILICAL CORD PROLAPSE

A. Description

1. Cord prolapse is descent of the umbilical cord into the vagina ahead of the fetal presenting part with resulting compression of the cord between the presenting part and the maternal pelvis.
2. Cord prolapse is an emergency situation; immediate delivery will be attempted to save the fetus.
3. It occurs in 1 of 200 pregnancies.

B. Etiology

1. This problem occurs most frequently in prematurity, rupture of membranes with the fetal presenting part unengaged, and shoulder or footling breech presentations.
2. It may follow rupture of the amniotic membranes because the fluid rush may carry the cord along toward the birth canal.

C. Pathophysiology.

Compression of the cord results in the compromise or cessation of fetoplacental perfusion.

D. Assessment findings

1. Associated findings
   a. Cord prolapse may be occult and occur at any time in the labor process, even when the amniotic membranes are intact.
   b. Client reports feeling the cord within the vagina.
2. Clinical manifestations
   a. Fetal bradycardia with deceleration during contraction
   b. The umbilical cord seen or felt during a vaginal examination

E. Nursing management

1. Identify prolapse of the cord and provide immediate intervention.
   a. ssess a laboring client often if the fetus is preterm or small for gestational age, if the fetal presenting part is not engaged, and if the membranes are ruptured.
   b. Periodically evaluate FHR, especially right after rupture of membranes (spontaneous or surgical), and again in 5 to 10 minutes.
   c. If cord prolapse is identified, notify the physician and prepare for emergency cesarean birth.
   d. If the client is fully dilated, the most emergent delivery route may be vaginal. In this case, encourage the client to push and assist with the delivery as follows:
      - Lower the head of the bed and elevate the client's hips on a pillow, or place the client in the knee-chest position to minimize pressure on the cord.
      - Apply oxygen at 10 to 12 L/minute.
      - Apply firm upward manual pressure to the presenting part of the fetus with a sterile gloved hand to elevate the fetus and relieve pressure from the cord.
      - Assess cord pulsations constantly.
      - Gently wrap gauze soaked in sterile normal saline solution around the prolapsed cord.

2. Provide physical and emotional support.
3. Provide client and family education.

VII. PROLONGED PREGNANCY

A. Description

1. A prolonged or postdate pregnancy is a pregnancy that extends beyond 42 weeks' gestation.
2. The incidence of prolonged pregnancy is approximately 10%.

B. Etiology. The actual physiologic cause of prolonged pregnancy is unknown. A suggested etiology is estrogen deficiency.

C. Pathophysiology. Pathophysiology includes excessively large infants with resultant birth trauma or small-for-gestational-age infants who are deprived of hydration and nutrition because of placental aging and dysfunction and decreased amniotic fluid.

D. Assessment findings

1. Clinical manifestations
   a. Weight loss and decreased uterine size (when the infant is suffering from placental dysfunction)
   b. Excessively large uterus
   c. Meconium-stained fluid
   d. Nonreassuring FHR patterns
2. **Laboratory and diagnostic study findings.** Ultrasound examination may be used to assist in determination of fetal size.

E. Nursing management

1. Carefully assess the fetus to identify risk.
   a. Perform a careful risk assessment upon admission.
   b. Closely monitor fetal status.
2. Prevent birth complications.
   a. Assist with induction of labor (see *Drug Chart* 13-1, pages 212 and 213).
   b. Prepare for a difficult delivery.
   c. Notify the pediatric staff of the potential for a birth-injured baby.
3. Provide physical and emotional support.
4. Provide client and family education.

VIII. DYSFUNCTIONAL LABOR

A. Description. Dysfunctional labor is difficult, painful, prolonged labor due to mechanical factors.

B. Etiology

1. Fetal factors (passenger) include unusually large fetus, fetal anomaly, malpresentation, and malposition.
2. Uterine factors (powers) include hypotonic labor, hypertonic labor, precipitous labor, and prolonged labor.

3. Pelvic factors (passage) include inlet contracture, midpelvis contracture, and outlet contracture.
4. "Psyche" factors include maternal anxiety and fear and lack of preparation.

C. Pathophysiology. Uterine contractions are ineffective secondary to muscle fatigue or overstretching.

D. Assessment findings. Clinical manifestations include irregular uterine contractions and ineffective uterine contractions in terms of contractile strength and duration.

E. Nursing management

1. **Optimize uterine activity.** Monitor uterine contractions for dysfunctional patterns; use palpation and an electronic monitor.
2. **Prevent unnecessary fatigue.** Check the client's level of fatigue and ability to cope with pain.
3. Prevent complications of labor for the client and infant.
   a. Assess urinary bladder; catheterize as needed.
   b. Assess maternal vital signs, including temperature, pulse, respiratory rate, and blood pressure.
   c. Check maternal urine for acetone (an indication of dehydration and exhaustion).
   d. Assess condition of fetus by monitoring FHR, fetal activity, and color of amniotic fluid.
4. Provide physical and emotional support.
   a. Promote relaxation through bathing and keeping the client and bed clean, back rubs, frequent position changes (side-lying), walking (if indicated), and by keeping the environment quiet.
   b. Coach the client in breathing and relaxation techniques.
5. Provide client and family education.

IX. SHOULDER DYSTOCIA

A. Description. In shoulder dystocia, the anterior shoulder of the baby is unable to pass under the maternal pubic arch.

B. Etiology. Shoulder dystocia is associated with advanced maternal age, diabetes, maternal obesity, large baby (macrosomia), postdate pregnancy, and multiparity.

C. Pathophysiology. The plane of the fetal shoulders aligns perpendicular to the pubis instead of at an angle. This causes the shoulder to become wedged under the pubic arch.

D. Assessment findings

1. **Associated findings.** The birth process may seem unnecessarily prolonged.
2. Clinical manifestations
   a. The fetal head retracts against the mother's perineum as soon as the head is delivered. This is known as the "turtle sign."
   b. External rotation does not occur.

E. Nursing management. Identify shoulder dystocia and assist with management.

1. Place the client in the McRobert's position (thighs pulled up against the abdomen with hips abducted).
2. Apply suprapubic pressure.

X. INDUCTION OF LABOR

A. Description

1. The deliberate initiation of labor before spontaneous contractions begin may be either mechanical (amniotomy [rupture of amniotic membranes]), physiologic (ambulation and nipple stimulation), or chemical (prostaglandins and oxytocin).
2. Artificial rupture of membranes (AROM) may be adequate stimulation to initiate contractions, or AROM may be done after oxytocin administration establishes effective contractions.
3. Induction and AROM are initiated when the cervix is soft, partially effaced, and slightly dilated, preferably when the fetal presenting part is engaged.
4. Oxytocin-induced labor must be done with careful, ongoing monitoring; oxytocin is a powerful drug. Hyperstimulation of the uterus may result in tetanic contractions prolonged to more than 90 seconds, which could cause fetal compromise due to impaired uteroplacental perfusion, abruptio placentae, laceration of the cervix, uterine rupture, or neonatal trauma.

B. Nursing management

1. Monitor for a safe labor and delivery process.
   a. AROM
   - Explain the procedure, and inform the client that labor usually follows within 6 to 8 hours of AROM.
   - Monitor fetal heart tones immediately before, during, and after the procedure.
   - Observe and record color, amount, and odor of amniotic fluid; time of procedure; cervical status; and maternal temperature.
   - Take and record the client's temperature every 2 hours to assess for infection.
   - Monitor for the onset of labor.

   b. Medication-induced labor (see *Drug Chart* 13-1, pages 212 and 213)
   - Review the hospital's policy relative to the amount, rate, and interval for increasing oxytocin or a prostaglandin-based preparation.
   - Use an infusion pump for precise regulation of the medication.
   - Observe for signs of hypertonicity, such as contractions exceeding 75 mm Hg (when using the internal pressure catheter) or 90 seconds, or closer together than 2 minutes. Be prepared to discontinue the medication immediately.
   - Initiate continuous internal or external fetal monitoring, and evaluate FHR for normal range of 110 to 160 beats/minute. If there is loss of variability, late decelerations, or persistent bradycardia (FHR less than 120 beats/minute), discontinue medication, administer oxygen, notify physician, reposition client to side-lying position, and perform a vaginal examination; fetal distress may result from rapid labor progress, descent of fetus, or cord prolapse.
   - Assess and record vital signs and FHR every 15 to 30 minutes, depending on stage of labor and risk status; assess for signs of impending delivery.
2. Provide physical and emotional support.

XI. UTERINE RUPTURE

A. Description

1. Uterine rupture is tearing of the uterus, either complete (rupture extends through entire uterine wall and uterine contents spill into the abdominal cavity) or incomplete (rupture extends through the endometrium and myometrium, but the peritoneum surrounding the uterus remains intact).
2. Small tears may be asymptomatic and may heal spontaneously, remaining undetected until the stress and strain of a subsequent labor.

B. Etiology

1. Traumatic uterine rupture may be caused by injury from obstetric instruments, such as uterine sound or curette used in abortion.
2. Rupture also may result from obstetric intervention, such as excessive fundal pressure, forceps delivery, violent bearing-down, tumultuous labor, and fetal shoulder dystocia.
3. Spontaneous uterine rupture is most likely to occur after previous uterine surgery or with grand multiparity combined with the use of oxytocic agents, cephalopelvic disproportion, malpresentation, or hydrocephalus.

C. Pathophysiology

1. The most common pathologic factor is a preexisting scar that results in a weakened or defective myometrium that does not stretch; this is most frequently identified in spontaneous uterine rupture.
2. Some episodes of rupture are due to traumatic disruption of the uterine surface.
3. More severe ruptures pose the risk of irreversible maternal hypovolemic shock or subsequent peritonitis, consequent fetal anoxia, and fetal or neonatal death.

D. Assessment findings. **Clinical manifestations** vary from mild to severe, depending on the site and extent of the rupture, degree of extrusion of the uterine contents, and intraperitoneal evidence or absence of spilled amniotic fluid and blood. They include:

1. Abdominal pain
2. Vaginal bleeding (is not always present)
3. Nonreassuring FHR pattern
4. Palpation of fetal parts under the skin
5. Signs of hypovolemic shock (with complete uterine rupture)

E. Nursing management

1. Monitor for the possibility of uterine rupture.
   a. In the presence of predisposing factors, monitor maternal labor pattern closely for hypertonicity or signs of weakening uterine muscle.
   b. Recognize signs of impending rupture, immediately notify the physician, and call for assistance.
2. Assist with rapid intervention.
   a. If the client has signs of possible uterine rupture, vaginal delivery is generally not attempted.
   b. If symptoms are not severe, an emergency cesarean birth may be attempted and the uterine tear repaired.
   c. If symptoms are severe, emergency laparotomy is performed to attempt immediate delivery of the fetus and then establish homeostasis.
   d. Implement the following preparations for surgery.

- Monitor maternal blood pressure, pulse, and respirations; also monitor fetal heart tones.
- If the client has a central venous pressure catheter in place, monitor pressure to evaluate blood loss and effects of fluid and blood replacement.
- Insert a urinary catheter for precise determinations of fluid balance.
- Obtain blood to assess possible acidosis.
- Administer oxygen, and maintain a patent airway.

3. Prevent and manage complications. **Take these steps in order to prevent or limit hypovolemic shock:**
   a. Oxygenate by providing 8 to 10 L/minute using a closed mask.
   b. Restore circulating volume using one or more intravenous lines.
   c. Evaluate the cause, response to therapy, and fetal condition.
   d. Remedy the problem by preparing the client for surgery and administering antibiotics.
4. Provide physical and emotional support.
   a. Provide support for the client's partner and family members once surgery has begun.
   b. Inform the partner and family how they will receive information about the mother and newborn.

XII. PLACENTA ACCRETA

A. Description. Placenta accreta is an uncommon condition in which the chorionic villa adhere to the myometrium. It can be exhibited as:

1. Placenta accreta — the placental chorionic villi adhere to the superficial layer of the uterine myometrium.
2. Placenta increta — the placental chorionic villi invade deeply into the uterine myometrium.
3. Placenta percreta — the placental chorionic villi grow through the uterine myometrium and often adhere to abdominal structures (such as the bladder or intestine).

B. Etiology. Predisposing factors are prior uterine surgery and placenta previa.

C. Pathophysiology. Implantation in an area of defective endometrium with no zone separation between the placenta and the myometrium

D. Assessment findings

1. **Associated findings.** Placenta accreta is usually diagnosed in the immediate postpartum period when the placenta fails to separate.
2. Clinical manifestations
   a. Placenta fails to separate
   b. Profuse hemorrhage may result depending on the portion of placenta involved

E. Nursing management

1. Identify placenta acreta in the client. Be aware of the client's risk status.
2. Assist with rapid treatment and intervention. Be prepared for a dilatation and curretage or hysterectomy.
3. **Provide physical and emotional support.**
4. **Provide client and family education.**

XIII. CESAREAN BIRTH

A. Description

1. In this surgical procedure, the newborn is delivered through the abdomen from an incision made through the maternal abdomen and the uterine myometrium.
2. The surgery may be preplanned (elective) or arise from an unanticipated problem.
3. Types of cesarean birth include the following.
   a. Classic or vertical. A vertical midline incision is made in the skin and the body of the uterus, permitting easier access to the fetus. This is indicated in emergency situations, when there are abdominal adhesions from previous surgeries, or when the fetus is in a transverse lie. Blood loss increases because large blood vessels of the myometrium are involved. Because the uterine musculature is weakened, there is greater possibility of rupture of the uterine scar in subsequent pregnancies.
   b. Transverse low segment. In this, the most common type, the incision is low ("bikini" or Pfannenstiel's incision), and the uterine incision is horizontal in the lower uterine segment. Blood loss is minimal, fewer postdelivery complications occur, and the incision is easy to repair, with less chance of rupture of uterine scar during future deliveries. The procedure takes longer to perform than the classic incision; therefore, it is not often used in emergencies.
4. In subsequent pregnancies and delivery, a trial of labor and vaginal birth is increasingly regarded as safe and appropriate as long as cephalopelvic disproportion does not exist and the previous incision was low transverse.
5. Elective, repeat cesarean birth may be performed in the absence of a specific indication for operative delivery when either the physician or the client is unwilling to attempt vaginal delivery.
6. Anesthesia may be general, spinal, or epidural; preoperative and postoperative care will vary accordingly.

B. Reasons for performing a cesarean birth

1. Maternal factors
   a. Cephalopelvic disproportion
   b. Active genital herpes or papilloma
   c. Previous cesarean birth by classic incision
   d. Presence of severe disabling hypertension or heart disease
2. Placental factors
   a. Placenta previa
   b. Abruptio placentae
3. Fetal factors
   a. Transverse fetal lie
   b. Extreme low birth weight
   c. Fetal distress
   d. Compound conditions, such as macrosomia and transverse lie

C. Nursing management

1. **Perform a complete maternal and fetal assessment.**
   a. Obtain a complete obstetric history.
   b. If the client presents with labor, determine frequency, duration, and intensity of contractions.

c. Determine the condition of the fetus through FHR, fetal monitoring, fetal scalp blood sample, fetal activity changes, and presence of meconium in amniotic fluid.

2. **Prepare the client for cesarean birth** in the same way whether the surgery is elective or emergency. Depending on hospital policy:
   a. Shave or clip pubic hair.
   b. Insert a retention catheter to empty the bladder continuously.
   c. As prescribed, insert intravenous lines, collect specimens for laboratory analysis, and administer preoperative medications.
   d. Also as prescribed, provide an antacid (to prevent vomiting and possible aspiration of gastric secretions) and prophylactic antibiotics (to prevent endometritis).
   e. Assist the client to remove jewelry, dentures, and nail polish, as appropriate.
   f. As needed, reinforce the obstetrician's explanation of the surgery, the expected outcome, and the anesthesiologist's explanation of the kind of anesthetics to be used (depending on the client's cardiopulmonary status).
   g. Make sure the client's signed informed consent is on file.
   ***h.* Continue assessing maternal and fetal vital signs in accordance with hospital policy until the client is transported to the operating room.**
   i. Notify other health care team members of the pending delivery.
   ***j.* Modify preoperative teaching to meet the needs of planned versus emergency cesarean birth; depth and breadth of instruction will depend on the circumstances and time available.**
   k. If there is time, begin explaining what the client can expect postoperatively. Discuss pain relief, turning, coughing, deep breathing, and ambulation.
   l. Inform the client that intraoperative and immediate postpartum care will be performed by the surgical and obstetric team, and that the newborn will receive care by the pediatrician and a nurse skilled in neonatal care procedures (resuscitation).
3. **Facilitate a family-centered cesarean birth** by including, when possible, such activities as:
   a. Preparing the partner for participation in the delivery.
   b. Reuniting the family as soon as possible following delivery.
   c. Providing for family time alone in the critical first hours after the mother and newborn are stabilized.
   d. Including the father and siblings (as possible) when demonstrating care of the newborn.
   e. Encouraging the mother's support person to remain with her as much as possible. In some cases, this person may accompany the client to the surgical suite and stay with her throughout the birth.
4. Provide physical and emotional support.
   a. Anticipate parental feelings of "failure" related to cesarean rather than "normal" birth. In such a situation, provide time for the client to relive and talk through the experience. Offer reassurance and support.
   b. Assist the family in planning for care of mother and newborn at home (*Client and Family Teaching* 13-1, page 222).

CLIENT AND FAMILY TEACHING 13-1

Planning for care of the mother and newborn at home after cesarean birth

Explain to the mother, her partner, and other family members that recovery from a surgical cesarean birth is slower, and often more painful, when compared with recovery from a normal vaginal birth. The following considerations must be taken into account:

- Need for increased rest (influenced by type of anesthesia, length of labor, and the type of abdominal or uterine incision)
- Need for increased pain medication and other pain-relieving techniques
- Inability to climb the stairs
- Inability to drive a car
- Difficulty with breast-feeding the newborn in certain positions (for example, cradle hold). Teach the mother the best positions to use and how to use pillows to cushion the incision site.
- Difficulty with normal activities of daily living (such as dressing, bathing, and toileting). Difficulty with providing normal newborn care (such as lifting, carrying, bathing, and dressing the newborn) and the need for assistance in caring for the newborn.

XIV. UTERINE INVERSION

A. Description. The uterus turns completely or partially inside out; it occurs immediately following delivery of the placenta or in the immediate postpartum period.

B. Etiology

1. Forced inversion is caused by excessive pulling of the cord or vigorous manual expression of the placenta or clots from an atonic uterus.
2. Spontaneous inversion is due to increased abdominal pressure from bearing down, coughing, or sudden abdominal muscle contraction.
3. Predisposing factors include straining after delivery of the placenta, vigorous kneading of the fundus to expel the placenta, manual separation and extraction of the placenta, rapid delivery with multiple gestation, or rapid release of excessive amniotic fluid.

C. Pathophysiology

1. The inverted uterus is unable to restore normal position or contract appropriately.
2. The women is placed at increased risk for bleeding and infection.

D. Assessment findings. Clinical manifestations include:

1. Excruciating pelvic pain with a sensation of extreme fullness extending into the vagina
2. Extrusion of the inner uterine lining into the vagina or extending past the vaginal introitus
3. Vaginal bleeding and signs of hypovolemia

E. Nursing management. Promptly identify and assist with the resolution of uterine inversion.

1. Recognize signs of impending inversion, and immediately notify the physician and call for assistance.
2. Immediate manual replacement of the uterus at the time of inversion will prevent cervical entrapment of the uterus; if reinversion is not performed immediately, rapid and extreme blood loss may occur, resulting in hypovolemic shock.
3. **Take steps to prevent or limit hypovolemic shock.**
   a. Insert a large gauge intravenous catheter for fluid replacement.

b. Measure and record maternal vital signs every 5 to 15 minutes to establish a baseline and document change.
c. Open an established intravenous line for optimal fluid replacement.
d. A fibrinogen level should be drawn to determine the risk of blood clot formation.
e. Prepare for anesthesia as needed.
f. Prepare to administer cardiopulmonary resuscitation, if required.

4. If manual reinversion is not successful, prepare the client and family for possible general anesthesia and surgery.

XV. EARLY POSTPARTUM HEMORRHAGE

A. Description

1. Early postpartum hemorrhage is defined as blood loss of 500 ml or more during the first 24 hours after delivery. (See Chapter 14 for a discussion of hemorrhage that occurs later in the postpartum period.)
2. Postpartum hemorrhage is the leading cause of maternal death worldwide and a common cause of excessive blood loss during the early postpartum period.
3. Approximately 5% of women experience some type of postdelivery hemorrhage.

B. Etiology

1. Major causes of postpartum hemorrhage are uterine atony (responsible for at least 80% of all early postpartum hemorrhages); laceration of cervix, vagina, or perineum; and retained placental fragments.
2. Predisposing factors include hypotonic contractions, overdistended uterus, multiparity, large newborn, forceps delivery, and cesarean birth.

C. Pathophysiology.
The uterus is unable to contract effectively and maintain hemostasis.

D. Assessment findings.
Clinical manifestations include:

1. Vaginal bleeding
2. Hypotonic uterus
3. Excessive blood loss, which may produce hypotension, thready pulse, pallor, restlessness, dyspnea, and chills

E. Nursing management

1. **Assist with appropriate treatment to prevent complications.**
   a. Determine the presence of uterine atony through frequent periodic assessment of uterine firmness and location and amount of vaginal bleeding immediately after delivery.
   b. Measure and record serial maternal vital signs after delivery — every 5 to 15 minutes until stable; increase or decrease the frequency of assessment relative to baseline and amount of bleeding.
   c. Notify the physician of abnormal assessment findings.
   d. Massage the fundus gently, taking care to support the uterus with one hand placed just above the symphysis pubis.
   e. Administer medications as prescribed.
   f. Keep an accurate pad count (100 ml per saturated pad).
   g. Assess condition of skin, urine output, and level of consciousness.
2. Provide physical and emotional support.
3. Provide client and family education.

Study questions

1. Which of the following may happen if the uterus becomes overstimulated by oxytocin during the induction of labor?
1. Weak contractions prolonged to more than 70 seconds
2. Tetanic contractions prolonged to more than 90 seconds
3. Increased pain with bright red vaginal bleeding
4. Increased restlessness and anxiety

2. When preparing a client for cesarean birth, which of the following key concepts should be considered when implementing nursing care?
1. Instruct the mother's support person to remain in the family lounge until after the delivery.
2. Arrange for a staff member of the anesthesia department to explain what to expect postoperatively.
3. Modify preoperative teaching to meet the needs of either a planned or emergency cesarean birth.
4. Explain the surgery, expected outcome, and kind of anesthetics that will be used.

3. Which of the following best describes preterm labor?
1. Labor that begins after 20 weeks' gestation and before 37 weeks' gestation
2. Labor that begins after 15 weeks' gestation and before 37 weeks' gestation
3. Labor that begins after 24 weeks' gestation and before 28 weeks' gestation
4. Labor that begins after 28 weeks' gestation and before 40 weeks' gestation

4. Following administration of a tocolytic agent for preterm labor, which of the following would the nurse report to the physician immediately?
1. FHR of 160 beats/minute
2. Maternal blood pressure 120/80 mm Hg
3. Maternal respiratory rate of 22 breaths/minute
4. Complaints of chest pain

5. When PROM occurs, which of the following provides evidence of the nurse's understanding of the client's immediate needs?
1. The chorion and amnion rupture 4 hours before the onset of labor.
2. PROM removes the fetus's most effective defense against infection.
3. Nursing care is based on fetal viability and gestational age.
4. PROM is associated with malpresentation and possibly incompetent cervix.

6. Which of the following factors is the underlying cause of dystocia?
1. Nutritional
2. Mechanical
3. Environmental
4. Medical

7. When uterine rupture occurs, which of the following would be the priority?
1. Limiting hypovolemic shock
2. Obtaining blood specimens
3. Instituting complete bed rest
4. Inserting a urinary catheter

8. Which of the following would alert the nurse to the possibility of uterine inversion?
1. Appearance of a large tissue mass within the vagina
2. Vaginal hemorrhage with hypervolemia
3. Dramatic increase in vaginal bleeding
4. Complaints of severe abdominal pain

9. Which of the following is the nurse's initial action when umbilical cord prolapse occurs?
1. Begin monitoring maternal vital signs and FHR
2. Place the client in a knee-chest position in bed

3. Notify the physician and prepare the client for delivery
4. Apply a sterile warm saline dressing to the exposed cord

10. All of the following are typical signs and symptoms of uterine rupture. Place them in the order in which they are most likely to occur:

1. Presence of a visible retraction ring
2. Presence of maternal hemorrhage
3. Severe pain during a contraction
4. Strong uterine contractions
5. Report of feeling a "tearing sensation"
6. Lack of cervical dilation

Answer key

1. The answer is 2.
Hyperstimulation of the uterus such as with oxytocin during the induction of labor may result in tetanic contractions prolonged to more than 90 seconds, which could lead to such complications as fetal distress, abruptio placentae, amniotic fluid embolism, laceration of the cervix, and uterine rupture. Weak contractions would not occur. Pain, bright red vaginal bleeding, and increased restlessness and anxiety are not associated with hyperstimulation.

2. The answer is 3.
A key point to consider when preparing the client for a cesarean birth is to modify the preoperative teaching to meet the needs of either a planned or emergency cesarean birth; the depth and breadth of instruction will depend on circumstances and time available. Allowing the mother's support person to remain with her as much as possible is an important concept, although doing so depends on many variables. Arranging for necessary explanations by various staff members to be involved with the client's care is a nursing responsibility. The nurse is responsible for reinforcing the explanations about the surgery, expected outcome, and type of anesthetic to be used. The obstetrician is responsible for explaining about the surgery and outcome and the anesthesiology staff is responsible for explanations about the type of anesthesia to be used.

3. The answer is 1.
Preterm labor is best described as labor that begins after 20 weeks' gestation and before 37 weeks' gestation. The other time periods are inaccurate.

4. The answer is 4.
Following tocolytic administration, the nurse would monitor for possible effects such as chest pain, decreased maternal blood pressure, dyspnea, and FHR greater than 180 beats/minute, which would require notification of the physician. An FHR of 160 beats/minute and a maternal respiratory rate of 22 breaths/minute are within normal parameters. A maternal blood pressure of 120/80 mm Hg may be within the normal range for the mother.

5. The answer is 2.
PROM can precipitate many potential and actual problems; one of the most serious is the fetus's loss of an effective defense against infection, This is the client's most immediate need at this time. Typically, PROM occurs about 1 hour, not 4 hours, before labor begins. Fetal viability and gestational age are less immediate considerations that affect the plan of care. Malpresentation and an incompetent cervix may be causes of PROM.

6. The answer is 2.
Dystocia is difficult, painful, prolonged labor due to mechanical factors involving the fetus (passenger), uterus (powers), pelvis (passage), or psyche. Nutritional, environmental,

and medical factors may contribute to the mechanical factors that cause dystocia.

7. The answer is 1.
With uterine rupture, the client is at risk for hypovolemic shock. Therefore, the priority is to prevent and limit hypovolemic shock. Immediate steps should include giving oxygen, replacing lost fluids, providing drug therapy as needed, evaluating fetal responses, and preparing for surgery. Obtaining blood specimens, instituting complete bed rest, and inserting a urinary catheter are necessary in preparation for surgery to remedy the rupture.

8. The answer is 3.
Once inversion occurs, the client may exhibit a dramatic increase in vaginal bleeding, accompanied by increasing pulse rate or other signs of hemorrhage. Rarely is the inverted uterus seen. The client does not become hypervolemic. Complaints of excruciating pelvic, not abdominal, pain and sensation of extreme fullness extending into the vagina are also associated with uterine inversion.

9. The answer is 2.
The immediate priority is to minimize pressure on the cord. Thus the nurse's initial action involves placing the client on bed rest and then placing the client in a knee-chest position or lowering the head of the bed, and elevating the maternal hips on a pillow to minimize the pressure on the cord. Monitoring maternal vital signs and FHR, notifying the physician and preparing the client for delivery, and wrapping the cord with sterile saline-soaked warm gauze are important, but these actions have no effect on minimizing the pressure on the cord.

10. The answer is 1 4 6 3 5 2.
Impending rupture is preceded by a pathologic retraction ring visible on the maternal abdomen. A rupture results when strong uterine contractions occur without increased cervical dilation. The woman experiences sudden severe pain and a "tearing sensation." Contractions stop, and overt or covert hemorrhage occurs. Although rupture of the uterus during labor is rare (1:1,500 births), it's always a possibility. A uterus will rupture when it undergoes more strain than it's able to sustain. Rupture occurs most commonly when a vertical scar from a previous cesarean birth or hysterotomy repair is torn. Contributing factors include prolonged labor, multiple gestation, unwise use of oxytocin, use of forceps or traction, and faulty presentation.

14 Postpartum Complications

I. ESSENTIAL CONCEPTS

A. Today, relatively short postpartum hospitalizations (for most clients, 24 to 72 hours) require the nurse to focus care on assisting parents to care effectively for themselves and their newborns.

B. Preexisting maternal health problems (such as anemia, pregnancy-induced hypertension, and diabetes) contribute to many postpartum complications.

C. Overall nursing objectives for high-risk postpartum clients include:

1. Assure prompt diagnosis and treatment of postpartum complications to minimize risk of morbidity, mortality, and dysfunctional effects.
2. Promote comfort and recovery through physical care measures, nutrition, and pain relief therapies.
3. Explore the emotional aspects of care of the high-risk newborn and family.
4. Minimize separation of mother and newborn, and assist in developing a bonding relationship through information, support, and encouragement of mother-newborn attachment.
5. Assist the client and family to deal with anxiety, anger, grief, and fear through self-expression and acceptance.

NURSING PROCESS OVERVIEW

II. THE WOMAN WITH POSTPARTUM COMPLICATIONS

A. Assessment

1. Health history
   a. Elicit a description of symptoms, including onset, duration, location, and precipitating factors. **Cardinal signs and symptoms** may include:
   - Altered bladder status and problems with voiding
   - Altered rest and sleep
   - Poor appetite, nutrition, and hydration
   - Tenderness, pain or discomfort (perineum, uterus, breasts, legs, and headache)
   - Poor, altered, or no response to the newborn
   - Altered response to maternal role
   - Poor or altered response to the partner

   b. Explore personal and family history for risk factors for postpartum complications.
2. Physical examination
   a. **Vital signs**
   - Measure temperature to detect patterns of temperature elevation.
   - Measure blood pressure to detect elevations.

   b. **Inspection**
   - Inspect the perineum for bruising, swelling, and characteristics of the episiotomy.
   - Assess the character of lochia for color, odor, and amount.
   - Inspect the legs for presence of edema or red streaks.
   - Inspect the breasts for reddened areas.
   - Inspect the nipples for cracks, blisters, and bleeding.

   c. **Palpation**
   - Palpate the uterus for bogginess, location, and tenderness.

- Palpate the legs for tenderness, warmth, lumps, and pain.
- Palpate the breasts for fullness, lumps, and tenderness.

3. Laboratory and diagnostic studies
   a. **Culture and sensitivity tests** (of wound sites, drainage, or urine) are used to diagnose infections.
   b. **Venography** is the most accurate method for the diagnosis of deep vein thrombosis (DVT).
   c. **Real-time and color Doppler ultrasound** are noninvasive diagnostic methods used to diagnose thrombophlebitis and thrombosis.

B. Nursing diagnoses.

(Both general and complication-specific are listed. Planning and outcome identification, implementation, and outcome evaluation are focused on general diagnoses.)

1. General diagnoses
   a. Pain
   b. Anxiety
   c. Fear
   d. Ineffective Individual Coping
   e. Altered Parenting
   f. Altered Family Processes
   g. Ineffective Family Coping: Compromised
   h. Knowledge Deficit
2. Complication-specific diagnoses
   a. Fluid Volume Deficit
   b. Risk for Infection
   c. Risk for Injury
   d. Impaired Tissue Integrity
   e. Impaired Physical Mobility
   f. Self-Care Deficit
   g. Urinary Retention

C. Planning and outcome identification

1. The client will make a full physical recovery from the complication.
2. The client and family will express grief and fear and will utilize appropriate coping and support mechanisms.
3. The parents and newborn will begin bonding.
4. The client and family will understand the complication and its expected course and treatment regimen.

D. Implementation

1. Promote a full physical recovery.
   a. Screen for and prevent additional complications.
   b. Provide effective pain relief.
   c. Assess vital signs.
   d. Collect specimens for laboratory testing.
   e. Administer prescribed medications.
   f. Provide physical care.
   g. Carry out the treatment regimen (such as sitz baths, medications, and dressings)
   h. Enhance fluid and food intake.

2. Assist the client and family to deal with physical and emotional stresses of postpartum complications.
   a. Support and communicate with the client and family members about the plan of care.
   b. Support and communicate with the client and family members during an emergency situation, thus enhancing cooperation with treatment efforts.
   c. Demonstrate self-care techniques as appropriate (such as fundal massage, assessing fundal height and consistency, and inspecting episiotomy and lacerations).
   d. Discuss the importance of rest and adequate nutrition.
   e. Encourage appropriate coping mechanisms.
   f. Encourage expressions of fear and sense of loss and grief.
3. Encourage parent-newborn bonding.
   a. Provide for maximum mother-newborn contact.
   b. Provide continuous information about the newborn.
   c. Promote father or partner interaction with the mother and newborn.
4. Provide client and family teaching.
   a. Explain and discuss the complication and its expected course and treatment regimen.
   b. Involve the client's partner in education about the complication, the newborn, and the mother's need for emotional support.

E. Outcome evaluation

1. The client fully recovers from the complication.
   a. The mother's vital signs are stable.
   b. The mother voids without difficulty.
   c. The mother remains symptom-free.
   d. The mother rests and sleeps well.
   e. The mother takes adequate fluids and food.
   f. The mother reports relief from pain and discomfort.
2. The client and family express grief and fear, and use appropriate coping and support mechanisms.
3. The parents and newborn begin bonding. The mother assumes as much caretaking of the newborn as her condition permits.
4. The client and family understand the complication and its expected course and treatment regimen.

III. POSTPARTUM HEMORRHAGE

A. Description. Postpartum hemorrhage is blood loss of more than 500 ml following the birth of a newborn.

B. Etiology

1. Early postpartum hemorrhage, which is usually due to uterine atony, lacerations, or retained placental fragments, occurs in the first 24 hours after delivery. (See Chapter 13 for information on nursing care related to early postpartum hemorrhage.)
2. Late postpartum hemorrhage occurs after the first 24 hours after delivery and is generally caused by retained placental fragments or bleeding disorders.

C. Pathophysiology. Delayed uterine atony or placental fragments prevent the uterus from contracting effectively. The uterus is unable to form an effective clot structure and bleeding ensues or continues.

D. Assessment findings. Common **clinical manifestations** include:

1. Vaginal bleeding, the obvious sign of postpartum hemorrhage; amount and character vary with cause
2. Signs of impending shock, including changes in skin temperature and color and altered level of consciousness

E. Nursing management

1. Prevent excessive blood loss and resulting complications.
   a. Massage the uterus, facilitate voiding, and report blood loss.
   b. Monitor blood pressure and pulse rate every 5 to 15 minutes.
   c. Prepare for intravenous infusion, oxytocin, and blood transfusion, if needed.
   d. Administer medications and oxygen as prescribed. (*Drug Chart* 14-1, page 232).
   e. Measure and record fluid intake and output.
   f. Be prepared for a possible dilatation and curettage.
2. **Assist the client and family in dealing with physical and emotional stress of postpartum hemorrhage.**

IV. SUBINVOLUTION

A. Description. Subinvolution is the delayed return of the uterus to its prepregnant size and shape.

B. Etiology. Subinvolution results from retained placental fragments and membranes, endometritis, or uterine fibroid tumor; treatment depends on the cause.

C. Pathophysiology. Uterine atony or placental fragments prevent the uterus from contracting effectively.

D. Assessment findings. **Clinical manifestations** include:

1. Prolonged lochial discharge
2. Irregular or excessive bleeding
3. Larger than normal uterus
4. Boggy uterus (occasionally)

E. Nursing management

1. Prevent excessive blood loss, infection, and other complications.
   a. Massage uterus, facilitate voiding, and report blood loss.
   b. Monitor blood pressure and pulse rate.
   c. Administer prescribed medications.
   d. Be prepared for a possible D&C. (See *Drug Chart* 14-1, page 232.)
2. **Assist the client and family in dealing with physical and emotional stress of the postpartum complications of subinvolution.**

DRUG CHART 14-1

Medications used for postpartum complications

Classifications	Used for	Selected interventions
Anticoagulants heparin sodium injection (Hepalean)	■ Blocks the conversion of prothrombin to thrombin and fibrinogen to fibrin thus decreasing clotting ability ■ Inhibits thrombus and clot formation	■ Give heparin I.V. as a "piggy back" infusion. ■ Give heparin S.C. into the abdomen; rotate sites, do not aspirate; apply pressure (do not massage). ■ Used to prevent and treat pulmonary embolism and thrombosis. ■ *Women receiving anticoagulants should not be given estrogen or aspirin.* ■ Obtain baseline coagulation studies. ■ Obtain serial coagulation studies while the client receiving therapy. ■ Keep protamine sulfate readily available in case of heparin overdose. ■ Assess client for bleeding from nose, gums, hematuria, blood in stool. ■ Observe color and amount of lochia. Institute a pad count. ■ Avoid I.M. injections to avoid formation of hematomas. ■ Inform client that this drug does not pass into breast milk. ■ Monitor client for hemorrhage, bruising, urticaria, and thrombocytopenia.
warfarin sodium (Coumadin, Warfilone)	■ Interferes with hepatic synthesis of vitamin K–dependent clotting factors (II, VII, IX, X)	■ *Women receiving anticoagulant therapy should not be given estrogen or aspirin.* ■ Obtain baseline coagulation studies. ■ Obtain serial coagulation studies while client is receiving therapy. ■ Keep AquaMEPHYTON (vitamin K) on hand in case of warfarin overdose. ■ Assess client for bleeding from nose, gums, hematuria, blood in stool. ■ Observe color and amount of lochia. Institute a pad count. ■ Avoid I.M. injections to avoid formation of hematomas. ■ Inform client that this drug passes into breast milk and its use is contraindicated during pregnancy. ■ Monitor client for the following side effects: hemorrhage, fever, nausea, and cramps.
Oxytoxic methylergonovin maleate (Methergine) (P.O., I.M., I.V.)	■ Directly stimulates uterine and vascular smooth muscle ■ Promotes uterine contraction ■ Prevents and treats postpartum or postabortion hemorrhage caused by uterine atony or subinvolution	■ Obtain a baseline calcium level. ■ Advise the client that this medication will cause menstrual-like cramps. ■ Assess for numb fingers and toes, cold, chest pain, nausea, vomiting, muscle pain, and weakness. ■ May cause decreased serum prolactin. ■ I.V. administration is used for emergency dosage only. Administer at a rate of 0.2 mg over at least 1 minute. ■ *Do not mix this drug with any other drug.* ■ Use solution only if it is clear and colorless, with no precipitate. May store at room temperature for 60 days. The drug deteriorates with age. ■ Monitor client for dyspnea, palpitations, diaphoresis, chest pain, hypotension, and headache.

V. PUERPERAL INFECTION

A. Description

1. Infection developing in the reproductive tract after delivery.
2. Puerperal infection is a major cause of maternal morbidity and mortality.
3. The incidence ranges from 1% to 8% of all deliveries; the incidence is higher in cesarean births.
4. A puerperal infection is always serious because, although it usually begins as a local infection, it can spread to involve the peritoneum or circulatory system.
5. Localized infections may affect the vagina, vulva, and perineum.
6. Endometritis, localized infection of the uterine lining, occurs 48 to 72 hours after delivery.

B. Etiology.

Etiology. Puerperal infection can be caused by poor sterile technique, delivery with significant manipulation, cesarean birth, or overgrowth of local flora.

C. Pathophysiology

1. Causative organisms
   a. Aerobic organisms include beta-hemolytic streptococci, *Escherichia coli, Klebsiella* organisms, *Proteus mirabilis, Pseudomonas, Staphylococcus aureus,* and *Neisseria* organisms.
   b. Anaerobic organisms include *Bacteroides, Peptostreptococcus,* and *Peptococcus* organisms, and *Clostridium perfringens.*
2. In parametritis (pelvic cellulitis), infection spreads by way of the lymphatics of the connective tissue surrounding the uterus.
3. Puerperal infection may extend to the peritoneum by way of the lymph nodes and uterine wall.

D. Assessment findings

1. Clinical manifestations
   a. Puerperal morbidity is marked by a temperature of 38° C (100.4° F) or higher after the first 24 hours postpartum on any two of the first 10 postpartum days.
   b. **Localized vaginal, vulval, and perineal infections** are marked by pain, elevated temperature, edema, redness, firmness and tenderness at the site of the wound; sensation of heat; burning on urination; and discharge from the wound.
   c. Manifestations of **endometritis** include a rise in temperature for several days. In severe endometritis, symptoms include malaise; headache; backache; general discomfort; loss of appetite; large, tender uterus; severe postpartum cramping; and brownish red, foul-smelling lochia.
   d. **Parametritis** (pelvic cellulitis) commonly produces a temperature of more than 38.6° C (101.5° F), chills, abdominal pain, subinvolution of uterus, tachycardia, and lethargy.
   e. Signs and symptoms of **peritonitis** include high fever, rapid pulse, abdominal pains, nausea, vomiting, and restlessness.

E. Nursing management

1. Promote resolution of the infectious process.
   a. Inspect the perineum twice daily for redness, edema, ecchymosis, and discharge.
   b. Evaluate for abdominal pain, fever, malaise, tachycardia, and foul-smelling lochia.
   c. Obtain specimens for laboratory analysis; report the findings.
   d. Offer a balanced diet, frequent fluids, and early ambulation.

e. Administer prescribed antibiotics or medications; document the client's response.

2. **Provide client and family teaching.**
   a. Describe and demonstrate self-care.
   b. Stress careful perineal hygiene and handwashing.
   c. Inform the client about the infection, its cause, and treatment.

VI. MASTITIS

A. Description

1. Mastitis is inflammation of the breast tissue that is usually caused by infection or by stasis of milk in the ducts.
2. An epidemic mastitis infection is derived from a nosocomial source, usually *Staphylococcus aureus,* and localizes in the lactiferous glands and ducts.
3. An endemic mastitis infection occurs randomly and localizes in the periglandular connective tissue.
4. Mastitis infections are largely preventable by prophylactic measures, such as good breast hygiene and effective handwashing.

B. Etiology. Injury to the breast is the primary predisposing factor (such as overdistention, stasis, or cracking of nipples).

C. Pathophysiology

1. The exact cause of stasis of milk in the ducts is not known; however, missed feedings, a bra that is too tight, or impaired infant suckling are contributory factors.
2. Introduction of an infectious organism from either the mother's hands following improper washing or from the infant's mouth is also contributory.
3. Cracked, blistered nipples also allow a port of entry for infectious agents.

D. Assessment findings. Because symptoms usually do not occur until the third or fourth postpartum week (or even months later), teach the client to recognize signs and symptoms of mastitis and to report them to her nurse or physician. **Clinical manifestations** include:

1. Elevated temperature, chills, general aching, malaise, and localized pain
2. Increased pulse rate
3. Engorgement, hardness, and reddening of the breasts
4. Nipple soreness and fissures
5. Swollen and tender axillary lymph nodes

E. Nursing management

1. **Promote resolution of the infectious process.**
   a. Observe for elevated temperature, chills, tachycardia, headache, and pain or tenderness, firmness, and redness of the breast.
   b. Administer antibiotics, and explain importance of following through with the prescribed regimen even when symptoms subside.
   c. Offer comfort measures, such as small side pillows, icecaps, or heat application over localized abscess.
2. Provide client and family teaching.
   a. Explain how to prevent infection through meticulous handwashing and prompt attention to blocked milk ducts.
   b. Encourage the mother to do the following:
      - Breast-feed frequently

- Perform adequate breast and nipple care (such as adequate around-the-clock nonconstrictive support of the breasts, gentleness during care, avoidance of harsh cleansing agents and decrusting the nipple, frequent breast pad changes, and intermittent exposure of nipples to the air)
- Recognize the signs and symptoms of infection

VII. THROMBOPHLEBITIS AND THROMBOSIS

A. Description

1. Thrombophlebitis is an inflammation of the vascular endothelium with clot formation on the vessel wall.
2. A thrombus forms when blood components (platelets and fibrin) combine to form an aggregate body (clot).
3. Pulmonary embolism occurs when a clot traveling through the venous system lodges within the pulmonary circulatory system, causing occlusion or infarction.
4. The incidence of postpartum thrombophlebitis is 0.1% to 1%; when not treated, 24% of this group develop pulmonary embolism, with a fatality rate of 15%.

B. Etiology. Predisposing risk factors include:

1. History of thrombophlebitis
2. Obesity
3. History of cesarean birth
4. History of forceps delivery
5. Maternal age older than 35
6. Multiparity
7. Lactation suppression with estrogens
8. Varicosities
9. Anemia and blood dyscrasias

C. Pathophysiology

1. The three major causes of thrombus formation and inflammation are venous stasis, hypercoagulable blood, and injury to the innermost layer of the blood vessel.
2. Both venous stasis (in the pelvis and lower extremities) and hypercoagulable blood are present during pregnancy.
3. The level of most coagulation factors (especially fibrinogen and factors III, VII, an X) increases during pregnancy. This increase is accompanied by a decrease in plasminogen and antithrombin III levels, which causes clots to disintegrate.
4. Injury to the innermost layer of the vessel is probably not contributory, in general, during pregnancy. However, the possibility exists if the birth is by cesarean birth.

D. Assessment findings

1. Common **clinical manifestations**
   a. Superficial thrombophlebitis within the saphenous vein system manifests as midcalf and pain, tenderness, redness, and warmth along the vein.
   b. DVT symptoms include muscle pain, the presence of Homans' sign (pain in the calf on passive dorsiflexion of the foot, possibly caused by DVT). However, the presence of Homans' sign is no longer believed to be conclusive because the pain may result from other causes, such as strained muscles or contusions.
   c. Pelvic thrombophlebitis, typically occurring 2 weeks after delivery, is marked by chills, fever, malaise, and pain.

d. Femoral thrombophlebitis, generally occurring 10 to 14 days after delivery, produces chills, fever, malaise, stiffness, and pain.

e. Pulmonary embolism is heralded by sudden intense chest pain with severe dyspnea followed by tachypnea, pleuritic pain, apprehension, cough, tachycardia, hemoptysis, and temperature above 38° C (100.4° F).

2. Laboratory and diagnostic study findings

a. **Venography** accurately diagnoses DVT. There are risks associated with the radiopaque dye that is used.

b. **Real-time and color Doppler ultrasound** diagnose deep venous thrombosis.

c. **Impedance plethysmography** measures changes in venous blood volume and flow.

E. Nursing management

1. Promote resolution of symptoms and prevent the development of embolus.

a. Assess vital signs.

b. Assess extremities for signs of inflammation, swelling, and the presence of Homans' sign.

c. Administer anticoagulant therapy as prescribed, and observe for signs of bleeding and allergic reactions. *Note:* Keep the antidote protamine sulfate available in case of a severe heparin overdose. Usually, protamine sulfate solution is administered intravenously at a rate no greater than 50 mg every 10 minutes.

d. *Caution:* Do not administer estrogens for lactation suppression because estrogens may encourage clot formation.

e. Prepare the client for diagnostic studies (venography and Doppler ultrasound), as indicated.

f. Implement measures to prevent complications of bed rest (such as bed placed in Trendelenburg position, use of footboard, passive or active range of motion exercises, frequent shifts in position, and adequate fluid intake and output).

2. Provide client and family teaching.

a. Explain strategies for preventing venous stasis (and thus thrombophlebitis) (*Client and Family Teaching* 14-1).

b. Provide information regarding the treatment regimen (such as anticoagulant therapy, analgesics, and bed rest).

3. Assist the client and family in dealing with physical and emotional stress of postpartum thrombophlebitis and thrombosis.

4. Encourage parent-newborn bonding.

CLIENT AND FAMILY TEACHING 14-1

Preventing venous stasis

- Ambulate early and change your position frequently when sitting.
- Avoid standing or sitting (with your knees bent sharply) for long periods of time.
- Avoid crossing your legs.
- When lying down, move your toes and lift your legs to improve circulation.
- If you are at risk for thrombophlebitis, talk to your physician about using support stockings during the postpartum period.

VIII. URINARY TRACT INFECTION (UTI)

A. Description

1. A UTI is indicated by more than 10^5 bacterial colonies/ml of urine in two consecutive clean, voided, midstream specimens.
2. Two common types of UTIs are cystitis (inflammation of the urinary bladder) and pyelonephritis (inflammation of the renal pelvis).
3. UTIs occur in about 5% of postpartum women; they occur in 15% of women who have undergone postpartum catheterization.

B. Etiology

1. Ascending bacterial infections account for most UTIs.
2. Another cause of UTIs is retention and residual urine due to overdistention and incomplete emptying of the bladder.
   a. Temporary urine retention may be due to decreased perception of the urge to void, resulting from perineal trauma and the effects of analgesia or anesthesia.
   b. Urinary stasis and residual urine provide a medium for bacterial growth, predisposing the client to cystitis and pyelonephritis.

C. Pathophysiology

1. Causative organisms in cystitis and pyelonephritis include *E. coli* (most common), *Proteus* and *Pseudomonas* organisms, *S. aureus*, and *Streptococcus faecalis.*
2. Consequences of not recognizing early symptoms of UTI include the extension of the infection upward with subsequent permanent loss of kidney function.

D. Assessment findings. **Clinical manifestations** depend on the type of infection.

1. Cystitis manifestations include frequency, urgency, dysuria, hematuria, nocturia, temperature elevation, and suprapubic pain.
2. Pyelonephritis manifestations include high fever, chills, flank pain, nausea, and vomiting.

E. Nursing management. **Recognize signs of infection and prevent the development of further complications.**

1. Determine if symptoms are present and if the woman had difficulty urinating after delivery.
2. Obtain specimens, report findings, and administer antibiotics and medications as prescribed.
3. Describe self-care related to regular emptying of bladder, proper perineal cleansing, and the need for increased fluids.
4. Insert intermittent or indwelling catheter as needed.
5. Observe and record the response to treatment.

IX. POSTPARTUM MOOD DISORDERS

A. Description

1. The *Diagnostic and Statistical Manual of Mental Disorders* contains official guidelines for the assessment and diagnosis of psychiatric illness. The disorders recognized during the postpartum period are:
   a. Postpartum blues
   b. Postpartum depression without psychotic features

  c. Postpartum depression with psychotic features (postpartum psychosis)
2. Between 50% and 80% of all new mothers report some form of postpartum blues.
3. The incidence of moderate or major postpartum depression or postpartum bipolar disorder ranges from 30 to 200 per every 1,000 live births; the incidence of brief psychotic disorder with postpartum onset is about 1 in every 1,000 live births.

B. Etiology

1. Predisposing factors include a history of puerperal psychosis, bipolar (formerly manic-depressive) disorder, delirium and hallucinations, rapid mood changes, agitation or confusion, and the potential for suicide or infanticide.
2. Postpartum depression with and without psychosis is being studied from three perspectives.
   - *a.* Biological theories include alteration in hypothalamic function, possibly related to altered hormonal influence.
   - *b.* Psychological theories include poor support systems, psychologic stress, and poor relationship with partner.
   - *c.* Sociocultural theories include low levels of social gratification, support, and control both at work and in the parenting role.

C. Assessment findings.

C. Assessment findings. Serious postpartum depression or psychosis usually does not occur until 3 to 5 days after delivery, at which time the client is usually discharged from the hospital or birthing center. Clinical manifestations depend on the type of mood disorder.

1. Postpartum blues manifestations include fatigue, weeping, anxiety, and mood instability with onset 1 to 10 days postpartum and lasting 2 weeks or less.
2. Postpartum depression without psychosis manifestations include confusion, fatigue, agitation, feelings of hopelessness and shame, and alterations in mood.
3. Postpartum depression with psychosis manifestations include symptoms of postpartum depression plus delusions, auditory hallucinations, and hyperactivity.

D. Nursing management

1. Identify postpartum mood disorders.
   - *a.* Be aware of signs and symptoms of postpartum mood disorders.
   - *b.* Teach the client and family about these disorders.
2. Support and treat the client and family.
   - *a.* Develop specific therapeutic goals.
   - *b.* Maintain the prescribed medication schedule.
   - *c.* Keep communication open with the health care providers; coordinate social services.
   - *d.* Include family participation and involvement in plans of care.
   - *e.* Make appropriate referrals.
3. Support efforts at parent-newborn bonding.
   - *a.* Provide support for the mother's continued care of the newborn, if appropriate and safe for the newborn.
   - *b.* Plan for continuity of care for the mother, newborn, and family.

Study questions

1. With today's shorter postpartum hospitalizations (24 to 72 hours), the focus of nursing revolves around which of the following essential concepts?

1. Promotion of comfort and recovery through physical care measures and pain relief therapies
2. Exploration of the emotional aspects of care of the high-risk newborn and the family
3. Parental assistance to care for themselves and their newborn safely and effectively
4. Client and family assistance to deal with anxiety effectively and completely.

2. Which of the following is most important when caring for high-risk postpartum clients?

1. Discussing hygiene and nutrition
2. Referring the mother to others for emotional support
3. Discussing complications and treatment
4. Promoting mother-newborn contact

3. Which of the following amounts of blood loss following birth marks the criterion for describing postpartum hemorrhage?

1. More than 200 ml
2. More than 300 ml
3. More than 400 ml
4. More than 500 ml

4. Which of the following best describes subinvolution?

1. Bleeding with an onset in the first 24 hours after delivery.
2. Delayed return of the enlarged uterus to normal size and function
3. Inflammation of the vascular endothelium with clot formation
4. Inability to form an effective clot structure, leading to continued bleeding

5. Which of the following best signals early puerperal infection?

1. Temperature elevation of 38° C (100.4° F) or higher after the first 24 hours postpartum.
2. Local infections of the vagina, vulva, and perineum after the first 24 hours postpartum.
3. Elevated temperature, dyspnea, hypovolemia, and malaise after the first 12 hours postpartum.
4. Lower abdominal pain, inability to void, and anxiety following the first postpartum week

6. Which of the following is the primary predisposing factor related to mastitis?

1. Epidemic infection from nosocomial sources localizing in the lactiferous glands and ducts
2. Endemic infection occurring randomly and localizing in the periglandular connective tissue
3. Temporary urine retention due to decreased perception of the urge to void
4. Breast injury caused by overdistention, stasis, and cracking of the nipples

7. Which of the following best describes thrombophlebitis?

1. Inflammation and clot formation that result when blood components combine to form an aggregate body
2. Inflammation and blood clots that eventually become lodged within the pulmonary blood vessels
3. Inflammation and blood clots that eventually become lodged within the femoral vein
4. Inflammation of the vascular endothelium with clot formation on the vessel wall

8. Which of the following assessment findings would the nurse expect if the client develops DVT?

1. Midcalf pain and tenderness and redness along the vein
2. Chills, fever, and malaise occurring 2 weeks after delivery
3. Muscle pain, the presence of Homans' sign, and swelling in the affected limb
4. Chills, fever, stiffness, and pain occurring 10 to 14 days after delivery

9. Which of the following are the most commonly assessed findings in cystitis?

1. Frequency, urgency, dehydration, nausea, chills, and flank pain
2. Nocturia, frequency, urgency, dysuria, hematuria, fever, and suprapubic pain
3. Dehydration, hypertension, dysuria, suprapubic pain, chills, and fever
4. High fever, chills, flank pain, nausea, vomiting, dysuria, and frequency

10. Which of the following best reflects the frequency of reported postpartum "blues"?

1. Between 10% and 40% of all new mothers report some form of postpartum blues.
2. Between 30% and 50% of all new mothers report some form of postpartum blues.
3. Between 50% and 80% of all new mothers report some form of postpartum blues.
4. Between 25% and 70% of all new mothers report some form of postpartum blues.

11. By definition, a postpartum hemorrhage is any blood loss from the uterus that is greater than how many milliliters?

Answer key

1. The answer is 3.
Because of shortened postpartum hospitalizations, nursing care focuses on assisting parents in caring for themselves and their newborn safely and effectively. Promoting comfort and recovery, exploring the emotional aspects, and assisting the client and family in dealing with anxiety are all important, but with shortened lengths of stay, the focus is on the overall situation of safe and effective parental and newborn care.

2. The answer is 4.
When caring for high-risk postpartum clients, care includes all of the routine measures plus minimizing the separation of mother and newborn and encouraging attachment. Because of the complication, the mother and newborn are often separated. Thus, measures to promote contact between them takes priority. Discussing hygiene and nutrition is part of the client's routine care. Providing emotional support and discussing complications and treatment are within the realm of appropriate nursing responsibilities, applicable to any client. Referring the mother to others for emotional support may be appropriate if the client needs additional help.

3. The answer is d.
Postpartum hemorrhage is defined as blood loss of more than 500 ml following birth. Any amount less than this is not considered postpartum hemorrhage.

4. The answer is 2.
Subinvolution is delayed return of the enlarged uterus to normal size and function, resulting from retained placental fragments and membranes, endometritis, or uterine fibroid tumor. Early postpartum hemorrhage occurs within the first 24 hours after delivery usually due to uterine atony, lacerations, or retained placental fragments. Inflammation of the vascular endothelium with clot formation describes thrombophlebitis. An inability to form an effective clot structure describes the mechanism underlying postpartum hemorrhage.

5. The answer is 1.
Puerperal infection is marked by a temperature of 38° C (100.4° F) or higher after the first 24 postpartum hours on any 2 of the first 10 postpartum days. Local infections of the vagina, vulva, and perineum; dyspnea; hypovolemia and malaise; lower abdominal pain; difficulty voiding; and anxiety all may be present with puerperal infection, but the temperature elevation is usually the first definitive sign.

6. The answer is 4.
With mastitis, injury to the breast, such as overdistention, stasis, and cracking of the nipples, is the primary predisposing factor. Epidemic and endemic infections are probable sources of infection for mastitis. Temporary urine retention due to decreased perception of the urge to void is a contributory factor to the development of urinary tract infection, not mastitis.

7. The answer is 4.
Thrombophlebitis refers to an inflammation of the vascular endothelium with clot formation on the wall of the vessel. Blood components combining to form an aggregate body describe a thrombus or thrombosis. Clots lodging in the pulmonary vasculature refers to pulmonary embolism; in the femoral vein, femoral thrombophlebitis.

8. The answer is 3.
Classic symptoms of DVT include muscle pain, the presence of Homans' sign, and swelling of the affected limb. Midcalf pain and tenderness and redness along the vein reflect superficial thrombophlebitis. Chills, fever, and malaise occurring 2 weeks after delivery reflect pelvic thrombophlebitis. Chills, fever, stiffness, and pain occurring 10 to 14 days after delivery suggest femoral thrombophlebitis.

9. The answer is 2.
Manifestations of cystitis include frequency, urgency, dysuria, hematuria, nocturia, fever, and suprapubic pain. Dehydration, hypertension, and chills are not typically associated with cystitis. High fever, chills, flank pain, nausea, vomiting, dysuria, and frequency are associated with pyelonephritis.

10. The answer is 3.
According to statistical reports, between 50% and 80% of all new mothers report some form of postpartum blues. The ranges of 10% to 40%, 30% to 50%, and 25% to 70% are incorrect.

11. The answer is 500.
Blood loss from the uterus greater than 500 ml is the traditional definition of postpartum hemorrhage. However, specific agencies may not consider blood loss from the uterus to be a hemorrhage until the amount reaches 1,000 ml. Hemorrhage is a major potential danger in the immediate postpartal period. The four main causes of postpartum hemorrhage are uterine atony, lacerations, retained placental fragments, and disseminated intravascular coagulation.

15 Neonatal Complications

I. ESSENTIAL CONCEPTS

A. Early identification of the high-risk newborn is the first step in detecting and managing complications to reduce morbidity and mortality.

B. Major neonatal complications covered in this chapter include:

1. Birth asphyxia
2. Complications related to gestational age, including preterm, small-for-gestational age (SGA), large-for-gestational age (LGA), and postterm
3. Complications related to maternal condition (such as diabetes)

C. Complications not covered extensively in this chapter include:

1. Birth injuries (such as fractures of skull, clavicle, humerus, or femur)
2. Infections — bacterial, viral, or protozoal
3. Hemolytic disease — Rh and ABO incompatibility
4. Central nervous system injuries (such as intracranial hemorrhage, brachial plexus injury, facial nerve injury, and phrenic nerve injury)
5. Maternal substance abuse (such as alcohol and other drugs)

NURSING PROCESS OVERVIEW

II. THE HIGH-RISK NEWBORN

A. Assessment

1. **Health history** should include both maternal and neonatal histories.
   a. Elicit a description of symptoms, including onset, duration, location, and precipitating factors. **Cardinal signs and symptoms** may include:
   - Problems identified during pregnancy (possible birth defects)
   - Respiratory distress
   - Ineffective thermoregulation
   - Maternal or neonatal infection
   - Cardiovascular difficulty in the neonate (persistent fetal circulation, low APGAR score)
   - Inability to take and retain fluids (such as breast milk, water, or formula)
   - Neonatal hypoglycemia, hyperbilirubinemia, anemia, pale to blue color, anorexia, and failure to thrive

   b. Explore personal and family history for **risk factors** for neonatal complications.
   - Personal risk factors include:
     - Alcohol use. Because the limit for safe ingestion of alcohol is unknown, newborns of mothers who use alcohol are at risk for fetal alcohol syndrome.
     - Abuse of substances (such as narcotics, cocaine, and nicotine). The newborn of a mother who is dependent on prescription or nonprescription substances may experience complications.
     - Poor maternal nutrition
   - Family risk factors include age, medical history (such as diabetes or cardiac problems) genetic history, obstetric history, onset and duration of prenatal care, and lifestyle choices.
     - Behavioral assessment should include observation of maternal-infant bonding, maternal care-giving activities, and concern for the infant's well-being.

2. **Physical examination**
   a. **Vital signs** are usually monitored continuously.
      - Place the newborn on a warmer (attach a skin probe to the neonate's abdomen).
      - Place the newborn on an apnea monitor.
      - Place the newborn on a blood pressure/pulse monitor.
      - Assess the newborn's weight daily.
      - Measure the newborn's length, chest, and head circumference.
   b. **Inspection**
      - Inspect the newborn's chest and abdomen for irregular breathing patterns and use of accessory muscles.
      - Inspect the newborn's skin for color changes (jaundice, cyanosis, and mottling).
      - Inspect the diaper for urination and defecation.
   c. **Palpation**
      - Palpate the fontanels as a measure of fluid excess or deficit.
      - Palpate the mucous membrane of the mouth as a measure of hydration status.
   d. **Auscultation**
      - Count the apical heart rate.
      - Listen to breath sounds to identify abnormal sounds (such as wheezes, rales, ronchi, and grunting).
      - Listen to bowel sounds to validate function.
3. **Laboratory and diagnostic studies**
   a. **Complete blood cell count (hematocrit)** is used to detect anemia.
   b. **Blood glucose tests** are used to determine the neonate's ability to regulate glucose metabolism.
   c. **Serum electrolyte studies** are used to ensure adequate fluid intake and acid-base status.
   d. **Serum bilirubin,** an indirect bilirubin level, measures the rate of red blood cell breakdown.
   e. **X-rays** are used to show areas of infiltration or consolidation in the lung, or to confirm necrotizing enterocolitis.
   f. **Arterial blood gas studies** are used to determine the effectiveness of ventilation and acid-base status.
   g. **Pulse oximetry** is used to measure oxygen saturation.

B. Nursing diagnoses

1. Ineffective Airway Clearance
2. Ineffective Breathing Pattern
3. Impaired Gas Exchange
4. Altered Cardiovascular Tissue Perfusion
5. Ineffective Thermoregulation
6. Risk for Infection
7. Risk for Altered Nutrition: Less than body requirements
8. Risk for Altered Parenting
9. Knowledge Deficit

C. Planning and outcome identification

1. The newborn will receive effective respiratory support.
2. A neutral thermal environment will be achieved in the newborn.
3. Infection will be prevented.
4. The newborn will receive adequate fluids and electrolytes and nutrition.

5. Parent-newborn attachment will occur.
6. The parents will receive education and emotional support.

D. Implementation

1. **Provide respiratory support** (providing airway clearance, maintaining gas exchange, promoting optimal breathing patterns, and maintaining adequate tissue perfusion).
   - *a.* Assess vital signs, breath sounds, respiratory effort, and oxygenation.
   - *b.* Maintain a patent airway.
   - *c.* Administer oxygen to keep oxygen saturation above 95%.
   - *d.* If the newborn experiences respiratory distress, discontinue oral feedings to prevent aspiration.
   - *e.* Administer prescribed medication to prevent or treat respiratory distress syndrome, if indicated (*Drug Chart* 15-1, page 246).
2. **Maintain a neutral thermal environment.**
   - *a.* Maintain body temperature between 97.6° and 98.6° F.
   - *b.* Provide appropriate heat-conserving mechanisms, including warming beds, heat pads, head coverings, and proper use of infant servo control probes.
   - *c.* Monitor isolette temperature or warmer temperature. Constant heater output is a sign of temperature instability.
   - *d.* Prevent unnecessary heat loss (such as working through isolette portholes and avoiding cold scales, bathing, and exposure to drafts).
   - *e.* Prevent cold stress, which increases metabolism, thereby rapidly consuming oxygen and glucose.
3. **Prevent infection.** Monitor the neonate for signs and symptoms of infection (temperature instability, apnea, cyanosis, decreased oxygen saturation, thrombocytopenia, and feeding intolerance).
4. **Provide adequate fluids and electrolytes and nutrition.**
   - *a.* Monitor the newborn for fluid volume deficits.
   - *b.* Precisely measure intake and output.
   - *c.* Measure the newborn's daily weight.
   - *d.* Assess serum electrolyte levels.
   - *e.* Minimize insensible water losses; cover the open warmers with plastic wrap, humidify oxygen, and close isolette ports.
   - *f.* Minimize the amount of blood withdrawn for laboratory tests.
   - *g.* Administer breast milk or formula as prescribed. Allow the newborn to breast-feed if stable.
   - *h.* Position the newborn on the right side after feeding to promote stomach emptying.
   - *i.* Measure the head circumference and plot growth on the chart.
   - *j.* Support conjugation and excretion of bilirubin. Initiate phototherapy as necessary.
5. **Promote parent-newborn attachment.**
   - *a.* Encourage early and frequent visits by the parents.
   - *b.* Place the newborn's name on the isolette.
   - *c.* Provide the parents with the unit phone number and names of staff caring for the newborn.
   - *d.* Give parents the opportunity to provide basic care for the newborn when appropriate.
   - *e.* Point out the newborn's unique characteristics.
6. **Provide education and emotional support.**
   - *a.* Explain the newborn's need for close observation and frequent blood tests.
   - *b.* Demonstrate and discuss newborn care.

DRUG CHART 15-1

Medications used for neonatal complications

Classifications	Used for	Selected interventions
Lung surfactant beractant (Survanta)	■ Restores naturally occurring lung surfactant to improve lung compliance ■ Prevents or treats respiratory distress syndrome in premature infant	■ The usual dose is 4 ml/kg intratracheally in four doses at least 6 hours apart in the first 48 hours of life. ■ Suction the infant's airway before administration and delay further suctioning as long as possible. ■ Assess the infant's respiratory rate, arterial blood gases (ABGs), and color before administration. ■ Change the infant's position every 2 hours to promote flow to both lungs. ■ Assess the infant's respiratory rate, color, and ABGs after administration. ■ Monitor the infant for adverse effects, which may include transient bradycardia or rales.
Recombinant human erythropoietin	■ Treats anemia caused by reduced endogenous erythropoietin production ■ Stimulates production of red blood cells (RBCs) in bone marrow ■ Reduces need for blood transfusions	■ Determine complete blood cell count, hematocrit, and hemoglobin. ■ Check for occult blood in stool (guaiac test). ■ Assess bowel sounds. ■ Measure ABGs.
Iron supplement	■ Treats iron deficiency resulting from inadequate iron stores	■ Observe for respiratory distress.
Folic acid	■ Increases RBC, white blood cell, and platelet formation	■ Observe for lethargy, hepatosplenomegaly, pallor, and tachycardia.
Vitamin E	■ Treats vitamin deficiency ■ Protects RBCs from destruction	■ Record amount of blood drawn for all specimens.
Newborn resuscitation		
– Atropine	■ Reduces bronchial secretions	■ Measure intake and output.
– Calcium chloride	■ Increases heart contractility	
– Dopamine	■ Increased systemic blood perfusion	
– Ephinephrine	■ Strengthens or initiates cardiac contractility	
– Lidocaine	■ Counteracts ventricular arrhythmias	
– Sodium bicarbonate	■ Corrects metabolic acidosis	■ Do not give unless ventilation is adequate because acidosis may increase.
– Nitric oxide	■ Potent vascular dilator; dilates capillaries next to alveoli, reduces pulmonary resistance	
– Liquid ventilation – Liquid fluorocarbon – Perflubron	■ Fills lungs, clings to alveoli; acts as an anti-inflammatory in the lung; prevents infection	■ Observe for pneumothorax or mucus plug.

CLIENT AND FAMILY TEACHING 15-1

Normal feelings and emotions after the birth of a newborn with a complication

Assure the parents and other family members that it is normal to experience a wide range of emotions after the birth of a child with a complication. Encourage them to discuss and work through their feelings with each other, with the health care team, and with professional counselors, if necessary. Explain that they may experience some or all of the following emotions at different times:

- Shock, disbelief, and denial
- Anger and searching self and others for causes
- Grief over loss of fantasized "perfect" newborn
- Grief over own inability to produce a "perfect" newborn
- Anticipatory worry over the loss of the newborn
- Desire for initiation of contact and bonding with the newborn
- Belief and desire that the newborn will live
- Feeling of readiness to establish a caretaking relationship

(Adapted from Reeder et al. [1997]. *Maternity Nursing: Family, Newborn, and Women's Health Care,* 18th ed. Philadelphia: Lippincott Williams & Wilkins, p. 1148.)

c. Explain the normal feelings and emotions that parents and other family members may experience (*Client and Family Teaching* 15-1).

d. Provide an opportunity for the mother to discuss her feelings and concerns.

E. Outcome evaluation

1. The newborn receives effective respiratory support and experiences no respiratory complications.
2. The newborn maintains a neutral thermal environment and experiences no stress from heat loss.
3. The newborn is free of infection.
4. The newborn receives adequate fluids and electrolytes and nutrition.
5. The parents demonstrate attachment to their newborn.
6. The parents state they have adequate knowledge about their newborn's condition, and that they are adjusting positively to the stressful experience.

III. BIRTH ASPHYXIA

A. Description. Birth asphyxia is characterized by hypoxemia (decreased PaO_2), hypercarbia (increased $PaCO_2$), and acidosis (lowered pH).

B. Etiology

1. Maternal causes include amnionitis, anemia, diabetes, pregnancy-induced hypertension, drugs, and infection.
2. Intrauterine causes include prolonged labor and abnormal fetal presentations.
3. Placental causes include placenta previa, abruptio placentae, and placental insufficiency.
4. Umbilical cord causes include cord prolapse and cord entanglement.
5. Fetal causes include cephalopelvic disproportion, congenital anomalies, difficult delivery, small for gestational age, low birth weight, and prematurity.

C. Pathophysiology

1. Unless vigorous resuscitation begins promptly, irreversible multisystem organ tissue changes will occur, possibly leading to permanent damage or death.

2. During the 24 hours after successful resuscitation, the newborn is vulnerable to post-asphyxial syndrome.

D. Assessment findings. Clinical manifestations include:

1. Poor response to resuscitative efforts
2. Hypoxia
3. Hypercarbia
4. Metabolic and or respiratory acidosis
5. Minimal or absent respiratory effort
6. Seizures
7. Altered cardiac function
8. Multisystem organ failure

E. Nursing management

1. **Observe the newborn who has been successfully resuscitated for the following constellation of signs.**
   a. Absence of spontaneous respirations
   b. Seizure activity in the first 12 hours after birth
   c. Decreased or increased urine output (which may indicate dehydration, inappropriate secretion of antidiuretic hormone or acute tubular necrosis)
   d. Metabolic alterations (such as hypoglycemia and hypocalcemia)
   e. Increased intracranial pressure marked by decreased or absent reflexes or hypertension
2. **Decrease noxious environmental stimuli.**
3. **Monitor the infant's level of responsiveness, activity, muscle tone, and posture.**
4. **Administer prescribed medications,** which may include anticonvulsants (such as phenobarbital), as prescribed.
5. **Provide respiratory support.**
6. **Monitor the newborn for complications.**
   a. Measure and record intake and output to evaluate renal function.
   b. Check every voiding for blood or protein, and monitor specific gravity, watching for renal injury.
   c. Check every stool for blood, which may indicate necrotizing enterocolitis (NEC), a condition in which the bowel develops necrotic patches that interfere with digestion and may cause paralytic ileus, perforation, and peritonitis.
   d. Take serial blood glucose determinations to detect hypoglycemia, and monitor serum electrolyte levels, as ordered.
7. **Administer and maintain intravenous fluids** to maintain hydration and fluid and electrolyte balance.
8. **Provide education and emotional support** for parents and supportive developmental care for the newborn.

IV. PRETERM NEWBORN

A. Description.
A preterm newborn is one born before 37 weeks' gestation.

B. Etiology

1. The etiology of preterm labor is poorly understood.
2. Possible factors include the following:
   a. Multiple gestation

b. Maternal history of preterm delivery
c. Hydramnios
d. Uterine anomalies
e. More than one second-trimester abortion
f. Incompetent cervix
g. Infection
h. Uterine structural anomalies
i. Premature rupture of membranes
j. Maternal substance abuse (especially cocaine)
k. Maternal age less than 18 years, poor nutrition, and lack of prenatal care

C. Pathophysiology. Preterm newborns exhibit anatomic and physiologic immaturity in all body systems; this immaturity hinders the adaptations to extrauterine life that the newborn must make.

D. Assessment findings

1. **Associated findings.** Altered parenting as evidenced by:
   a. Decreased or absent parental visits
   b. Parental resistance or refusal to participate in newborn care
   c. Denial of severity of newborn illness
   d. Resistance or refusal to touch newborn
   e. Persistent verbalization of guilt.
2. **Clinical manifestations.** There is a higher risk of the following manifestations in a newborn with a younger gestational age.
   a. Respiratory manifestations include tachypnea, grunting, nasal flaring, retractions, cyanosis, decreased oxygen saturation, decreased oxygen levels, and abnormal arterial blood gas values.
   b. Cardiovascular manifestations include poor tissue perfusion, hypotension, and patent ductus arteriosus.
   c. GI manifestations include feeding intolerance, gastric reflux, vomiting, and gastric residuals.
   d. Altered fluid status may be manifested by fluid excess or fluid deficit.
   - Fluid excess is indicated by edema and heart failure.
   - Fluid deficit is indicated by tachycardia, poor skin turgor, decreased urine output, abnormal electrolyte levels, and decreased blood pressure.

   e. Iatrogenic anemia caused by blood sampling may be present. It is exhibited by tachycardia, pallor, decreased blood pressure, increasing oxygen requirements, and apnea. (See *Drug Chart* 15-1, page 246.)
   f. Infection may occur.
   g. Hypoglycemia or hyperglycemia may be present.
   h. Ineffective temperature control may be observed and is exhibited by an inability to maintain core body temperature.
   i. Neuromuscular system manifestations include decreased suck and swallow reflex, hypotonia, and altered state transition.
   j. Hyperbilirubinemia is characterized by rapid destruction of red blood cells, jaundice, and lethargy. Kernicterus is the deposition of unconjugated bilirubin in the brain cells and is associated with mental retardation.

E. Nursing management

1. **Provide respiratory support** (see *Drug Chart* 15-1, page 246).
2. **Perform the following assessments:**

  a. Assess heart sounds for presence of murmurs.
  b. Assess pulse and perfusion.
  c. Monitor blood pressure, heart rate, and pulse pressures.
3. **Provide adequate fluids and electrolytes and nutrition.**
4. **Maintain a neutral thermal environment.**
5. **Prevent infection.**
6. **Assess for readiness for selected interventions.**
  a. Provide stimulation when appropriate to infant state and readiness.
  b. Encourage flexion in the supine position by using blanket rolls.
  c. Provide the newborn with body boundaries through swaddling or using blanket rolls against the newborn's body and feet.
7. **Promote parent-newborn attachment.**
8. **Initiate phototherapy as required.**

V. SMALL-FOR-GESTATIONAL-AGE NEWBORN

A. Description

1. A small-for-gestational-age (SGA) infant is one whose length, weight, and head circumference are below the 10th percentile of the normal variation for gestational age as determined by neonatal examination.
2. The SGA infant may be preterm, term, or postterm.

B. Etiology

1. Maternal conditions associated with SGA babies include:
  a. Hypertension (chronic or pregnancy-induced)
  b. Cardiac, pulmonary, or renal disease
  c. Diabetes mellitus (classes D, E, F, and R)
  d. Poor nutrition
  e. Use of alcohol, tobacco, or drugs
  f. Age
  g. Multiple gestation
  h. Placental insufficiency
  i. Placental fetal abnormalities
  j. Pregnancy that occurred at high altitudes
2. Fetal conditions associated with SGA infants include:
  a. Normal genetically small infant
  b. Chromosomal abnormality
  c. Malformations
  d. Congenital infections, especially rubella and cytomegalovirus
3. The effect of these factors on the fetus is dependent on the stage of fetal development. Early gestation is a time of rapid cell proliferation. An insult at this time results in organs that contain normal size cells, but they are fewer in number. Infants are symmetrical (their heads and bodies grew proportionately) but their organs are smaller. Usually these infants have a poor prognosis and may never catch up.
4. Later in gestation, growth of the fetus results from an increase in cell size. An insult at this time results in organs with a normal number of cells that are smaller in size and causes asymmetrical growth. These infants have appropriate-sized heads and body lengths, but their weight and organ sizes are decreased. These infants usually have a

better prognosis because they have an adequate number of cells. Their growth catches up if they are provided with good nutrition postnatally.

C. Assessment findings

1. **Clinical manifestations**
   a. Soft tissue wasting and dysmaturity
   b. Loose, dry, and scaling skin
   c. Perinatal asphyxia (from a small placenta that is less efficient in gas exchange)
   d. Polycythemia, respiratory distress, and central nervous system (CNS) aberrations and persistent acrocyanosis
   e. Congenital anomalies (occurring in as many as 35% of SGA infants who suffered insults early in gestation)
2. **Laboratory and diagnostic study findings**
   a. Glucose testing will reveal decreased glycogen stores, which increase the potential for hypothermia and hypoglycemia.
   b. Hematocrit level may be increased (65%), which indicates polycythemia as a result of chronic fetal hypoxia.

D. Nursing management

1. **Provide adequate fluid and electrolytes and nutrition.**
   a. Provide a high-calorie formula for feeding (more than 20 calories per ounce) to promote steady weight gain (15 to 30 g per day; growth plotted on curves shows a normal growth rate).
   b. If the infant is breast-feeding, add human milk fortifier to expressed breast milk.
2. **Decrease metabolic demands when possible.**
   a. Provide small frequent feedings.
   b. Provide gavage feedings if the infant does not have a steady weight gain.
   c. Provide a neutral thermal environment.
   d. Decrease iatrogenic stimuli.
3. **Prevent hypoglycemia.**
   a. Monitor glucose screening.
   b. Provide early feedings.
   c. Provide frequent feedings (every 2 to 3 hours).
   d. Administer I.V. glucose if blood glucose level does not normalize with oral feedings.
4. **Maintain a neutral thermal environment.**
5. **Monitor serum hematocrit** (normal is 45% to 65%).
   a. If an initial high hematocrit was obtained by heel stick capillary sample, a follow-up sample should be done by venipuncture.
   b. Observe for the following signs, symptoms, and complications of polycythemia:
      - Ruddy appearance
      - Cyanosis
      - Lethargy, jitteriness, and seizures
      - Jaundice.
   c. Provide adequate hydration to prevent hyperviscosity.
6. **Assess the prenatal history** for possible toxoplasmosis, rubella, cytomegalovirus, or herpes simplex infections during pregnancy. Assess maternal and infant antibody titers. Use isolation precautions when congenital infections are suspected.
7. **Provide education and emotional support.**
   a. Explain the possible causes of intrauterine growth retardation.
   b. Inform parents of the infant's goal weight for discharge.

c. Provide instruction on managing the infant at home.
- Explain how to prepare a high-calorie formula or fortify breast milk.
- Explain the importance of follow-up with a developmental specialist who will screen for milestone achievements.

VI. LARGE-FOR-GESTATIONAL-AGE NEWBORN

A. Description

1. A large-for-gestational-age (LGA) newborn is one who weighs more than 4,000 g, is above the 90th percentile, or is two standard deviations above the mean.
2. The LGA infant can be preterm, term, or postterm.

B. Etiology. Predisposing factors include:

1. Genetic predisposition
2. Excessive maternal weight gain during pregnancy
3. Poorly controlled maternal diabetes secondary to a high level of maternal glucose that crosses the placental barrier during pregnancy

C. Pathophysiology

1. Infants who are large for gestational age have been subjected to an overproduction of growth hormone in utero. This most frequently happens with infants of diabetic mothers who are poorly controlled. It may also occur in multiparous pregnancies because with each pregnancy babies tend to grow larger.
2. Other associated conditions include transposition of the great vessels, Beckwith syndrome, and congenital anomalies.

D. Assessment findings. Clinical manifestations include:

1. Complications associated with maternal diabetes (see section VII)
2. Birth injuries due to size of newborn disproportionate to size of birth passageway
   a. Fractured clavicle
   b. Facial nerve injury
   c. Erb-Duchenne palsy or brachial plexus paralysis
   d. Klumpke paralysis
   e. Phrenic nerve palsy
   f. Possible skull fracture.

E. Nursing management

1. **If an infant of a diabetic mother, observe for potential complications** (see section VII).
2. **Monitor the newborn for, and manage, birth injuries and complications of birth injuries.**
   a. Clavicle fracture
   - Confirm by X-ray.
   - Assess the infant for crepitus, hematoma, or deformity over the clavicle; decreased movement of arm on the affected side; and asymmetrical or absent Moro reflex.
   - Limit arm motion by pinning the infant's sleeve to the shirt.
   - Manage the pain.

   b. Facial nerve injury
   - Assess for asymmetry of mouth while crying.
   - Wrinkles are deeper on the unaffected side.
   - The paralyzed side is smooth, with a swollen appearance.

- The nasolabial fold is absent.
- If the eye is affected, protect it with patches and artificial tears.

c. Erb-Duchenne palsy and Klumpke paralysis
- Erb-Duchenne palsy. Assess for adduction of the affected arm with internal rotation and elbow extension. The Moro reflex is absent on the affected side. The grasp reflex is intact.
- Klumpke paralysis. Assess for absent grasp on the affected side. The hand appears claw-shaped.
- Management includes:
  - X-ray studies of the shoulder and upper arm to rule out bony injury
  - Examination of the chest to rule out phrenic nerve injury
  - Delay of passive movement to maintain range of motion of the affected joints until the nerve edema resolves (7 to 10 days)
  - Possible splinting to prevent wrist and digit contractures on the affected side

d. Phrenic nerve palsy
- Assess for respiratory distress with diminished breath sounds.
- X-ray usually shows elevation of the diaphragm on the affected side.
- Provide pulmonary toilet to avoid pneumonia during the recovery phase (1 to 3 months).

e. Skull fracture. Assess for soft-tissue swelling over fracture site, visible indentation in scalp, cephalhematoma, positive skull X-ray, and CNS signs and symptoms with intracranial hemorrhage (such as lethargy, seizures, apnea, and hypotonia).

VII. INFANT OF A DIABETIC MOTHER

A. Description. An infant of a diabetic mother (IDM) may be SGA or LGA, with or without congenital anomalies and with or without birth injury

B. Etiology. IDM is caused by chronic hyperglycemia in the mother (such as gestational diabetes mellitus or long-term diabetes mellitus with or without vascular changes).

C. Pathophysiology

1. Hyperglycemia in the mother *without* vascular changes causes large amounts of amino acids, free fatty acids, and glucose to be transferred to the fetus, but maternal insulin does not cross the placental barrier.

   a. The fetal response to these transferred substances includes:
   - Islet cells of the pancreas enlarge (hypertrophy).
   - Hypertrophic cells produce large volumes of insulin, which acts as a growth hormone, and protein synthesis accelerates.
   - Fat and glycogen are deposited in fetal tissue, and the fetus grows large (macrosomia), especially if maternal blood glucose levels are not well controlled in the third trimester.

   b. Various unknown factors also may contribute to changes.

2. In maternal long-term diabetes *with* vascular changes, the newborn may be SGA because of compromised placental blood flow, maternal hypertension, or pregnancy-induced hypertension, which restricts uteroplacental blood flow.
3. Associated complications in IDM include:

   a. Fractures and nerve damage — May occur from birth trauma if the infant is LGA.

b. Congenital anomalies (such as heart, kidney, vertebral, and CNS) — Three to five times more common, with incidence decreasing if maternal blood glucose level remains controlled and normal during the first trimester.

c. Risk of respiratory distress syndrome — Increases (high insulin levels interfere with production of pulmonary surfactant).

d. Hypoglycemia — May result after birth from lack of glucose from the mother but continued production of insulin by the newborn.

e. Hypocalcemia — May result from decreased parathyroid hormone production.

f. Polycythemia (hematocrit exceeding 65%) — May result from placental insufficiency causing chronic fetal hypoxia and increased fetal erythropoietin production.

g. Organ damage — May result from decreased blood flow and renal vein thrombosis.

h. Hyperbilirubinemia — May result from breakdown of excess red blood cells after birth.

D. Assessment findings

1. Clinical manifestations

a. Congenital anomalies are more likely in IDMs who are SGA than in other SGA newborns.

b. Size differences and variations are more common in IDMs who are LGA than in other LGA newborns.

- Greater size results from fat deposits and hypertrophic liver, adrenal glands, and heart.
- Length and head size are usually within normal range for gestational age.

c. Observation shows characteristic appearance of a round, red face and an obese body.

d. Possible signs and symptoms of hypoglycemia include jitteriness, irritability, diaphoresis, and blood glucose level less than 45 mg/dl.

e. Possible signs and symptoms of hypocalcemia include jitteriness, twitching, and a high-pitched cry.

2. Laboratory and diagnostic study findings.

a. Blood glucose evaluation at 30 and 60 minutes and at 2, 4, 6, and 12 hours after birth as directed by nursery protocol

- If results are abnormal, repeat testing every 30 to 60 minutes until newborn achieves stable level; also test before each feeding for 24 hours.
- If reagent strips indicate blood glucose level less than 40 mg/dl, findings should be verified by laboratory and reported to pediatrician.

b. Serum electrolyte studies may reveal hypocalcemia (total serum calcium 6 to 12 mg/dl).

c. Hematocrit level may be elevated, indicating polycythemia.

E. Nursing management

1. Establish an initial database.

a. Review the mother's health history and history of the pregnancy.

b. Complete an initial newborn examination and assess for birth injuries.

2. Monitor the newborn for complications.

a. Monitor the newborn for signs and symptoms of hypoglycemia (see section VII, D, 1, d).

- Measure the newborn's glucose level according to nursery protocol.
- Feed the newborn early according to nursery protocol to prevent or treat hypoglycemia.
- If signs and symptoms continue after feeding, observe for other complications.

b. Monitor the newborn for signs and symptoms of hypocalcemia (see section VII, D, 1, e).
c. Obtain hematocrit value; report the findings to the physician.
d. Observe for signs of respiratory distress (such as nasal flaring, grunting, retractions, and tachypnea).
e. Initiate gavage feeding if the newborn cannot suck well or if the respiratory rate exceeds normal (30 to 60 breaths per minute).

3. **Maintain a neutral thermal environment.**
4. **Provide education and emotional support.**

VIII. POSTTERM NEWBORN

A. Description. A postterm pregnancy is one that extends beyond 42 weeks' gestation. The postterm infant may be LGA, appropriate for gestational age, SGA, or dysmature, depending on placental function.

B. Etiology. The cause of prolonged pregnancy is unknown. Factors associated with postmaturity include anencephaly and trisomy 16 to 18.

C. Pathophysiology

1. If the placenta continues to function well, the fetus will continue to grow, which results in an LGA infant who may manifest such problems as birth trauma and hypoglycemia.
2. If placental function decreases, the fetus may not receive adequate nutrition. The fetus will utilize its subcutaneous fat stores for energy. Wasting of subcutaneous fat occurs, resulting in fetal dysmaturity syndrome. There are three stages of fetal dysmaturity syndrome.
   a. **Stage 1** — Chronic placental insufficiency
   - Dry, cracked, peeling, loose, and wrinkled skin
   - Malnourished appearance
   - Open-eyed and alert baby

   b. **Stage 2** — Acute placental insufficiency
   - First two features of stage 1
   - Meconium staining
   - Perinatal depression

   c. **Stage 3** — Subacute placental insufficiency
   - Findings of stage 1 and 2 except that baby is not open-eyed and alert
   - Green staining of skin, nails, cord, and placental membrane
   - A higher risk of fetal intrapartum or neonatal death
3. The newborn is at increased risk for developing complications related to compromised uteroplacental perfusion and hypoxia (such as meconium aspiration syndrome [MAS])
4. Chronic intrauterine hypoxia causes increased fetal erythropoietin and red blood cell production, resulting in polycythemia.
5. Postterm infants are susceptible to hypoglycemia because of the rapid use of glycogen stores.

D. Assessment findings. Clinical manifestations include:

1. A long, thin newborn with wasted appearance, parchment-like skin, and meconium-stained skin, nails, and umbilical cord. Fingernails are long and lanugo is absent.
2. Signs and symptoms of MAS (fetal hypoxia, meconium staining of amniotic fluid, respiratory distress at delivery, and meconium-stained vocal cords).

E. Nursing management

1. **Manage MAS.**
   a. Suction the infant's mouth and nares while the head is on the perineum and before the first breath is taken to prevent aspiration of meconium that is in the airway.
   b. Once the infant is dry and on the warmer, intubate with direct tracheal suctioning.
   c. Perform chest physiotherapy with suctioning to remove excess meconium and secretions.
   d. Provide supplemental oxygen and respiratory support as needed.
2. **Obtain serial blood glucose measurements.**
3. **Provide early feeding to prevent hypoglycemia,** if not contraindicated by respiratory status.
4. **Maintain skin integrity.**
   a. Keep the skin clean and dry.
   b. Avoid the use of powders, creams, and lotions.
   c. Avoid the use of tape.

Study questions

1. Which of the following is the **most** important concept associated with all high-risk newborns?
1. Support the high-risk newborn's cardiopulmonary adaptation by maintaining an adequate airway.
2. Identify complications with early intervention in the high-risk newborn to reduce morbidity and mortality.
3. Assess the high-risk newborn for any physical complications that may interfere with parental bonding.
4. Support the mother and significant others in their quest toward adaptation to the high-risk newborn.

2. Which of the following would the nurse expect to find in a newborn with birth asphyxia?
1. Hyperoxemia
2. Hypocarbia
3. Acidosis
4. Ketosis

3. When planning and implementing care for the newborn who has been successfully resuscitated, which of the following would be important to assess?
1. Muscle flaccidity
2. Decreased intracranial pressure
3. Hypoglycemia
4. Spontaneous respirations

4. When describing a preterm newborn, the nurse would describe the newborn as being born at which of the following?
1. Before 25 weeks' gestation
2. After 25 weeks' gestation
3. After 37 weeks' gestation
4. Before 37 weeks' gestation

5. Which of the following assessment findings would the nurse expect in the preterm newborn?
1. Tachypnea, decreased or absent parental visits, constant return to fetal position, hyperpnea
2. Tachypnea, abnormal arterial blood gas (ABG) values, decreased sucking reflex, temperature instability
3. Cyanosis, abnormal ABG values, unstable body core temperature, increased gag and sucking reflexes
4. Hyperpnea, unstable body core temperature, bradycardia, cyanosis, arching behaviors with hyperextension

6. Which of the following would the nurse identify as characteristic of an SGA newborn?
1. Weight above 10th percentile on standard growth chart

2. Maternal history of malnutrition or premature placental aging
3. Stable temperature control
4. Small anterior fontanel

7. When implementing supportive measures for airway clearance for the preterm newborn, the nurse would plan to do which of the following?
1. Assess for hypoglycemia and other complications, such as fractures and Bell's palsy
2. Perform suctioning as needed, positioning the newborn to facilitate chest expansion
3. Observe for hypercalcemia, respiratory distress, polycythemia, and altered parenting
4. Provide chest physiotherapy before feedings, assessing for potential respiratory distress

8. Which of the following characteristics is most commonly associated with an LGA newborn?
1. Weight under 4,000 g
2. Dysmorphic features
3. Risk for birth injury
4. Hypothermia

9. When assessing a postterm newborn, which of the following would the nurse expect?
1. Meconium-stained skin
2. Round, red face
3. Hypoglycemia
4. Poor feeding

10. Brain damage as a result of kernicterus in the preterm infant may occur when the indirect serum bilirubin level reaches mg/dl?

Answer key

1. The answer is 2.
Early identification of complications in the high-risk newborn is the first step toward intervening to reduce morbidity and mortality. Supporting cardiopulmonary status, assessing for physical complications, and supporting the mother and significant others are all aspects of high-risk newborn care depending on the newborn's specific problem.

2. The answer is 3.
Birth asphyxia is a condition characterized by hypoxemia, hypercarbia, and acidosis. Ketosis is not present.

3. The answer is 3.
Following successful resuscitation of a newborn, the nurse should observe for the following: absence of spontaneous respirations, seizure activity in the first 12 hours after birth, decreased or increased urine output (which may indicate acute tubular necrosis or syndrome of inappropriate antidiuretic hormone), metabolic alterations (such as hypoglycemia and hypocalcemia), and increased intracranial pressure marked by decreased or absent reflexes or hypertension. Seizures, not muscle flaccidity; increased, not decreased, intracranial pressure; and the absence of spontaneous respirations would be important signs.

4. The answer is 4.
The preterm newborn is one who is born before 37 weeks' gestation. A newborn born after 37 weeks' gestation is considered a term newborn.

5. The answer is 2.
Tachypnea, abnormal ABG values, decreased sucking reflex, and temperature instability are all assessment findings typically seen in the preterm newborn. Constant return to fetal position, hyperpnea, and increase in the gag and sucking reflexes would not be seen.

6. The answer is 2.
Maternal history of malnutrition or premature placental aging is a predisposing factor for an SGA newborn. Additionally, the SGA

newborn exhibits a weight below the 10th percentile on standard growth charts, unstable temperature control with temperature swings, and a large anterior fontanel.

7. The answer is 2.
Clearing the newborn's airway by suctioning as needed and positioning to facilitate chest expansion are key interventions for maintaining airway patency in a preterm newborn. Assessing for hypoglycemia or hypercalcemia, other complications, respiratory distress, polycythemia, and altered parenting, although important assessments, have no effect on maintaining airway patency. Chest physiotherapy aids in mobilizing secretions but not maintaining the airway patency.

8. The answer is 3.
Because of its size, an LGA newborn is typically at risk for birth injuries, such as fractured clavicle, Bell's palsy, Erb-Duchenne palsy, and possible skull fracture. The LGA newborn weighs over 4,000 g and exhibits hyperthermia from increased amounts of fatty tissue serving as insulation. Dysmorphic features are associated with SGA newborns.

9. The answer is 3.
When assessing the postterm newborn, one born after 42 weeks' gestation, the nurse would expect to find meconium-stained skin. Round, red face is typically seen in infants of diabetic mothers (IDMs). Hypoglycemia would be seen in IDMs and also in LGA and SGA newborns. Poor feeding is common in SGA newborns.

10. The answer is 12.
Immaturity of the preterm newborn's liver predisposes the infant to several problems. One of these is the inability to conjugate and excrete bilirubin. Thus, bilirubin levels increase more rapidly and reach higher levels than in the full-term infant. Clinical assessment of jaundice associated with hyperbilirubinemia is more difficult in preterm newborns because they lack subcutaneous fat. The indirect bilirubin level rises rapidly as red blood cells are destroyed and indirect bilirubin is released. Indirect bilirubin is fat-soluble and cannot be excreted from the body. Under normal circumstances, the liver enzyme glucuronyl transferase converts indirect bilirubin to direct bilirubin. Direct bilirubin is water-soluble and combines with bile for excretion in the feces. The preterm infant is unable to make this conversion; therefore, serum bilirubin levels increase. Kernicterus is the invasion of brain cells by bilirubin, causing irreversible brain damage.

COMPREHENSIVE TEST: QUESTIONS

1. For the client who is using oral contraceptives, the nurse informs the client about the need to take the pill at the same time each day to accomplish which of the following?
1. Decrease the incidence of nausea
2. Maintain hormonal levels
3. Reduce side effects
4. Prevent drug interactions

2. When teaching the client who is receiving medroxyprogesterone (Depo-Provera) contraceptive injections, at which of the following times would the nurse instruct the client to return to the clinic for follow-up?
1. Twelve weeks for a subsequent injection
2. Six months for a Papanicolaou smear
3. One year for an annual gynecologic examination
4. Five years for reevaluation of family planning goals

3. When teaching a client about contraception, which of the following would the nurse include as the **most** effective method for preventing sexually transmitted infections?
1. Spermicides
2. Diaphragm
3. Condoms
4. Vasectomy

4. When preparing a woman who is 2 days postpartum for discharge, recommendations for which of the following contraceptive methods would be avoided?
1. Diaphragm
2. Female condom
3. Hormonal contraceptives
4. Rhythm method

5. Which of the following would the nurse identify as the most important factor in choosing a contraceptive method?
1. Financial expense
2. Compliance with cultural expectations
3. Noncontraceptive benefits
4. Correct and consistent use

6. For which of the following clients would the nurse expect that an intrauterine device would not be recommended?
1. Woman over age 35
2. Nulliparous woman
3. Promiscuous young adult
4. Postpartum client

7. When discussing contraceptive choices with a client who has a history of thrombophlebitis, the nurse would keep in mind that which of the following would be contraindicated?
1. Intrauterine device
2. Subdermal implants
3. Intramuscular injections
4. Hormonal contraceptives

8. Which of the following would be the nurse's best response to a pregnant client asking if she can have a "social drink" with her clients 2 to 3 times a week?
1. "It is best to avoid all alcoholic beverages during pregnancy."
2. "After the first trimester, you may have 3 drinks per week."
3. "Beer is safer to drink because it has less alcohol."
4. "If you're used to drinking alcohol, you may continue during pregnancy."

9. A client in her third trimester tells the nurse, "I'm constipated all the time!" Which of the following should the nurse recommend?

1. Daily enemas
2. Laxatives
3. Increased fiber intake
4. Decreased fluid intake

10. Which of the following would the nurse use as the basis for the teaching plan when caring for a pregnant teenager concerned about gaining too much weight during pregnancy?
1. 10 pounds per trimester
2. 1 pound per week for 40 weeks
3. $^1/_2$ pound per week for 40 weeks
4. A total gain of 25 to 30 pounds

11. The client tells the nurse that her last menstrual period started on January 14 and ended on January 20. Using Nägele's rule, the nurse determines her estimated date of delivery to be which of the following?
1. September 27
2. October 21
3. November 7
4. December 27

12. The nurse should anticipate which of the following screening tests will be ordered for a pregnant African-American woman that would not be routinely ordered for a Caucasian pregnant woman?
1. Sickle cell screen
2. Alpha fetoprotein
3. Diabetes screen
4. Blood type and Rh

13. When taking an obstetric history on a pregnant client who states, "I had a son born at 38 weeks' gestation, a daughter born at 30 weeks' gestation, and I lost a baby at about 8 weeks," the nurse should record her obstetric history as which of the following?
1. G3 T2 P0 A0 L2
2. G4 T1 P1 A0 L2
3. G3 T2 P0 A1 L2
4. G4 T1 P1 A1 L2

14. When preparing to listen to the fetal heart rate at 12 weeks' gestation, the nurse would use which of the following?
1. Stethoscope placed midline at the umbilicus
2. Doppler placed midline at the suprapubic region
3. Fetoscope placed midway between the umbilicus and the xiphoid process
4. External electronic fetal monitor placed at the umbilicus

15. When developing a plan of care for a client newly diagnosed with gestational diabetes, which of the following instructions would be the **priority?**
1. Dietary intake
2. Medication
3. Exercise
4. Glucose monitoring

16. A client at 24 weeks' gestation has gained 6 pounds in 4 weeks. Which of the following would be the **priority** when assessing the client?
1. Glycosuria
2. Depression
3. Edema of the hands or face
4. Dietary intake

17. A client at 12 weeks' gestation comes to the emergency department with abdominal cramping and moderate vaginal bleeding. Speculum examination reveals 2- to 3-cm cervical dilation. The nurse would document these findings as which of the following?
1. Threatened abortion
2. Imminent abortion
3. Complete abortion
4. Missed abortion

18. Which of the following would be the **priority** nursing diagnosis for a client with an ectopic pregnancy?
   1. Risk for infection
   2. Pain
   3. Knowledge Deficit
   4. Anticipatory Grieving

19. A client who is 14 weeks pregnant and Rh negative experienced a complete spontaneous abortion. The nurse would anticipate administering which of the following?
   1. Antibiotics
   2. Rubella vaccine
   3. RhoGAM
   4. Iron supplements

20. Which of the following statements by a client with hyperemesis indicates effective teaching about the postdischarge management plan?
   1. "I'm glad I won't ever have to be hospitalized again for this!"
   2. "I need to eat small, frequent meals to maintain my weight."
   3. "I hope the doctor will give me medicine to stop this nausea."
   4. "Prenatal vitamins are making me sick. I need to quit taking them."

21. Which of the following would be **most** important to include in the discharge teaching plan for a client who had a suction curettage evacuation of the uterus for hydatidiform molar pregnancy?
   1. Continuation of prenatal vitamins for 6 weeks
   2. Psychological support for grief counseling
   3. Importance of follow-up care
   4. Hormonal contraceptives to prevent pregnancy

22. Before assessing the postpartum client's uterus for firmness and position in relation to the umbilicus and midline, which of the following should the nurse do **first?**
   1. Assess the vital signs
   2. Administer analgesia
   3. Ambulate the client in the hall
   4. Assist the client to urinate

23. When caring for a client in the postpartum "taking-in" psychosocial adaptation phase, the nurse should plan to do which of the following?
   1. Promote self-care activities
   2. Expect control of elimination functions
   3. Provide nourishment and rest
   4. Teach newborn care skills

24. When assisting a postpartum client to the bathroom to urinate, the nurse determines that the client needs further teaching on the technique for perineal care when the nurse observes the client doing which of the following?
   1. Wiping the perineum from front to back
   2. Avoiding touching the inside of the perineal pad
   3. Washing her hands before and after elimination
   4. Directing the perineal wash between separated labia

25. Which of the following should the nurse do when a breast-feeding primipara tells the nurse that she has sore nipples?
   1. Tell her to breast-feed more frequently
   2. Administer an opioid before breast-feeding
   3. Encourage her to wear a nursing bra
   4. Use soap and water to clean the nipples

26. During assessment of the perineum, the nurse identifies three medium-blue, soft, painful hemorrhoids. Which of the following would be the nurse's **best initial** action?
   1. Instruct the client to ambulate 3 times a day
   2. Encourage the client to use the sitz bath

3. Teach the client about foods high in fiber
4. Administer a stool softener

27. The nurse assesses the vital signs of a client 4 hours postpartum. They are as follows: blood pressure 90/60; temperature 100.4° F; pulse 100 weak, thready; respirations 20 per minute. Which of the following should the nurse do **first?**

1. Report the temperature to the physician
2. Recheck the blood pressure with another cuff
3. Assess the uterus for firmness and position
4. Determine the amount of lochia

28. The nurse assesses the postpartum vaginal discharge (lochia) on four clients. Which of the following assessments would warrant notification of the physician?

1. A dark red discharge on a 2-day postpartum client
2. A pink to brownish discharge on a client who is 5 days postpartum
3. Almost colorless to creamy discharge on a client 2 weeks after delivery
4. A bright red discharge 5 days after delivery

29. A postpartum client has a temperature of 101.4° F, with a uterus that is tender when palpated, remains unusually large, and is not descending as normally expected. Which of the following should the nurse assess next?

1. Lochia
2. Breasts
3. Incision
4. Urine

30. Which of the following microorganisms would the nurse expect to be the **most** common cause of mastitis?

1. *Escherichia coli*
2. *Streptococcus pneumoniae*
3. *Staphylococcus aureus*
4. *Neisseria gonorrhoeae*

31. Two hours after delivery, the nurse is massaging the uterus of a client experiencing uterine atony leading to excessive bleeding. The nurse anticipates the immediate administration of which of the following medications?

1. Promethazine
2. Oxytocin
3. Meperidine
4. Magnesium sulfate

32. Which of the following is the **priority** focus of nursing practice considering the current trend of early postpartum discharge?

1. Promoting comfort and restoration of health
2. Exploring the emotional status of the family
3. Facilitating safe and effective self-care and newborn care
4. Teaching about the importance of family planning

33. A client with deep vein thrombosis is started on intravenous fluids with heparin. Which of the following agents would the nurse expect to have readily available?

1. Naloxone
2. Glucagon
3. Calcium gluconate
4. Protamine sulfate

34. A postpartum client's husband calls the nurse's desk and tells the nurse, "My wife has terrible chest pain and difficulty getting her breath!" Upon arrival at the client's room, the nurse notes a diaphoretic woman, who is very apprehensive, holding her right chest at the costovertebral area, and crying with pain. Which of the following would the nurse immediately suspect?

1. Myocardial infarction
2. Pulmonary embolism
3. Acute pneumonia
4. Panic attack

35. The home health nurse visits a client 3 weeks after delivery. The single mother cries and tells the nurse, "I just can't seem to be able to take care of myself and the baby, too. I'm not a good mother. The baby cries a lot and gets on my nerves! I'm always so sad and irritable!" Which of the following nursing diagnoses would be **most** appropriate?

1. Hopelessness
2. Ineffective individual coping
3. Powerlessness
4. Altered parenting

36. Which of the following observable behaviors indicates that the client outcome of "will demonstrate positive bonding behaviors" has been met?

1. Placing the infant across the knees or on the bed
2. Handling the infant for feeding and diaper changes
3. Asking few questions about newborn care
4. Touching the unwrapped infant with palms of hands

37. Which of the following actions would be **least** effective in maintaining a neutral thermal environment for the newborn?

1. Placing infant under a radiant warmer after bathing
2. Covering the scale with a warmed blanket prior to weighing
3. Placing crib close to nursery window for family viewing
4. Covering the infant's head with a knit stockinette

38. A newborn who has an asymmetrical Moro reflex response should be further assessed for which of the following?

1. Talipes equinovarus
2. Fractured clavicle
3. Congenital hypothyroidism
4. Increased intracranial pressure

39. During the first 4 hours after a male circumcision, assessing for which of the following is the **priority?**

1. Infection
2. Hemorrhage
3. Discomfort
4. Dehydration

40. The mother asks the nurse, "What's wrong with my son's breasts? Why are they so enlarged?" Which of the following would be the **best** response by the nurse?

1. "The breast tissue is inflamed from the trauma experienced with birth."
2. "A decrease in maternal hormones present before birth causes enlargement."
3. "You should discuss this with your doctor. It could be a malignancy."
4. "The tissue hypertrophied while the baby was in the uterus."

41. Immediately after birth, the nurse notes the following on a male newborn: respirations 78, apical heart rate 160 beats per minute, nostril flaring, mild intercostal retractions, and grunting at the end of expiration. Which of the following should the nurse do?

1. Call the assessment data to the physician's attention
2. Start oxygen per nasal cannula at 2 L/minute
3. Suction the infant's mouth and nares
4. Recognize this as normal first period of reactivity

42. The nurse hears a mother telling a friend on the telephone about umbilical cord care. Which of the following statements by the mother indicates effective teaching?

1. "Daily soap and water cleansing is best."
2. "Alcohol helps it dry and kills germs."
3. "An antibiotic ointment applied daily prevents infection."
4. "He can have a tub bath each day."

43. A newborn weighing 3,000 grams and feeding every 4 hours needs 120 calories/kg of body weight every 24 hours for proper growth and development. How many ounces of 20-calories/ounce formula should this newborn receive at each feeding to meet nutritional needs?

1. 2 ounces
2. 3 ounces
3. 4 ounces
4. 6 ounces

44. A neonate delivered to a mother who is HIV seropositive would be expected to have which of the following?

1. HIV antibodies
2. Hepatosplenomegaly
3. Opportunistic infection
4. Elevated white blood cell count

45. A newborn weighing 7 lb and 40 weeks' gestation was successfully resuscitated for birth asphyxia secondary to cord compression. Which of the following should be included in the plan of care?

1. Antibiotic administration
2. Daily bathing
3. Nothing by mouth for 24 to 48 hours
4. 100% oxygen via oxyhood

46. While nipple-feeding a preterm newborn (32 weeks' gestation, 4 lb), the nurse notes evidence of exhaustion, increased respirations and pulse, and a dusky color. The nurse should stop the feeding and do which of the following?

1. Notify the physician
2. Gavage-feed the remainder
3. Position the infant on the left side
4. Administer oxygen via nasal cannula

47. A 3-day-old neonate of 40 weeks' gestation has a serum bilirubin level of 15 mg/dl and is to receive phototherapy. Which of the following would the nurse include in the neonate's plan of care?

1. Monitoring body temperature every hour
2. Shielding the eyes from the light source
3. Restricting fluids to prevent diarrhea
4. Dressing infant in diaper and shirt

48. Which of the following nursing diagnoses would take **priority** when caring for the infant of a diabetic mother?

1. Ineffective thermoregulation
2. Impaired gas exchange
3. Risk for injury
4. Risk for infection

49. The postterm neonate with meconium-stained amniotic fluid needs care designed to especially monitor him for which of the following?

1. Respiratory problems
2. GI problems
3. Integumentary problems
4. Elimination problems

50. Which of the following would the nurse expect to assess in a neonate with fetal alcohol syndrome, whose mother consistently abused alcohol throughout the pregnancy?

1. Lethargy
2. Weight more than 9 pounds
3. Hypoglycemia
4. Craniofacial anomalies

51. The nurse instructs the client who selects the basal body temperature method of contraception to take her temperature daily at which of the following times?
1. Before arising
2. After breakfast
3. Before bedtime
4. After lunch

52. When measuring a client's fundal height, which of the following techniques denotes the correct method of measurement used by the nurse?
1. From the xiphoid process to the umbilicus
2. From the symphysis pubis to the xiphoid process
3. From the symphysis pubis to the fundus
4. From the fundus to the umbilicus

53. A client with severe preeclampsia is admitted with a blood pressure of 160/110, proteinuria, and severe pitting edema. Which of the following would be **most** important to include in the client's plan of care?
1. Daily weight measurement
2. Seizure precautions
3. Right lateral positioning
4. Stress reduction

54. A postpartum primipara asks the nurse, "When can we have sexual intercourse again?" Which of the following would be the nurse's **best** response?
1. "Anytime you both want to."
2. "As soon as you choose a contraceptive method."
3. "When the discharge has stopped and the incision is healed."
4. "After your examination at 6 weeks."

55. The home health nurse visits a client 7 days postpartum who tells her, "My incision is still very painful." Upon inspection of the episiotomy, the nurse notes redness, edema, unapproximated edges, and a yellowish discharge. Which of the following should the home health nurse do?
1. Recommend twice-daily sitz baths
2. Suggest use of an ice pack for discomfort
3. Administer anti-inflammatory medications
4. Notify the client's physician

56. When preparing to administer the vitamin K injection to a neonate, the nurse would select which of the following sites as appropriate for the injection?
1. Deltoid muscle
2. Anterior femoris muscle
3. Vastus lateralis muscle
4. Gluteus maximus muscle

57. Which of the following factors would the nurse keep in mind as being associated with preterm labor?
1. Grand multiparity
2. Maternal infections
3. First pregnancy
4. Trisomy

58. When performing a pelvic examination, the nurse observes a red, swollen area on the right side of the client's vaginal orifice. The nurse would document this as enlargement of which of the following?
1. Clitoris
2. Parotid gland
3. Skene's gland
4. Bartholin's gland

59. On inspection of the client's perineum, the nurse identifies the raised longitudinal folds of pigmented adipose tissue containing hair and extending from the mons veneris. The nurse identifies these as which of the following?
1. Labia minora
2. Labia majora
3. Mons pubis
4. Vestibule

60. The physician documented gynecoid pelvis after a pelvic exam of a client. The nurse knows that this refers to which of the following?

1. A typical female pelvis with a rounded inlet
2. A normal pelvis with a heart-shaped inlet
3. An apelike pelvis with an oval inlet
4. A flat female pelvis with a transverse oval inlet

61. To differentiate as a female, the hormonal stimulation of the embryo that must occur involves which of the following?

1. Increase in maternal estrogen secretion
2. Decrease in maternal androgen secretion
3. Secretion of androgen by the fetal gonad
4. Secretion of estrogen by the fetal gonad

62. A client at 8 weeks' gestation calls complaining of slight nausea in the morning hours. Which of the following client interventions should the nurse question?

1. Taking 1 teaspoon of bicarbonate of soda in an 8-ounce glass of water
2. Eating a few low-sodium crackers before getting out of bed
3. Avoiding the intake of liquids in the morning hours
4. Eating six small meals a day instead of three large meals

63. Which of the following responses would be **best** when a client asks about when she will gain the most weight during her pregnancy?

1. "Weight is gained equally in the three trimesters."
2. "Most weight is gained equally in the first two trimesters."
3. "Most women gain too much the first trimester."
4. "About 1 pound a week is gained during the last two trimesters."

64. Which of the following findings during a prenatal exam should the nurse report to the physician for further evaluation?

1. Breast tenderness
2. Increased areola pigmentation
3. Nodularity in the upper-left outer quadrant
4. Prominent superficial veins

65. The nurse documents positive ballottement in the client's prenatal record. The nurse understands that this indicates which of the following?

1. Contractions palpable on the abdomen
2. Passive movement of the unengaged fetus
3. Fetal kicking felt by the client
4. Enlargement and softening of the uterus

66. During a pelvic exam, the nurse notes a purple-blue tinge of the cervix. The nurse documents this as which of the following?

1. Braxton Hicks sign
2. Chadwick's sign
3. Goodell's sign
4. McDonald's sign

67. The obstetric conjugate is measured at 10 cm, indicating to the nurse that the anteroposterior diameter is which of the following?

1. Within normal limits for a vaginal delivery
2. Too narrow for a normal vaginal delivery
3. Extremely large
4. Marginal for a vaginal delivery

68. When describing to a client how a pregnancy test works, the nurse understands that which of the following hormones is being evaluated?

1. Human chorionic gonadotropin
2. Estrogen
3. Follicle-stimulating hormone
4. Progesterone

69. A couple attending a childbirth class asks the nurse why back massage against the sacral area soothes the laboring woman. Which of the following would be the nurse's **best** response?

1. "The pressure of massage counters the pressure from inside the woman, easing discomfort."
2. "This pressure helps the baby rotate during its passage down the birth canal."
3. "If the baby is in the posterior position, it helps the baby turn around to the anterior."
4. "Lying in bed during labor makes the mother's back hurt."

70. During a prenatal class, the nurse explains the rationale for breathing techniques during preparation for labor based on the understanding that breathing techniques are **most** important in achieving which of the following?

1. Eliminating pain and giving the expectant parents something to do
2. Reducing the risk of fetal distress by increasing uteroplacental perfusion
3. Facilitating relaxation, possibly reducing the perception of pain
4. Eliminating pain so that less analgesia and anesthesia are needed

71. The nurse instructs a client that a radiopaque material will be inserted into her uterus and fallopian tubes to assess tubal patency. The nurse is describing which of the following?

1. Uterotubal insufflation
2. Laparoscopy
3. Culdoscopy
4. Hysterosalpingography

72. A couple has been unable to conceive after 5 years of marriage with no use of birth control. They use lubrication with petroleum jelly for additional pleasure during intercourse three to four times a week. The lab report shows a lower than normal sperm count, but other assessment data appear to be within normal limits. Which of the following recommendations should the nurse make?

1. Eliminate the additional lubrication
2. Reduce intercourse to twice weekly
3. Have consistency in how they perform intercourse
4. Clarify their degree of sexual satisfaction

73. To differentiate as a male, the embryo must do which of the following?

1. Receive increased estrogen from the mother
2. Increase its own secretion of estrogen
3. Decrease its production of androgen
4. Increase its production of androgen

74. Which of the following would the nurse identify as the leading cause of maternal death after delivery throughout the world?

1. Puerperal infection
2. Thrombophlebitis
3. Postpartum hemorrhage
4. Uterine inversion

75. Which of the following correctly identifies the theory explaining the onset of labor caused by a release of a complex cascade of bioactive chemical agents into the amniotic fluid?

1. Oxytocin theory
2. Prostaglandin theory
3. Progesterone deprivation theory
4. Uterine decidua activation theory

76. One hour after delivery, assessment reveals the client's uterus is one fingerbreadth below the umbilicus and deviated to the right of midline. Which of the following would be the nurse's **priority** action at this time?

1. Assist the mother to void.
2. Vigorously massage the fundus.
3. Administer additional oxytocin to contract the uterus.
4. Give a tocolytic drug intravenously.

77. After 4 hours of active labor, the nurse notes that the contractions of a primigravid client are not strong enough to dilate the cervix. Which of the following would the nurse anticipate doing?
1. Obtaining an order to begin I.V. oxytocin infusion
2. Administering a light sedative to allow the patient to rest for several hours
3. Preparing for a cesarean birth for failure to progress
4. Increasing the encouragement to the patient when pushing begins

78. When augmenting labor with oxytocin, which of the following would be the **priority** assessment?
1. Maternal vital signs
2. Fetal heart rate
3. Urinary output
4. Contraction characteristics

79. The nurse would anticipate which of the following for a client who has been in true labor for 12 hours and is diagnosed with borderline pelvic measurements?
1. Ultrasonography
2. Cesarean birth
3. Radiographic pelvimetry
4. Manual internal measurements

80. A multigravida at 38 weeks' gestation is admitted with painless, bright red bleeding and mild contractions every 7 to 10 minutes. Which of the following assessments should be avoided?
1. Maternal vital signs
2. Fetal heart rate
3. Contraction monitoring
4. Cervical dilation

81. Which of the following would be the nurse's **most** appropriate response to a client who asks why she must have a cesarean birth if she has a complete placenta previa?
1. "You will have to ask your physician when he returns."
2. "You need a cesarean to prevent hemorrhage."
3. "The placenta is covering most of your cervix."
4. "The placenta is covering the opening of the uterus and blocking your baby."

82. A postpartum client was in labor for 30 hours and had ruptured membranes for 24 hours. For which of the following would the nurse be alert?
1. Endometritis
2. Endometriosis
3. Salpingitis
4. Pelvic thrombophlebitis

83. A 37-week gestation multigravida is admitted with a blood pressure of 90/60, pulse 110, and respirations 28. She has been having a sharp abdominal pain for the last hour and states she was involved in a "minor fender-bender" car accident earlier in the afternoon. The nurse questions the client about any vaginal bleeding, based on the knowledge that, with these symptoms, blood loss is usually which of the following?
1. Unobserved
2. Minimal
3. Greater than observed
4. Less than observed

84. Which of the following physician orders should take **priority** when caring for a client with abruptio placentae?
1. Type and crossmatching for whole blood
2. Assessment of maternal vital signs every 15 minutes
3. Assessment of fetal heart rate by continuous electronic monitoring
4. Measurement of fundal height

85. A patient presents with signs of abruptio placentae following a motor vehicle accident. She has no external injuries but reports extreme abdominal pain. Her abdomen is rigid on palpation. Fetal monitoring indicates acute fetal distress. Which of the following interventions would be **most** appropriate?
1. Monitoring maternal urine output and hydration status
2. Monitoring maternal and fetal physiologic status
3. Providing emotional support regarding potential fetal demise
4. Administering a tocolytic to stop labor

86. The nurse understands that the fetal head is in which of the following positions with a face presentation?
1. Completely flexed
2. Completely extended
3. Partially extended
4. Partially flexed

87. With a fetus in the left-anterior breech presentation, the nurse would expect the fetal heart rate would be **most** audible in which of the following areas?
1. Above the maternal umbilicus and to the right of midline
2. In the lower-left maternal abdominal quadrant
3. In the lower-right maternal abdominal quadrant
4. Above the maternal umbilicus and to the left of midline

88. The amniotic fluid of a client has a greenish tint. The nurse interprets this to be the result of which of the following?
1. Lanugo
2. Hydramnio
3. Meconium
4. Vernix

89. A patient is in labor and has just been told she has a breech presentation. The nurse should be particularly alert for which of the following?
1. Quickening
2. Ophthalmia neonatorum
3. Pica
4. Prolapsed umbilical cord

90. Which of the following pieces of data gathered on an initial infertility work-up would suggest a tubal cause for the infertility?
1. Use of an intrauterine device for contraception
2. History of polycystic ovary
3. Repeated vaginal yeast infections
4. Use of diethylstilbestrol by client's mother

91. When reviewing assisted methods of reproduction, the nurse would understand that surrogate embryo transfer would be a viable reproductive alternative for which of the following?
1. A couple in which the woman is unable to carry a fetus to viability
2. A woman with damaged fallopian tubes but who still ovulates regularly
3. A couple in which the male partner is infertile and the woman is fertile
4. A woman unable to produce normal mature follicles with a fertile male partner

92. When describing dizygotic twins to a couple, on which of the following would the nurse base the explanation?
1. Two ova fertilized by separate sperm
2. Sharing of a common placenta
3. Each ova with the same genotype
4. Sharing of a common chorion

93. Which of the following **best** describes the basic pattern of single gene inheritance that includes cystic fibrosis?
1. X-linked dominant
2. X-linked recessive
3. Autosomal dominant
4. Autosomal recessive

94. A client is considered a habitual aborter because she has lost three previous pregnancies during the first 2 months. Her progesterone level is determined to be low. The nurse understands that this is the result of a problem with which of the following?
1. Placenta
2. Chromosome
3. Corpus luteum
4. Spermatozoa

95. Which of the following refers to the single cell that reproduces itself after conception?
1. Chromosome
2. Blastocyst
3. Zygote
4. Trophoblast

96. In the late 1950s, consumers and health care professionals began challenging the routine use of analgesics and anesthetics during childbirth. Which of the following was an outgrowth of this concept?
1. Labor, delivery, recovery, postpartum (LDRP)
2. Nurse-midwifery
3. Clinical nurse specialist
4. Prepared childbirth

97. A client has a midpelvic contracture from a previous pelvic injury due to a motor vehicle accident as a teenager. The nurse is aware that this could prevent a fetus from passing through or around which structure during childbirth?
1. Symphysis pubis
2. Sacral promontory
3. Ischial spines
4. Pubic arch

98. When teaching a group of adolescents about variations in the length of the menstrual cycle, the nurse understands that the underlying mechanism is due to variations in which of the following phases?
1. Menstrual phase
2. Proliferative phase
3. Secretory phase
4. Ischemic phase

99. The Maternal and Infant Care projects were established in 1964 by which amendment to the Public Health Service Act?
1. The Sheppard-Towner Act
2. The Women, Infants and Children program
3. Title V
4. Title XIX

100. When teaching a group of adolescents about male hormone production, which of the following would the nurse include as being produced by the Leydig cells?
1. Follicle-stimulating hormone
2. Testosterone
3. Luteinizing hormone
4. Gonadotropin-releasing hormone

101. A 39-year-old pregnant woman is seen in the clinic at 16 weeks' gestation. It is decided that an amniocentesis should be performed. The nurse knows that an amniocentesis can be used to identify which of the following? Select all that apply:
1. Fetal lung maturity
2. Gestational diabetes
3. Polyhydramnios
4. Sex of the fetus
5. Presence of neural tube defects
6. Presence of chromosomal defects

102. In the third stage of labor, which of the following are anticipated signs of placental separation? Select all that apply:
1. The uterus rises in the abdomen.
2. The cervix is completely effaced and dilated.
3. There is an increase in the length of the umbilical cord.
4. The presenting part is at zero station.
5. There is a trickle or spurt of blood from the vagina.
6. The uterus changes shape from discoid to globular.

103. Gestational diabetes can be determined by a blood test called a 3-hour-glucose tolerance test. This blood test requires the pregnant woman to ingest an oral solution containing ________ grams of glucose.

104. The nurse is about to administer vitamin K (AquaMEPHYTON) to a newborn following birth. A 0.5-mg dose is to be given to the newborn. The medication comes in a concentration of 2 mg/ml. How many milliliters of medication should the infant receive?

105. The recovery nurse is palpating the fundus of a woman who delivered 12 hours ago. Place an X on the drawing of the abdomen where the nurse would expect to palpate the fundus at this time.

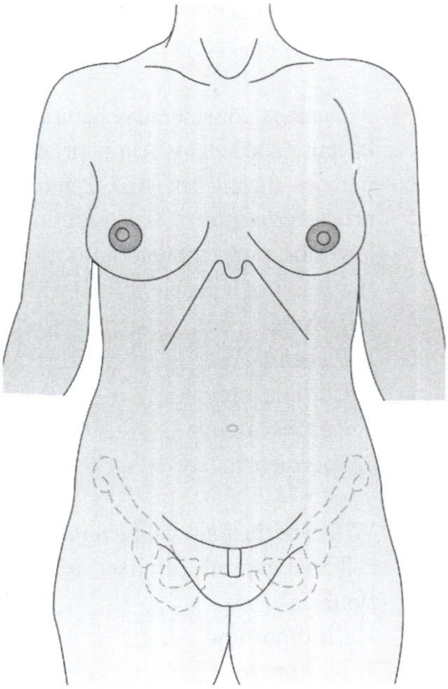

COMPREHENSIVE TEST: ANSWERS

1. The answer is 2.
Regular timely ingestion of oral contraceptives is necessary to maintain hormonal levels of the drugs to suppress the action of the hypothalamus and anterior pituitary leading to inappropriate secretion of follicle-stimulating hormone and luteinizing hormone. Therefore, follicles do not mature, ovulation is inhibited, and pregnancy is prevented. The estrogen content of the oral contraceptive may cause the nausea, regardless of when the pill is taken. Side effects and drug interactions may occur with oral contraceptives regardless of the time the pill is taken.

2. The answer is 1.
Medroxyprogesterone (Depo-Provera) injections are administered every 12 weeks and may be continued as long as there are no serious adverse effects. In the absence of an abnormal cytology report, Papanicolaou smears are recommended yearly for all women. Women receiving hormonal contraception should receive an annual gynecologic examination. However, because the injection must be given every 12 weeks, this client cannot wait 1 year to return to the clinic. Subdermal implants, not injections, are reevaluated as a method of contraception in 5 years.

3. The answer is 3.
Condoms, when used correctly and consistently, are the most effective contraceptive method or barrier against bacterial and viral sexually transmitted infections. Although spermicides kill sperm, they do not provide reliable protection against the spread of sexually transmitted infections, especially intracellular organisms such as human immunodeficiency virus. Insertion and removal of the diaphragm along with the use of the spermicides may cause vaginal irritations, which could place the client at risk for infection transmission. Male sterilization eliminates spermatozoa from the ejaculate, but it does not eliminate bacterial or viral microorganisms that can cause sexually transmitted infections.

4. The answer is 1.
The diaphragm must be fitted individually to ensure effectiveness. Because of the changes to the reproductive structures during pregnancy and following delivery, the diaphragm must be refitted, usually at the 6-weeks examination following childbirth or after a weight loss of 15 pounds or more. In addition, for maximum effectiveness, spermicidal jelly should be placed in the dome and around the rim. However, spermicidal jelly should not be inserted into the vagina until subinvolution has occurred at approximately 6 weeks. Use of a female condom protects the reproductive system from the introduction of semen or spermicides into the vagina and may be used after childbirth. Hormonal contraceptives may be started within the first postpartum week to ensure suppression of ovulation. For the couple who has determined the female's fertile period using the rhythm method, avoidance of intercourse during this period is safe and effective.

5. The answer is 4.
To achieve the maximum effectiveness from a contraceptive, it must be used correctly and consistently. It should also be safe, have few adverse effects, and be easy to use. Although cost may be a factor, it is not the most important factor. The most economical contraceptive may not be acceptable, convenient, or afford maximum sexual pleasure. In choosing a contraceptive method, the client needs to consider social, religious, and cultural beliefs and values. However, this is not the priority. Although noncontraceptive benefits are important in assisting the client in deciding between two or more suitable methods, this is not the most important aspect of selection.

6. The answer is 3.
An intrauterine device (IUD) may increase the risk of pelvic inflammatory disease, especially in women with more than one sexual partner, because of the increased risk of sexually transmitted infections. An IUD should not be used if the woman has an active or chronic pelvic infection, postpartum infection, endometrial hyperplasia or carcinoma, or uterine abnormalities. Age is not a factor in determining the risks associated with IUD use. Most IUD users are over the age of 30. Although there is a slightly higher risk of infertility in women who have never been pregnant, the IUD is an acceptable option as long as the risk-benefit ratio is discussed. IUDs may be inserted immediately after delivery, but this is not recommended because of the increased risk and rate of expulsion at this time.

7. The answer is 4.
Hormonal contraceptives contain exogenous estrogen capable of activating blood-clotting mechanisms. Women with a history of blood clots are at risk for future coagulation problems, and hormonal contraceptives would be contraindicated. An intrauterine device may precipitate excessive uterine bleeding, but it does not cause blood clots. Subdermal implants and intramuscular injections contain only progesterone, which does not precipitate blood clots.

8. The answer is 1.

The safest recommendation to women is total abstinence during pregnancy. It has been estimated that 11% of women who drink moderately during the first trimester (1 to 2 ounces of alcohol per day) have infants with fetal alcohol syndrome. Although alcohol consumption in the first trimester causes the most damage to the fetus, abstinence throughout pregnancy is recommended. Alcohol in any vehicle or amount can be damaging to the fetus. Abstinence is best. Alcohol consumption in the early weeks of pregnancy is the most damaging to the fetus because it may affect nutritional intake, decrease maternal resistance to infection, and cause bone marrow suppression or liver disease—all potentially harmful to a fetus.

9. The answer is 3.

During the third trimester, the enlarging uterus places pressure on the intestines. This coupled with the effect of hormones on smooth-muscle relaxation causes decreased intestinal motility (peristalsis). Increasing fiber in the diet will help fecal matter pass more quickly through the intestinal tract, thus decreasing the amount of water that is absorbed. As a result, stool is softer and easier to pass. Enemas could precipitate preterm labor or electrolyte loss and should be avoided. Laxatives may cause preterm labor by stimulating peristalsis and may interfere with the absorption of nutrients. Use for more than 1 week also can lead to laxative dependency. Liquid in the diet helps provide a semisolid, soft consistency to the stool. Eight to ten glasses of fluid per day are essential to maintain hydration and promote stool evacuation.

10. The answer is 4.

To ensure adequate fetal growth and development during the 40 weeks of a pregnancy, a total weight gain of 25 to 30 pounds is recommended: 1.5 pounds in the first 10 weeks; 9 pounds by 30 weeks; and 27.5 pounds by 40 weeks. The pregnant woman should gain less weight in the first and second trimesters than in the third. During the first trimester, the client should only gain 1.5 pounds in the first 10 weeks, not 1 pound per week. A weight gain of 0.5 pound per week would be 20 pounds for the total pregnancy, less than the recommended amount.

11. The answer is 2.

To calculate the estimated date of delivery by Nägele's rule, add 7 days to the first day of the last menstrual period (LMP) and count back 3 months, changing the year appropriately. To obtain a date of September 27, 7 days have been added to the last day of the LMP (rather than the first day of the LMP); in addition, 4 months (instead of 3 months) were counted back. To obtain the date of November 7, 7 days have been subtracted (instead of added) from the first day of the LMP. November indicates counting back 2 months (instead of 3 months) from January. To obtain the date of December 27, 7 days were added to the last day of the LMP (rather than the first day of the LMP) and December indicates counting back only 1 month (instead of 3 months) from January.

12. The answer is 1.

Sickle cell disease is found primarily in the African American population or among persons whose ancestors come from the Mediterranean area, Middle East, or parts of India. Thus, a sickle cell screen would be performed routinely for a pregnant woman of African American heritage but not for a Caucasian pregnant woman. Alpha fetoprotein is recommended for all pregnant women to detect the presence of fetal neural tube defects. All pregnant women are screened for diabetes at 26 to 28 weeks to detect the presence of gestational diabetes. The blood type and Rh of all pregnant women must be determined in anticipation of future complications.

13. The answer is 4.
The client has been pregnant four times, including current pregnancy (G). Birth at 38 weeks' gestation is considered full term (T), while birth from 20 weeks to 38 weeks is considered preterm (P). A spontaneous abortion occurred at 8 weeks (A). She has two living children (L).

14. The answer is 2.
At 12 weeks' gestation, the uterus rises out of the pelvis and is palpable above the symphysis pubis. The doppler intensifies the sound of the fetal pulse rate so it is audible. The uterus has merely risen out of the pelvis into the abdominal cavity and is not at the level of the umbilicus. The fetal heart rate (FHR) at this age is not audible with a stethoscope. The uterus at 12 weeks is just above the symphysis pubis in the abdominal cavity, not midway between the umbilicus and the xiphoid process. At 12 weeks, the FHR would be difficult to auscultate with a fetoscope. Although the external electronic fetal monitor would project the FHR, the uterus has not risen to the umbilicus at 12 weeks.

15. The answer is 1.
Although all of the choices are important in the management of diabetes, diet therapy is the mainstay of the treatment plan and should always be the priority. Women diagnosed with gestational diabetes generally need only diet therapy without medication to control their blood glucose levels. Exercise is important for all pregnant women, especially diabetic women, because it burns up glucose, thus decreasing blood glucose level. However, dietary intake, not exercise, is the priority. All pregnant women with diabetes should have periodic monitoring of serum glucose. However, those with gestational diabetes generally do not need daily glucose monitoring. The standard of care recommends a fasting and 2-hour postprandial blood glucose level every 2 weeks.

16. The answer is 3.
After 20 weeks' gestation, when there is a rapid weight gain, preeclampsia should be suspected, which may be caused by fluid retention manifested by edema, especially of the hands and face. The three classic signs of preeclampsia are hypertension, edema, and proteinuria. Although urine is checked for glucose at each clinic visit, this is not the priority. Depression may cause either anorexia or excessive food intake, leading to excessive weight gain or loss. This is not, however, the priority consideration at this time. Weight gain thought to be caused by excessive food intake would require a 24-hour diet recall. However, excessive intake would not be the primary consideration for this client at this time.

17. The answer is 2.
Cramping and vaginal bleeding coupled with cervical dilation signifies that termination of the pregnancy is inevitable and cannot be prevented. Thus, the nurse would document an imminent abortion. In a threatened abortion, cramping and vaginal bleeding are present, but there is no cervical dilation. The symptoms may subside or progress to abortion. In a complete abortion, all the products of conception are expelled. A missed abortion is early fetal intrauterine death without expulsion of the products of conception.

18. The answer is 2.
For the client with an ectopic pregnancy, lower abdominal pain, usually unilateral, is the primary symptom. Thus, pain is the priority. Although the potential for infection is always present, the risk is low in ectopic pregnancy because pathogenic microorganisms have not been introduced from external sources. The client may have a limited knowledge of the pathology and treatment of the condition and will most likely experience grieving, but this is not the priority at this time.

19. The answer is 3.
Because the blood type of the fetus is unknown and a small amount of the fetal blood may have entered the mother's circulation during the abortion, isoimmunization with resultant Rh antibody production may have occurred. RhoGAM prevents antibody formation and complications with future pregnancies. Unless signs of infection are present, antibiotics are not administered with a spontaneous complete abortion. If the rubella titer is low, vaccine could be administered at this time. However, this would not be the most important action. Unless an excessive amount of blood loss occurred, iron supplements are not essential.

20. The answer is 2.
The goal of prenatal care for the woman with hyperemesis gravidarum is that she will maintain a dietary and fluid intake that will provide adequate nutritional components for a healthy pregnancy. Eating small, frequent meals facilitates food retention, which will help maintain her weight. Women with hyperemesis gravidarum may have to be hospitalized multiple times for fluid and electrolyte replacement. Generally, antiemetic medications are not prescribed for hyperemesis gravidarum because of the potential teratogenic risks to the fetus. Prenatal vitamins taken at bedtime cause less nausea. They should be continued throughout pregnancy if possible.

21. The answer is 3.
Follow-up care is extremely important following the diagnosis of a hydatiform molar pregnancy. Weekly determination of human chorionic gonadotropin (hCG) levels for 3 months, then monthly for 1 year is essential to monitor the disorder. A pelvic examination also is necessary every 2 weeks for 3 months to palpate uterine and ovarian size to detect complications. Vitamin supplementation is not necessary after termination of the pregnancy. Although the nurse should assess the woman's feelings about the loss of the pregnancy and help her deal with the grief, this is not the most important area of teaching. Hormonal contraceptives are not recommended, because they suppress pituitary luteinizing hormone, which may interfere with serum hCG measurements.

22. The answer is 4.
Before uterine assessment is performed, it is essential that the woman empty her bladder. A full bladder will interfere with the accuracy of the assessment by elevating the uterus and displacing it to the side of the midline. Vital sign assessment is not necessary unless an abnormality in uterine assessment is identified. Uterine assessment should not cause acute pain that requires administration of analgesia. Ambulating the client is an essential component of postpartum care, but is not necessary prior to assessment of the uterus.

23. The answer is 3.
During the first 1 to 2 days after birth, the taking-in phase, the mother is passive, dependent, and focused on her own needs, primarily food and rest, to restore her mental and physical energy. During the taking-in phase, the new mother typically needs assistance with activities of daily living. Elimination functions return to normal about the 2nd to 3rd day during the taking-hold phase of psychosocial adjustment. During the taking-in phase, the woman's energies are focused on her own bodily functions and she is not ready to focus on learning new skills.

24. The answer is 4.
Separation of the labia with nonsterile perineal rinse directed toward the vaginal orifice may predispose the client to infection. The labia should not be separated when rinsing the perineum after urination and defecation, to prevent introduction of bacteria. Wiping the perineum from front to back decreases contamination with mi-

croorganisms from the anus to the vaginal and urinary orifices. The surface of the perineal pad that will be placed against the vaginal orifice and the episiotomy should be kept free of microorganisms. Therefore, touching the inside of the pad should be avoided. Handwashing before and after toileting is the single most important action to prevent the introduction of microorganisms onto the perineal area.

25. The answer is 1.

Feeding more frequently, about every 2 hours, will decrease the infant's frantic, vigorous sucking from hunger and will decrease breast engorgement, soften the breast, and promote ease of correct latching-on for feeding. Opioids given before breast-feeding are passed through the breast milk to the infant, causing excessive sleepiness. Nipple soreness is not severe enough to warrant opioid analgesia. All postpartum clients, especially lactating mothers, should wear a supportive bra with wide cotton straps. This does not, however, prevent or reduce nipple soreness. Soaps are drying to the skin of the nipples and should not be used on the breasts of lactating mothers. Dry nipple skin may lead to cracks and fissures, which can become sore and painful.

26. The answer is 2.

Because the hemorrhoids are painful, this client problem should receive priority. A sitz bath promotes relaxation and comfort. Although ambulation will increase peristalsis, it will not decrease the hemorrhoidal pain. Teaching the client to eat foods high in fiber will prevent constipation and reduce straining but will not decrease the immediate problem of pain. Administration of a stool softener will decrease the chances of constipation but does not address the immediate priority problem of pain.

27. The answer is 4.

A weak, thready pulse elevated to 100 beats per minute may indicate impending hemorrhagic shock. An increased pulse is a compensatory mechanism of the body in response to decreased fluid volume. Thus the nurse should check the amount of lochia present. Temperatures up to 100.4° F in the first 24 hours after birth are related to the dehydrating effects of labor and are considered normal. Although rechecking the blood pressure may be a correct choice of action, it is not the first action that should be implemented in light of the other data. The data indicate a potential impending hemorrhage. Assessing the uterus for firmness and position in relation to the umbilicus and midline is important, but the nurse should check the extent of vaginal bleeding first. Then it would be appropriate to check the uterus, which may be a possible cause of the hemorrhage.

28. The answer is 4.

Any bright red vaginal discharge would be considered abnormal, but especially 5 days after delivery, when the lochia is typically pink to brownish. Lochia rubra, a dark red discharge, is present for 2 to 3 days after delivery. Bright red vaginal bleeding at this time suggests late postpartum hemorrhage, which occurs after the first 24 hours following delivery and is generally caused by retained placental fragments or bleeding disorders. Lochia rubra is the normal dark red discharge occurring in the first 2 to 3 days after delivery and containing epithelial cells, erythrocytes, leukocytes, and decidua. Lochia serosa is a pink to brownish serosanguineous discharge occurring from 3 to 10 days after delivery that contains decidua, erythrocytes, leukocytes, cervical mucus, and microorganisms. Lochia alba is an almost colorless to yellowish discharge occurring from 10 days to 3 weeks after delivery and containing leukocytes, decidua, epithelial cells, fat, cervical mucus, cholesterol crystals, and bacteria.

29. The answer is 1.
The data suggest an infection of the endometrial lining of the uterus. The lochia may be decreased or copious, dark brown in appearance, and foul smelling, providing further evidence of a possible infection. All the client's data indicate a uterine problem, not a breast problem. Typically, transient fever (usually a temperature of 101° F) may be present with breast engorgement. Symptoms of mastitis include influenza-like manifestations. Localized infection of an episiotomy or cesarean birth incision rarely causes systemic symptoms, and uterine involution would not be affected. The client data do not include dysuria, frequency, or urgency, symptoms of urinary tract infections, which would necessitate assessing the client's urine.

30. The answer is 3.
Derived from nosocomial sources, *Staphylococcus aureus* is most commonly introduced in breast-feeding women through cracked nipples, localizing in the lactiferous glands and ducts and causing mastitis. *Escherichia coli, Streptococcus pneumoniae,* or *Neisseria gonorrhoeae* is rarely a cause of mastitis.

31. The answer is 2.
Oxytocin increases the excitability of the uterine muscle cell to increase the strength of contraction and facilitate hemostasis. Promethazine is an antiemetic administered to control nausea and vomiting. Meperidine is an opioid analgesic, which would precipitate muscle relaxation. Magnesium sulfate is a tocolytic, which interferes with muscle contractility to facilitate relaxation.

32. The answer is 3.
Because of early postpartum discharge and limited time for teaching, the nurse's priority is to facilitate the safe and effective care of the client and newborn. Although promoting comfort and restoration of health, exploring the family's emotional status, and teaching about family planning are important in postpartum and newborn nursing care, they are not the priority focus in the limited time presented by early postpartum discharge.

33. The answer is 4.
Protamine sulfate is an antithromboplastin that prolongs clotting time and neutralizes the anticoagulant activity of heparin. It should be readily available in case the client develops bleeding. Naloxone is an opioid antagonist, which blocks the effects of opiates. Glucagon mobilizes glucose to counteract the hypoglycemic effect of insulin. Calcium gluconate is the antidote for magnesium sulfate.

34. The answer is 2.
Based on the assessment, the nurse would suspect a pulmonary embolism. Symptoms of pulmonary embolism include dyspnea, tachypnea, cough, tachycardia, pleuritic chest pain, and a feeling of impending catastrophe or doom. Although the client is exhibiting some of the symptoms of a myocardial infarction, the chest pain is at the costovertebral area of the right chest, not in the substernal area of the left side of the chest. Symptoms of pneumonia develop over several hours or days, not suddenly, and include fever, malaise, and more generalized chest pain. Symptoms of panic attack include apprehension, tachycardia, and tachypnea, but not acute chest pain.

35. The answer is 2.
Based on the client's statements and events during the past several weeks, the most appropriate nursing diagnosis would be Ineffective individual coping. Ineffective individual coping is a state in which an individual experiences an inability to manage internal or environmental stressors adequately because of inadequate resources (physical, psychological, behavioral, or cognitive). Hopelessness refers to a sustained emotional state in which an individual sees no alternatives or personal choices avail-

able to solve problems or to achieve what is desired. Powerlessness refers to a state in which an individual perceives a lack of personal control over certain events or situations. Altered parenting refers to a state in which the caregiver experiences a real or potential inability to provide a constructive environment that nurtures the growth and development of a child.

36. The answer is 4.
A parent who does not unwrap the infant and uses only fingertip touch without progressing to using palms on the trunk or drawing the infant toward her body does not display positive bonding behaviors. Snuggling the infant to the parent's face and neck demonstrates positive bonding, but holding the infant away from the parent's body, such as across the knees or on the bed, does not. A parent with adaptive bonding behaviors handles and holds the baby at times other than when giving direct care. The parent who is bonding with the infant will ask questions about the characteristics and behaviors of the infant, as well as infant care after discharge.

37. Theanswer is 3.
Heat loss by radiation occurs when the infant's crib is placed too near cold walls or windows. Thus, placing the newborn's crib close to the viewing window would be least effective. Body heat is lost through evaporation during bathing. Placing the infant under the radiant warmer after bathing will help rewarm the infant. Covering the scale with a warmed blanket prior to weighing prevents heat loss through conduction. A knit cap prevents heat loss from the head, a large body surface area of the newborn's body.

38. The answer is 2.
A fractured clavicle would prevent the normal Moro response of symmetrical sequential extension and abduction of the arms followed by flexion and adduction. In talipes equinovarus (clubfoot), the foot is turned medially, and in plantar flexion, with the heel elevated. The feet are not involved with the Moro reflex. Congenital absence of thyroid function is detectable at birth only by laboratory testing. Hypothyroidism has no effect on the primitive reflexes. Absence of the Moro reflex is the most significant single indicator of central nervous system status, but it is not a sign of increased intracranial pressure.

39. The answer is 2.
Hemorrhage is a potential risk following any surgical procedure. Although the infant has been given vitamin K to facilitate clotting, the prophylactic dose is often not sufficient to prevent bleeding. Although infection is a possibility, signs will not appear within 4 hours after the surgical procedure. The primary discomfort of circumcision occurs during the surgical procedure, not afterward. Although feedings are withheld before the circumcision, the chances of dehydration are minimal.

40. The answer is 2.
The presence of excessive estrogen and progesterone in the maternal-fetal blood followed by prompt withdrawal at birth precipitates breast engorgement, which will spontaneously resolve in 4 to 5 days after birth. The trauma of the birth process does not cause inflammation of the newborn's breast tissue. Newborns do not have breast malignancy. This reply by the nurse would cause the mother to have undue anxiety. Breast tissue does not hypertrophy in the fetus or newborn.

41. The answer is 4.
The first 15 minutes to 1 hour after birth is the first period of reactivity involving respiratory and circulatory adaptation to extrauterine life. The data given reflect the normal changes during this time period. The infant's assessment data reflect normal adaptation. Thus, the physician does not need to be notified and oxygen is not needed. The data do not indicate the pres-

ence of choking, gagging, or coughing, which are signs of excessive secretions. Suctioning is not necessary.

42. The answer is 2.

Application of 70% isopropyl alcohol to the cord minimizes microorganisms (germicidal) and promotes drying. The cord should be kept dry until it falls off and the stump has healed. Antibiotic ointment should only be used to treat an infection, not a prophylaxis. Infants should not be submerged in a tub of water until the cord falls off and the stump has completely healed.

43. The answer is 2.

To determine the amount of formula needed, do the following calculation: 3 kg × 120 calories/kg/day = 360 calories/day; feeding q 4 hours = 6 feedings/day = 60 calories/feeding; 60 calories/feeding with formula 20 calories/ounce = 3 ounces/feeding. Based on the calculation, 2, 4, and 6 ounces are incorrect.

44. The answer is 1.

Virtually every baby born to a mother who is seropositive for human immunodeficiency virus (HIV) will have HIV antibodies at birth. Pregnant women infected with HIV produce immunoglobulin G antibodies, which cross the placental barrier to the fetus; therefore, cord blood is positive for HIV antibodies. Less than half of the infants are actually infected with the virus. Only infants infected with the HIV virus will manifest symptoms, such as hepatosplenomegaly, before 1 year of age. The average age of onset for an opportunistic infection is 3 to 6 months of age in infants who become infected with HIV. Elevation of the white blood cell count occurs with bacterial infections. HIV is a virus.

45. The answer is 3.

Because of the newborn's status, the intestinal tract should be kept in a resting state for 24 to 48 hours. Bowel sounds should be monitored to detect signs of necrotizing enterocolitis. Infection has not been manifested. Prophylactic antibiotics are not necessary. The postasphyxial newborn should be disturbed as little as possible and allowed to rest and recover. Oxygen is not routinely administered (especially at 100%) unless the infant is symptomatic of hypoxemia.

46. The answer is 2.

Calories are important for growth and maintenance of bodily functions. Gavage-feeding the remainder of the carefully calculated quantity of milk is passive and requires no effort for the infant. Preterm infants often become exhausted during feedings. This does not require physician notification. The infant needs the rest of the feeding by some method. Infants should be placed on their right side after feedings to facilitate gastric emptying. Although the infant has increased respirations and a dusky color, currently there is no indication for the administration of oxygen.

47. The answer is 2.

For the infant receiving phototherapy, the eyes must be protected with an impermeable shield to prevent retinal damage. Unless the infant has an alteration in body temperature, the temperature only needs to be monitored every 4 hours. Although diarrhea is a common occurrence with phototherapy, fluid intake must be increased to compensate for the insensible water loss. The effectiveness of the phototherapy depends on the light contacting the skin, which converts the bilirubin to a water-soluble state for elimination. The infant's skin needs to be exposed.

48. The answer is 3.

An infant of a diabetic mother (IDM) is at increased risk for a traumatic birth with resultant injuries. The infant should be monitored 30 minutes after birth and thereafter per protocol for hypoglycemia and should be fed as soon as possible to prevent low blood glucose level and potential brain injury. The IDM is not at additional risk for alteration in temperature. Although maternal glucose and cortisol levels may lead to decreased lung maturity, this is not the most common problem. The IDM is not at additional risk for infection.

49. The answer is 1.
Intrauterine anoxia may cause relaxation of the anal sphincter and emptying of meconium into the amniotic fluid. At birth, some of the meconium fluid may be aspirated, causing mechanical obstruction or chemical pneumonitis. The infant is not at increased risk for GI problems. Even though the skin is stained with meconium, it is noninfectious (sterile) and nonirritating. The postterm meconium-stained infant is not at additional risk for bowel or urinary problems.

50. The answer is 4.
Alcohol is a teratogen, which affects the morphogenesis of the developing fetus, with the possibility of multiple structural anomalies, especially craniofacial, including short palpebral fissures, flat midface, flat upper lip groove, thin upper lip, and low nasal bridge. Newborns with fetal alcohol syndrome (FAS) exhibit common behaviors not unlike the drug-exposed infant with irritability, tremors, and hypersensitivity to stimuli. Infants with FAS are smaller at birth. Head circumference and weight are most commonly affected. Infants born with FAS are not especially prone to hypoglycemia.

51. The answer is 1.
The basal body temperature is the lowest body temperature of a healthy person that is taken immediately after waking and before getting out of bed. The temperature may be taken orally or rectally, but always before arising, not at the middle or end of a day of activity, which would increase the temperature and give a false reading.

52. The answer is 3.
The nurse should use a nonelastic, flexible, paper measuring tape, placing the zero point on the superior border of the symphysis pubis and stretching the tape across the abdomen at the midline to the top of the fundus. The xiphoid and umbilicus are not appropriate landmarks to use when measuring the height of the fundus (McDonald's measurement).

53. The answer is 2.
Women hospitalized with severe preeclampsia need decreased central nervous system stimulation to prevent a seizure. Seizure precautions provide environmental safety should a seizure occur. Because of edema, daily weight is important but not the priority. Preeclampsia causes vasospasm and therefore can reduce utero-placental perfusion. The client should be placed on her left side to maximize blood flow, reduce blood pressure, and promote diuresis. Interventions to reduce stress and anxiety are very important to facilitate coping and a sense of control, but seizure precautions are the priority.

54. The answer is 3.
Cessation of the lochial discharge signifies healing of the endometrium. Risk of hemorrhage and infection is minimal 3 weeks after a normal vaginal delivery. Telling the client anytime is inappropriate because this response does not provide the client with the specific information she is requesting. Choice of a contraceptive method is important, but not the specific criterion for safe resumption of sexual activity. Culturally, the 6-weeks examination has been used as the time frame for resuming sexual activity, but it may be resumed earlier.

55. The answer is 4.
The nurse's assessment reveals signs of an acute infection that will require systemic antibiotics. The physician needs to be informed so that appropriate treatment can

be instituted. Sitz baths increase the circulation, cleanse the area, and facilitate healing. However, sitz baths alone will not manage the acute infection. An ice pack will decrease the discomfort but will not manage the acute infection. Anti-inflammatory medications might help the discomfort but will not manage the acute infection.

56. The answer is 3.
The middle third of the vastus lateralis muscle is the preferred injection site for vitamin K administration because it is free of blood vessels and nerves and is large enough to absorb the medication. The deltoid muscle of a newborn is not large enough for an I.M. injection. Injections into this muscle in a small child might cause damage to the radial nerve. The anterior femoris muscle is the next safest muscle to use in a newborn but is not the safest. Because of the proximity of the sciatic nerve, the gluteus maximus muscle should not be used until the child has been walking for 2 years.

57. The answer is 2.
Infections outside the uterus (most commonly urinary tract infections) are thought to cause preterm labor by a mechanism involving the production of interleukins and tumor necrosis factor by maternal macrophages, which trigger the reduction of prostaglandin by the amnion. Genital tract infections are strongly associated with premature rupture of membranes, especially in pregnancies less than 30 weeks' gestation. Grand multiparity, first pregnancies, and trisomy are factors more commonly associated with postterm labor than preterm labor.

58. The answer is 4.
Bartholin's glands are the glands on either side of the vaginal orifice. The clitoris is female erectile tissue found in the perineal area above the urethra. The parotid glands open into the mouth. Skene's glands open into the posterior wall of the female urinary meatus.

59. The answer is 2.
Labia majora are raised longitudinal folds of adipose tissue containing hair and extending from the mons veneris. Labia minora are soft longitudinal folds of skin. The mons pubis is a mound of fatty tissue over the symphysis pubis. The vestibule is the almond-shaped area between the labia minora.

60. The answer is 1.
A gynecoid pelvis is a typical female pelvis with a rounded inlet. An android pelvis refers to a normal pelvis with a heart-shaped inlet. An anthropoid pelvis refers to an apelike pelvis with an oval inlet. A platypelloid pelvis is a flat female pelvis with a transverse oval inlet.

61. The answer is 4.
The fetal gonad must secrete estrogen for the embryo to differentiate as a female. An increase in maternal estrogen secretion does not effect differentiation of the embryo, and maternal estrogen secretion occurs in every pregnancy. Maternal androgen secretion remains the same as before pregnancy and does not effect differentiation. Secretion of androgen by the fetal gonad would produce a male fetus.

62. The answer is 1.
Using bicarbonate would increase the amount of sodium ingested, which can cause complications. Eating low-sodium crackers would be appropriate. Because liquids can increase nausea, avoiding them in the morning hours when nausea is usually the strongest is appropriate. Eating six small meals a day would keep the stomach full, which often decreases nausea.

63. The answer is 4.
Weight gain of approximately 1 lb per week during the last two trimesters is the ideal weight gain during pregnancy. Weight is

not gained equally in the three trimesters, nor is it gained equally in the first two trimesters. The first trimester is the time of least weight gain.

64. The answer is 3.
Nodularity, although possibly normal, should be reported to the physician for further evaluation because a great number of cancerous breast lumps are found in this portion of the breast. Breast tenderness, increased areolar pigmentation, and prominent superficial veins are normal findings.

65. The answer is 2.
Ballottement indicates passive movement of the unengaged fetus. Ballottement is not a contraction. Fetal kicking felt by the client represents quickening. Enlargement and softening of the uterus is known as Piskacek's sign.

66. The answer is 2.
Chadwick's sign refers to the purple-blue tinge of the cervix. Braxton Hicks contractions are painless contractions beginning around the 4th month. Goodell's sign indicates softening of the cervix. Flexibility of the uterus against the cervix is known as McDonald's sign.

67. The answer is 2.
The obstetric conjugate should measure at least 11 cm for a normal vaginal delivery. A measurement of 10 cm is not within normal limits for a vaginal delivery, indicating too narrow a passageway. 10 cm is not an extremely large obstetric conjugate, and it is not considered a marginal anteroposterior diameter.

68. The answer is 1.
Human chorionic gonadotropin is the hormone present during a pregnancy and is the basis for the pregnancy test. Estrogen, follicle-stimulating hormone, and progesterone are not the basis for pregnancy tests.

69. The answer is 1.
Back massage against the sacral area provides counterpressure, thus easing the woman's discomfort. It does not rotate the baby or help a posterior baby turn to the anterior. Lying in bed contributes to the backache, but this response does not address the couple's question as to why back massage soothes the laboring woman.

70. The answer is 3.
Breathing techniques can raise the pain threshold and reduce the perception of pain. They also promote relaxation. Breathing techniques do not eliminate pain, but they can reduce it. Positioning, not breathing, increases uteroplacental perfusion.

71. The answer is 4.
A hysterosalpingography is a test involving the insertion of radiopaque material into a client's uterus and fallopian tubes to assess tubal patency. A laparoscopy involves a small abdominal incision to inspect the abdominal and pelvic areas. No radiopaque dye is used. A culdoscopy involves the insertion of a tube into the posterior fornix and does not use a radiopaque dye.

72. The answer is 1.
Petroleum jelly has been shown to be spermicidal and should be eliminated. Rather, if additional lubrication is needed, a water-soluble lubricant such as K-Y jelly should be used. Reducing the frequency of intercourse will not increase the probability of conception. There is nothing to support that consistency is a factor in their inability to conceive. Clarifying the degree of sexual satisfaction does not have a bearing on their inability to conceive.

73. The answer is 4.
For an embryo to differentiate as a male, it must increase its production of androgen. Increased estrogen by the mother will not influence differentiation. Secretion of estrogen by the fetal gonad is necessary to

differentiate as a female. Decreasing androgen production will not influence differentiation.

74. The answer is 3.
The leading cause of maternal death after delivery throughout the world is postpartum hemorrhage. The incidence of puerperal infection is less than that of hemorrhage. Thrombophlebitis may lead to pulmonary embolism, but the incidence of death is still less than that from hemorrhage. Uterine inversion is a rare cause of maternal death.

75. The answer is 4.
The onset of labor caused by a release of a complex cascade of bioactive chemical agents into the amniotic fluid describes the uterine decidua activation theory for the onset of labor. According to the oxytocin theory, the uterus becomes more sensitive to oxytocin as pregnancy advances. The prostaglandin theory poses that lipids trigger steroids and release precursors that increase the synthesis of prostaglandin. Decreased production of progesterone by the placenta is the basis for the progesterone deprivation theory.

76. The answer is 1.
A distended bladder will elevate and displace the uterus to the right. Therefore, the nurse should assist the mother to void. A displaced uterus is usually caused by a full bladder. Vigorous massage of the fundus will not correct this and may cause unnecessary discomfort. Oxytocin would be used if the uterus was not contracting. There are no data to suggest a need for that at this time. A tocolytic would be used if the uterus required relaxation, such as in premature labor.

77. The answer is 1.
The client's labor is hypotonic. The nurse should call the physician and obtain an order for an infusion of oxytocin, which will help the uterus contract more forcefully in an attempt to dilate the cervix. Administering a light sedative would be done for hypertonic uterine contractions. Preparing for cesarean birth is unnecessary at this time. Oxytocin would increase the uterine contractions and hopefully progress labor before a cesarean birth would be necessary. It is too early to anticipate client pushing with contractions.

78. The answer is 4.
Oxytocin can overstimulate the uterus. Therefore, it is essential to monitor contraction frequency, duration, and intensity. Maternal vital signs, fetal heart rate, and urine output are important assessments, but they are not the priority at this time.

79. The answer is 3.
For this client at this time, radiographic pelvimetry will give the most accurate measurements. Ultrasonography will only show soft tissue, not pelvic measurements. Further evaluation must be done before a cesarean birth is performed. Manual internal measurements are not as accurate as pelvimetry and would have been previously done to determine the borderline status.

80. The answer is 4.
The signs indicate placenta previa; therefore, a vaginal exam to determine cervical dilation would not be done because it could cause hemorrhage. Assessing maternal vital signs can help determine maternal physiologic status. Fetal heart rate is important to assess fetal well-being and should be done. Monitoring the contractions will help evaluate the progress of labor.

81. The answer is 4.
A complete placenta previa occurs when the placenta covers the opening of the uterus, thus blocking the passageway for the baby. This response explains what a complete previa is and the reason the baby cannot come out except by cesarean birth. Telling the client to ask the physician

is a poor response and would increase the patient's anxiety. Although a cesarean birth would help to prevent hemorrhage, the statement does not explain why the hemorrhage could occur. With a complete previa, the placenta is covering all the cervix, not just most of it.

82. The answer is 1.
Endometritis is an infection of the uterine lining and can occur after prolonged rupture of membranes. Endometriosis does not occur after a long labor and prolonged rupture of membranes. Salpingitis is a tubal infection and could occur if endometritis is not treated. Pelvic thrombophlebitis involves clot formation, but it is not a complication of prolonged rupture of membranes.

83. The answer is 3.
The client's symptoms suggest abruptio placentae with possible concealed hemorrhage, indicating blood loss greater than that which is observed. Blood loss is present vaginally and is typically more than minimal.

84. The answer is 1.
Since blood loss is often greater than observed, replacement is the priority. Type and crossmatching would be the first nursing action when the orders are received. Assessment of maternal vital signs is very important, but if blood needs replacing, it is not the highest priority action. Assessing fetal heart rate also is very important but won't solve the problem of blood loss being greater than observed if replacement is not available. Measuring fundal height could aid in determining if there is blood accumulation but won't solve the problem of blood replacement if needed.

85. The answer is 2.
Continued monitoring is necessary to promote survival and decrease the risk of morbidity. Both mother and fetus should be monitored. Monitoring urine output is but one component of the maternal assessment. Emotional support is always important, but potential fetal demise should not be the focus at the present time. Tocolytics are contraindicated with abruptio placentae.

86. The answer is 2.
With a face presentation, the head is completely extended. With a vertex presentation, the head is completely or partially flexed. With a brow (forehead) presentation, the head would be partially extended.

87. The answer is 4.
With this presentation, the fetal upper torso and back face the left upper maternal abdominal wall. The fetal heart rate would be most audible above the maternal umbilicus and to the left of the midline. The other positions would be incorrect.

88. The answer is 3.
The greenish tint is due to the presence of meconium. Lanugo is the soft, downy hair on the shoulders and back of the fetus. Hydramnios represents excessive amniotic fluid. Vernix is the white, cheesy substance covering the fetus.

89. The answer is 4.
In a breech position, because of the space between the presenting part and the cervix, prolapse of the umbilical cord is common. Quickening is the woman's first perception of fetal movement. Ophthalmia neonatorum usually results from maternal gonorrhea and is conjunctivitis. Pica refers to the oral intake of nonfood substances.

90. The answer is 1.
Patients who use an intrauterine device for contraception have an increased risk of pelvic inflammatory disease, which is a prominent cause of tubal scarring. Polycystic ovary is an ovarian cause of infertility and is not related to tubal problems. Repeated vaginal yeast infections are a vagi-

nal cause of infertility, not tubal. Use of diethylstilbestrol by the client's mother is a cervical cause of infertility, not tubal.

91. The answer is 4.
A woman unable to produce normal mature follicles but having a fertile male partner describes the classic couple that can use surrogate embryo transfer, a process in which the donor is inseminated with the male partner's sperm. Several days later, the fertilized ovum is washed from the donor uterus and implanted in the female partner's uterus. The couple in which the woman is unable to carry a fetus to viability would not be candidates for surrogate embryo transfer because the woman must be able to carry a fetus to viability. Surrogate embryo transfer would not be needed if the woman ovulates regularly because the woman has the ability to produce ova. The male partner needs to be fertile to use surrogate embryo transfer.

92. The answer is 1.
Dizygotic (fraternal) twins involve two ova fertilized by separate sperm. Monozygotic (identical) twins involve a common placenta, same genotype, and common chorion.

93. The answer is 4.
Cystic fibrosis is considered an autosomal recessive inheritance. Hypophosphatemia is an example of an X-linked dominant disorder. Hemophila A is an example of an X-linked recessive disorder. Marfan syndrome and Huntington's disease are examples of autosomal dominant disorders.

94. The answer is 3.
The corpus luteum supplies most of the progesterone necessary for maintenance of a pregnancy in the first 2 months. The placenta is forming during the first 2 months and does not take over production of progesterone in amounts needed to maintain a pregnancy until after the 10th to 12th week of gestation. The chromosome and the spermatozoa have nothing to do with progesterone supply.

95. The answer is 3.
The zygote is the single cell that reproduces itself after conception. The chromosome is the material that makes up the cell and is gained from each parent. Blastocyst and trophoblast are later terms for the embryo after zygote.

96. The answer is 4.
Prepared childbirth was the direct result of the 1950s' challenging of the routine use of analgesics and anesthetics during childbirth. The labor,delivery, recovery, postpartum approach was a much later concept and was not a direct result of the challenge to routine use of analgesics and anesthetics during childbirth. Roles for nurse-midwives and clinical nurse specialists did not develop from this challenge.

97. The answer is 3.
The ischial spines are located in the midpelvic region and could be narrowed because of the previous pelvic injury. The symphysis pubis, sacral promontory and pubic arch are not part of the midpelvis.

98. The answer is 2.
Variations in the length of the menstrual cycle are due to variations in the proliferative phase. The menstrual, secretory, and ischemic phases do not contribute to this variation.

99. The answer is 3.
Title V of the Public Health Service Act established the Maternal and Infant Care projects. The Sheppard-Towner act is not an amendment to the Public Health Service Act but did provide funds for maternal-child health programs. The Women, Infants, and Children program was not established until 1975 and is not an amendment to the Public Health Service Act. Title XIX provided funds to the Medicaid program to fa-

cilitate care for pregnant women and young children.

100. The answer is 2.
Testosterone is produced by the Leydig cells in the seminiferous tubules. Follicle-stimulating hormone and luteinizing hormone are released by the anterior pituitary gland. The hypothalamus is responsible for releasing gonadotropin-releasing hormone.

101. The answer is 4, 5, 6.
Amniocentesis done in early pregnancy can identify chromosomal and neural tube defects. It can also be used to identify the sex of the fetus. During the last trimester, amniocentesis can be used to determine fetal lung maturity. It can also be used to treat polyhydraminos by removing excess fluid.

102. The answer is 1, 3, 5, 6.
After the infant is born and the umbilical cord is cut and clamped, the birth attendant observes for the following signs of placental separation: the uterus rises upward in the abdomen as the placenta settles into the lower uterine segment; the length of umbilical cord protruding from the vagina increases as the placenta moves downward; there is a visible trickle or spurt of blood from the vagina; and the shape of the uterus changes from discoid to globular. The condition of the cervix changes during the first stage of labor to completely dilated and effaced to accommodate the birth. The presenting part at zero station signifies that the fetus is settled into the maternal pelvis.

103. The answer is 100.
During a client's pregnancy, a 1-hour, 50-gram oral glucose tolerance test reveals a plasma level of 130 to 140 mg/dl, indicating the need for further diagnostic testing. The actual diagnosis is based on a 3-hour, 100-gram oral glucose tolerance test, performed as follows: A fasting plasma glucose level is drawn. A 100-gram glucose solution is administered to the mother, and blood is drawn at 1, 2, and 3 hours. Gestational diabetes is diagnosed if two or more of the following values are met or exceeded: Fasting—95 mg/dl; 1 hour—180 mg/dl; 2 hour—155 mg/dl; 3 hour—140 mg/dl

104. The answer is 0.25.
The following formula applies:

Dose on hand/Quantity on hand = desired dose/X

The formula then becomes:

2 mg/1 ml = 0.5 mg/X
X = 0.25 ml

105. Answer: Uterine involution begins immediately after the birth. The fundus may be palpated through the abdominal wall halfway between the umbilicus and the symphysis pubis within a few minutes after birth. However, 1 hour later, it has risen to the level of the umbilicus, where it remains for the next 24 hours. Thereafter, it will decrease in size by one fingerbreadth (1 cm) each day. By day 9 or 10, the fundus will again be behind the symphysis pubis and will no longer be palpable.

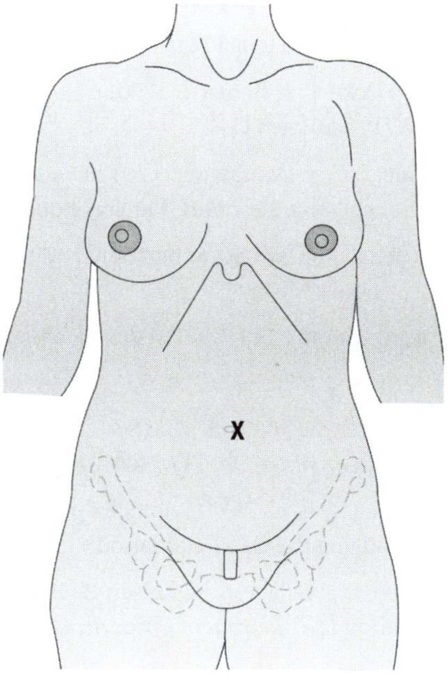

BIBLIOGRAPHY

_____. (2003). *AWHOON Standards and Guidelines* (6th ed.).

_____. (1999). *Journal watch: Women's health.* Waltham, Mass.: Massachusetts Medical Society. 4(12), 89.

_____. (2004). *NCLEX-RN 250 new format questions: Preparing for the revised NCLEX-RN.* Philadelphia: Lippincott Williams & Wilkins.

_____. (2004). *Nursing drug reference.* St. Louis: Mosby.

_____. (1997). *Taber's cyclopedic medical dictionary* (18th ed.). Philadelphia: F.A. Davis.

_____. (2002). *World almanac and book of facts.* New York: World Almanac Books.

American Diabetes Association. (2002). Position statement: Gestational diabetes mellitus. *Diabetes Care,* 25, S94-S96.

Ball, J. & Bindler, R. (1999). *Pediatric nursing: Caring for children* (2nd ed.). Stamford, Conn.: Appleton & Lange.

Beck, C.T. (1998). A checklist to identify women at risk for developing postpartum depression. *Journal of Obstetric, Gynecologic, and Neonatal Nursing,* 27(1), 39.

Belew, C. (1999). Herbs and the childbearing woman: Guidelines for midwives. *Journal of Nurse-Midwifery,* 44(3), 231-246.

Bobak, I. & Lagerquist, S. (1998). *Maternal-newborn core content at-a-glance.* Philadelphia: Lippincott Williams & Wilkins.

Brooks, C. (1997). Neonatal hypoglycemia. *Neonatal Network,* 16(2), 16.

Boushey, C., Edmonds, W., & Welshimer, K. (2001). Estimates of the effects of folic-acid fortification and folic-acid bioavailability for women. *Nutrition,* 17(10), 873-879.

Cady, R. (1999). Legal issues in the treatment of infertility. *Maternal Child Nursing,* 24(5), 264.

Chernecky, C. & Berger, B. (2001). *Laboratory tests and diagnostic procedures* (3rd ed.). Philadelphia: W.B. Saunders Co.

Cifalo, R.C. & Dominguez, J.A. (2003). *A multicultural approach to patients. A continuing education monograph.* New York Medical Education Collaborative and Creative 4 Media, Inc.

Collier, I., McCash, K., & Bartram, J. (1996). *Writing nursing diagnoses: A critical thinking approach.* St Louis: Mosby.

Cunningham, F.G. (1997). *Williams obstetrics* (20th ed.). Stamford, Conn.: Appleton & Lange.

Green, C. & Wilkinson, J. (2004). *Maternal newborn nursing careplans.* St. Louis: Mosby.

Grimes, D. A., Hanson, V., & Sondheimer, S. (2001). New approaches to emergency contraception. *Contemporary OB/GYN,* 46(6), 89-99.

Hatcher, R., et al. (2000). *A pocket guide to managing contraception* (2nd ed.). Dawsonville, Ga.: Bridging the Gap Foundation.

Jensen, D., Wallace, S., & Kelsay, P. (1994). LATCH: A breast feedings charting system and documentation tool. *Journal of Obstetric, Gynecologic, and Neonatal Nursing,* 23(1), 27.

Johnson, B. (1997). *Psychiatric-mental health nursing* (4th ed.). Philadelphia: Lippincott Williams & Wilkins.

Letko, M. (1996). Understanding the Apgar score. *Journal of Obstetric, Gynecologic, and Neonatal Nursing,* 25(4), 299.

Lowdermilk, D. & Perry, S. (2004). *Maternity & women's health care* (8th ed.). St. Louis: Mosby.

Malone, F. & Dalton, M. (1997). Drugs in pregnancy: Anticonvulsants. *Seminars in Perinatology,* 21(2), 114.

Mandeville, L. & Troiano, N. (1999). *High risk and critical care: Intrapartum nursing* (2nd ed.). Philadelphia: Lippincott Williams & Wilkins.

Mathews, T. J., Menacker, F., & MacDorman, M. F. (2002). Infant mortality statistics for the 2000 period. Linked birth/infant death data set. *National Vital Statistics Report,* 50(12), 1-27.

Matteson, P. S. (2001). *Women's health during the childbearing years: A community-based approach.* St. Louis: Mosby.

Montgomery, K. (1996). Caring for the pregnant woman with sickle cell disease. *MCN, The American Journal of Materna/Child Nursing,* 21(5), 224.

Nardi, D. (1999). Parenting education as family support. *Journal of Psychosocial Nursing,* 37(7), 11.

Nilson, L. (1990). *A child is born.* New York: Dell Publishing.

Olds, S., London, M., Ladewig, P., & Davidson, M. (2004). *Maternal-newborn nursing & women's health care* (7th ed.) Upper Saddle River, N.J.: Pearson/Prentice Hall.

Pagana, K. & Pagana, T. (1999). *Mosby's diagnostic and laboratory test reference* (4th ed.). St Louis: Mosby.

Payton, R. & Brucker, M. (1999). Drugs and uterine motility. *Journal of Obstetric, Gynecologic, and Neonatal Nursing,* 28(6), 628.

Pepper, G. (1999). Pharmacology of antihypertensive drugs. *Journal of Obstetric, Gynecologic, and Neonatal Nursing,* 28(6), 649.

Pilliteri, A. (2003). *Maternal and child health nursing: Care of the childbearing and childrearing family* (4th ed.). Philadelphia: Lippincott Williams & Wilkins.

Reece, E. & Erikson, U. (1996). The pathogenesis of diabetes associated with congenital malformations. *Obstetrics and Gynecology Clinics of North America,* 23(1), 29.

Reifsnider, E. & Gill, S.L. (2000). Nutrition for the childbearing years. *Obstetric, Gynecologic, and Neonatal Nursing,* 29, 43-55.

Simpson, K. & Creehan, P. (1996). *Perinatal nursing.* Philadelphia: Lippincott Williams & Wilkins.

Skidmore-Roth, L. (2001). *Mosby's handbook of herbs and natural supplements.* St. Louis: Mosby.

Stone, M. H., Westley, E., & Cullin, V. E. (2002). Emergency contraception: America's best kept secret. *Contemporary OB/GYN,* 47(3), 106-116.

Urdang, L. & Swallow, H. (eds). (1998). *Mosby's medical and nursing dictionary.* St. Louis: Mosby.

Zieman, M. (2001). Transdermal contraception. *The Female Patient,* (12), 22-25.

Other resources

American Botanical Council
http://www.herbalgram.org/

American Diabetes Association
http://www.diabetes.org/

American Holistic Nurses' Association
P.O. Box 2130
Flagstaff, AZ 86003-2130
http://www.ahna.org/

Association of Maternal and Child Health Programs
1220 19th St., NW, Suite 801
Washington, DC 20036
http://www.amchp.org/

Association of Women's Health Obstetric, and Neonatal Nurses
http://www.awhonn.org/

Breast Cancer Information Center
http://www.awarebse.com/

Genetic Alliance
http://www.geneticalliance.org

Georgetown University National Center for Cultural Competence
http://www.gucdc.georgetown.edu/nccc/topic4.html

Health Literacy Toolbox 2000
http://www.prenataled.com/healthlit/hlt2k/script/index.asp

Healthy People 2010
http://www.health.gov/healthypeople

Infertility Resources
http://www.ihr.com/infertility/index.html

Institute for Women's Policy Research
1400 20th St., NW, Suite 104
Washington, DC 20036
http://www.iwpr.org/

International Society of Nurses in Genetics (ISONG)
http://www.isong.org/

March of Dimes
http://www.modimes.org/

National Center for Complementary and Alternative Medicine (NCCAM)
P.O. Box 8218
Silver Spring, MD 20907-8218
http://www.altmed.od.nih.gov/nccam

National Coalition Against Domestic Violence
P.O. Box 34103
Washington, D.C. 20043-4301
http://www.ncadv.org/

The National Multicultural Institute
http://www.ncmi.org/

Nutrient Data Laboratory
http://www.nal.usda.gov/fnic/foodcomp

NuvaRing
http://www.nuvaring.com/

Office of Minority Health
P.O. Box 37337
Washington, DC 20013-7337
http://www.omhrc.gov/

INDEX

Page numbers followed by c indicate charts; those followed by f indicate figures; those followed by t indicate tables.

B

C

Page numbers followed by c indicate charts; those followed by f indicate figures; those followed by t indicate tables.

Page numbers followed by c indicate charts; those followed by f indicate figures; those followed by t indicate tables.

D

E

F

G

Page numbers followed by c indicate charts; those followed by f indicate figures; those followed by t indicate tables.

Page numbers followed by c indicate charts; those followed by f indicate figures; those followed by t indicate tables.

KL

M

Page numbers followed by c indicate charts; those followed by f indicate figures; those followed by t indicate tables.

N

Page numbers followed by c indicate charts; those followed by f indicate figures; those followed by t indicate tables.

O

P

Page numbers followed by c indicate charts; those followed by f indicate figures; those followed by t indicate tables.

Page numbers followed by c indicate charts; those followed by f indicate figures; those followed by t indicate tables.

Page numbers followed by c indicate charts; those followed by f indicate figures; those followed by t indicate tables.

QR

S

Page numbers followed by c indicate charts; those followed by f indicate figures; those followed by t indicate tables.

Page numbers followed by c indicate charts; those followed by f indicate figures; those followed by t indicate tables.

WXYZ

About the CD-ROM

Lippincott's Review Series CD-ROMs provide a convenient way to assess readiness for academic tests and licensure exams. Over 200 carefully selected, multiple-choice, and alternative-format questions are provided for study and simulated testing.

Minimum system requirements

- Windows 98
- Pentium 166
- 128 MB RAM
- 8 MB of free hard-disk space
- SVGA monitor with high color (16-bit)
- CD-ROM drive

Installation

Place the CD in your CD-ROM drive. After a few moments, the install process will automatically begin. *Note:* If the install process doesn't automatically begin, click the Start button and select Run. At the command line, type *D:\setup.exe.* (Note: The letter D represents the CD-ROM drive. If your drive is designated by a different letter, use your drive letter instead.) Click OK. Follow the installation instructions.

Technical support

For technical support, call toll-free 1-800-638-3030, Monday through Friday, 8:30 a.m. to 5 p.m. Eastern Time. You may also write to Lippincott Williams & Wilkins Technical Support, 351 W. Camden Street, Baltimore, MD 21201-2436, or e-mail us at techsupp@lww.com.